A Compleat History OF MAGICK, SORCERY, AND WITCHCRAFT

Volumes I & II

by
Richard Boulton

1716

A Compleat History OF MAGICK, SORCERY, AND WITCHCRAFT; CONTAINING,

I. The most Authentick and best attested RELATIONS of Magicians, Sorcerers, Witches, Apparitions, Spectres, Ghosts, Dæmons, and other preternatural Appearances.

II. A Collection of several very scarce and valuable TRYALS of Witches, particularly that famous one, of the WITCHES of Warboyse.

III. An Account of the first Rise of Magicians and Witches; shewing the Contracts they make with the Devil, and what Methods they take to accomplish their Infernal Designs. IV. A full Confutation of all the Arguments that have ever been produced against the Belief of Apparitions, Witches, &c. with a Judgment concerning Spirits, by the late Learned Mr. JOHN LOCKE.

by
Richard Boulton
1716

VOLUME I.

THE PREFACE TO THE READER.

THE following Sheets containing a History of Magick, Sorcery, Witchcraft, Apparitions, Spectres, &c. we think it requisite to give the Reader a brief Account of the Nature and Usefulness of our Design in the first place; and (since they may fall into the Hands both of the Learned and Unlearned, some of which are apt to question Truths, though most sacred and never so well attested,) having represented the Design and Usefulness of this Treatise, we shall in the next Place offer something to confirm the Belief and Credit of Histories so well attested.

And First to represent the Nature of our Design we shall briefly lay down the Method we have taken in this History, and give the Reader a short Account of what he may expect to find in the ensuing Sheets. First then, we have given the Reader a compendious Account of the Origin and Rise of the Art of Magick and Witchcraft, as an Introduction to the following History, that he might have at once in View, a general Notion of the Diabolical Arts practised by such wretched Persons, and the Manner how they make their abominable Contracts with the Devil, and bring wicked Spirits under their Command, to put their ill Designs in Practice; from whence we proceed to give an Historical Account of the mischievous Proceedings and Actions of those Instruments of the Devil, Magicians and Witches, and what untimely and disgraceful Ends such wicked Practices have brought such Persons to at the last.

And for as much as several Tracts have been published upon these Subjects, several of which are too prolix, and intermix'd with long and tedious Relations, which are less worthy our Notice, as they are less authentick and not so well attested, and are intermix'd with tedious Disputes, which are scarce necessary to prove Truths which are so apparent; in this Work we have taken Notice only of such as appear to be of undoubted Credit and Authority, and may be entertaining and diverting as well as useful. As for the Usefulness of this Treatise, the Histories contained in it, being collected from the best Authors who have wrote upon those Subjects; they not only serve to put us in Mind of the Delusions of Satan, and the ill Consequences that attend such who serve so bad a Master as the Devil; but also, since from these Histories it appears that the Devil hath not equal Power to execute his ill Purposes on all Persons indifferently, but only on such as God Almighty pleases to permit; they may put us in Mind to arm our selves both against the Temptations of the Devil, and to implore God Almighty's Assistance, that the Devil may have no Power over us: And as Divinity teaches us how to serve God, and to withstand the Temptations of so bad a Master; so the Reading of these Histories may increase our Horror of so great an Enemy of our Salvation, in shewing, us by Examples, how he constantly endeavours to disturb our Quiet, and ruin our Souls; and may also incline us to serve God, who is our Saviour and Protector from this grand Adversary, with the greater Courage and Zeal.

Having thus briefly represented the Design and Usefulness of this Work, we shall in the next Place, for the Sake of those who are less apt to believe Truths of this Kind, though never so well attested, offer something to confirm the Belief and Credit of Histories which are so well testified. And as in the following Histories, we make use of the Authority of the most approved Writers, Ancient and Modern, and take Notice of none, but those of undoubted Credit, and very well attested; so in this Matter we shall recite the Opinions of the best Authors, and Men of most Repute to strengthen the Belief and Probability of these Histories.

To shew then what may be suggested by Reason, concerning the Existence of Spirits and their Operations, we shall first offer what Kircher in his Epist. Parænet. prefixed to his Obeliscus Pamphilius writes on this Occasion; says he, 'We know a threefold Demonstration hath been always used by the unanimous Consent of Philosophers in the Acquisition of Science; Mathematical, Physical, and Moral: Mathematical Demonstration, as it enquires into the Effects and Properties of Quantity, by Principles known by the Light of Nature, of eternal

Truth, and void of all Deceit; so it begets a certain, and properly called Science, all Scruples of Doubt being removed. Physical Demonstration, as it comes, by Experiments of Things, to the secret Knowledge of Causes, it begets indeed Science, but by Reason of the Experiment, which for the most Part is exposed to the false Representations of the Senses, it is not void of Deception, nor does it arrive at the Certainty of the Former. Moral Demonstration, as it depends on the Experience of Human Actions, begets indeed Science, but such as the Nature of moral Things admit, which is called Human Faith, and for the most Part relies on the Authority of the Relater: And for the same Cause the Authority of the Revealer begets divine Faith, more certain than all Science. Human Authority is a Kind of Imitation of this, on which we must rely, unless we will make void, and annihilate the Histories of all past Things. I speak not here of the Authority and Histories of suspected Credit, but of those which have the clear Prescription of many Ages for their Authority.'

Upon this fundamental Thesis we shall add what a learned Author says, viz. 'Laying this before us, it is to be noted, That Christian Divines do not pretend to a Methematical or Physical Demonstration of the Existence of Spirits; for their Existence can not be demonstrated from their Essence, or the Effects ascribed to them; not from the First, because it's not from the Nature of Spirits, nor from that of any other Creatures that they exist: for God so freely created all Beings, that he might have left them uncreated: Nor from their Effects, because the Concourse of God alone, or other Causes might be conceived to suffice for such Effects; but Christian Divines build chiefly on Divine Revelation, which is superior to all Science, and on the constant Tradition of all Christian Divines, from the first Ages of Christianity; and all they pretend to, as Physiologers, in what they say concerning Spirits, is, that there is nothing in it which implies a Contradiction, or is inconsistent with Reason: And as there have been, and are many Phænomena in the World, which it hath concerned Philosophers to account for, the Doctrine of the Existence of Spirits hath been Hypothetically introduced into the

World, and backed by as great Men among the Gentiles as the World hath had; and though other Philosophers have set up other Hypotheses to explain those Phænomena; yet I think it would be a strange Rashness in any Person, owning the Law of Moses or Christ, to lay aside an Hypothesis, backed by Divine Revelation; or rather introduced by the most Learned of the Gentiles, consonant to it; and to adhere to any other Hypothesis, contrived only by the Wit of Man; and which does not so fairly account for Phænomena, as the other does, or shamefully to deny Facts which are to be accounted for; as I know not with what unbounded Confidence some even amongst Christians have done; whereas Vanini, who died a Martyr to Atheism, and Pomponatius, who hath been looked upon by some to be of the same Opinion; and many others freely own the Facts, which they found uncontestably manifested to them by Experience and Testimonies, though they did not think fit to explain them by the Agency of Spirits.'

For the reasonableness of the Hypothesis of Spirits, Plutarch introduces Gleombrotus, thus expressing himself: As those say very well, who hold that Plato having describ'd that Element, whence Qualities spring and are ingendred, which is sometimes called the first Matter, and sometimes Nature; hath freed the Philosophers from many Difficulties; so it seems to me, that those who have introduced the Nature of Dæmons, betwixt that of the Gods and Men, have resolved more Doubts and Difficulties, and greater, together, as it were, our Society and Communication with them; whether this Opinion came from the ancient Magi and Zoroastres, or from Thracia and Orpheus, or from Ægpyt is doubtful, we rather conjecture from Phrygia, considering the Sacrifices that are made in those Countries. Father le Brun having set forth many odd Discouries of hidden Things, made by the Conjuring Wand, examines the Causes of its Turning, in order to Discoveries; and having validly refuted all natural Causes, which others have pretended to assign for it, he concludes it is done by the Agency of Evil Spirits; the Existence of which he proves as follows.

If there are Effects which cannot be produced by Bodies, there must necessarily be in the World other Beings than Bodies: And if amongst these prodigious Effects, there are some that do not carry Men to God, and make them fall into Error and Illusion; it's a further invincible Argument, that we must acknowledge other Beings, than the Being absolutely perfect, and Bodies: So those extraordinary Effects which can neither be called in Doubt, nor be attributed to God nor Bodies, are an incontestable Proof that we must admit created Spirits capable of amusing Men, and seducing them by Deceits. Though therefore the Scriptures had not clearly taught us the Existence of Spirits separated from Bodies, I dare say, that extraordinary Effects, such as the Discovery of many hidden Things, by the Turning of the Conjuring Wand, would give a strong Proof that there are wicked Spirits. But their Existence is clear enough in the Scriptures; and certainly it is the best established of any Article of our Faith, the least contested, and the most universally spread through the World. Maimonides, in his More Nevochim proves, with much Learning and Judgment; that before Moses, the Sabæans, Ægyptians and Chaldeans, knew good and evil Spirits; all the ancient Poets and Philosophers owned this Truth. And we find in the History of the Conversion of the People, that it hath always been found established amongst the remote Nations; nor can it be said that this is a Stupidness of some Nations, for the most polite People differ not in this from those they call Barbarians: And we may see in the Works of Prophyrius, Jamblicus, and Clemens Alexandrinus, how much the Doctrine of the Greeks was like that of the Ægyptians, concerning the Existence of Spirits.

The new converted Christians of the Primitive Times, who, being disabused of the Follies of Paganism, were watchful over the Gentiles, to discover their Practices, owned that sometimes Prodigies were wrought by the Dæmons. Minutius Fælix, who lived in the second Century, hath very well set forth what the Sense of the Christians of those Times was, concerning the Nature and Operations of those Dæmons, whom the Gentiles worshiped. Tertullian and Origen, and almost all the Writers of the three first Centuries, have delivered the same, with all the Assurance that Truth may give: And what these great Men have said, is a very good Answer to what is sometimes objected, that Christ destroyed the Kingdom of Satan, and that the Prince of this World is now judged; Job xvi. 11. St. Peter, St. Paul and St. John, Men well instructed in the Words of Christ, and in the Sense that ought to be given them, tell us, that the Devil as a roaring Lion goes about to deceive us; that we ought to have Recourse to Prayer, to keep us firm in Faith, to preserve us from his Artifices, and the Snares he lays for us. The Devil therefore is not out of the World, so as to act no longer, but is driven from a great many Places where he had Rule. It's a Truth of our Faith, that God hath left some Power to Devils; and he permits them on many Occasions to put it in Execution. The frequent Possessions in the first Ages of the Church are authentick Testimonies of it, and the best averred Histories since Christ; and a Thousand superstitious Practices, producing extraordinary Effects, furnish us with incontestible Proofs of the Operation of Dæmons: And is there any Ecclesiastical Writer, who hath not either proved or supposed this Truth? The learned Gerson tells us what we ought to believe in this Case; and whence it is that this Truth makes so little Impression on the Spirits of many Persons, saying, certainly it is an Impiety and Error, directly contrary to the Scriptures, to deny that Dæmons are the Authors of many surprizing Facts; and those that look upon all that is said of it as a Fable, and make a Mock of Divines for ascribing Effects to. Dæmons, deserve a severe Correction. Sometimes even the Learned fall into this Error, because they let their Faith be weaken'd, and their natural Light be darkened. Their Souls being all possessed with sensible Things, refer all to Bodies, and cannot raise themselves to Spirits detach'd from Matter. It's what Plato hath said, that nothing so much hinders the finding of Truth, as to refer all Things to what the Senses present us with: Cicero, St. Austin, Albertus Magnus, Gulielmus Parisiensis, and above all, Experience, have taught us the same; we may see a Proof of it in the Sadduces and the Epicureans, who admitting nothing but what is corporeal, find themselves amongst those senseless Persons, of whom Solomon speaks in Ecclesiastes, and the Book of Wisdom, who have pushed their Folly so far, that they cannot own they have a Soul, and Effects that cannot be produced but by Spirits. I wish there were no more Persons of that Mind; but we shall always find some, who will tell us in cold Blood, that they cannot believe Prodigies nor Miracles, because they have seen nothing extraordinary. Dispute not with such Persons: When a Man will be incredulous, he will be so in the midst of Prodigies and Miracles; there are always found People tempered like Celsus and Lucian, who will have all Things to be Fable, Illusion, and Imposture. Many Persons measure all Things by what they ordinarily see, and hold all for false that surpass the Bounds of Nature. They believe Facts while they appear natural; convince them that they cannot so be, and you shall see them presently conclude them Impostures.

It is manifest that we conceive but two Sorts of Beings, Spirits and Bodies; and since we can reason but according to our Ideas, we ought to ascribe to Spirits, what cannot be ascribed to Bodies.'

The Author of the Republick of Learning, having proposed a Draught for Writing a good Tract upon Witchcraft, which he looks upon as a Desideratum; amongst other Things, writes, that since this Age is well stored with good Systems, he wonders none should be contrived concerning the Commerce that may be betwixt Dæmons and Men.

To which Father le Brun thus answers, 'Doubtless here the Author complies with the Language of a great many Persons, who for Want of Attention and Light, would have us put all Religion in Systems. Whatever Regard I ought to have for many of these Persons, I must not be afraid to say. That there is no Systems to be made of those Truths, which we ought to learn distinctly by Faith, because we must advance nothing here but what we receive from the Oracle. We must make Systems to explain the Loadstone, the Ebbing and Flowing of the Sea, the Motion of the Planets; the Cause of these Effects being not evidently signified to us, and many being to be conceived by us; and to determine us we have Need of a great Number of Observations, which an exact Induction may lead us to a Cause, that may satisfie all the Phænomena. It is not the same in the Truths of Religion, we come not at them by Groping; and it were to be wished Men spoke not of them but after a decisive and infallible Authority. It's thus we should speak of the Power of Dæmons, and of the Commerce they have with Men. It's of Faith that they have Power, and that they attack Men, and try to seduce them several Ways. We find it in Job and Tobit, and in a Thousand other Places in Scripture and Tradition. It's certain also, that the Power they have, depends not on us, that they have it over the Just, since they may tempt them as they did Christ; though they have it not ordinarily, but over those that want Faith, or fear not to partake of their Works; and to these last, particularly these disordered Intelligences, try to make what they wish exactly succeed; inspiring them to have Recourse to certain Practices, by which those seducing Spirits enter in Commerce with Men: All this is discovered without System.' So far Le Brun.

As for those Philosophers, who chiefly reject Spirits, because they say they can have no Notion of such a Thing as a spiritual Substance, I think the late Mr. Locke, in his Elaborate Essay on Human Understanding, hath fairly made it out, that Men

Page 13

have as clear a Notion of a spiritual Substance, as they have of any corporeal Substance, Matter or Body; and that there is as much Reason for the Existence of the one as of the other; so that if they don't admit the Latter, it is but Humour in them to deny the Former: He Reasons thus: 'If a Man will examin himself, concerning his Notion of pure Substance in general, he will find he hath no other Ideas of it, but by a Supposition of he knows not what Support of such Qualities, which are capable of producing simple Ideas in us, which Qualities are commonly called Accidents; thus, if we talk or think of any particular corporeal Substance, as Horse, Stone, &c. though the Idea we have of either of them, be but the Complication, or Collection of those several simple Ideas, or sensible Qualities, which we use to find united in the Thing called Horse or Stone; yet because we cannot conceive how they should subsist alone, nor one in another, we suppose them to exist in, and to be supported by some common Subject; which Support we denote by the Name of Substance, though it be certain we have no clear or distinct Idea of that Thing we suppose a Support.

The same happens concerning the Operations of our Mind, viz. Thinking, Reasoning, Fearing, &c. which we concluding not to subsist of themselves, and not apprehending how they can belong to Body, we are apt to think these the Actions of some Substance we call Spirit; whereby it is evident, that having no other Notion of Matter, but something wherein these many sensible Qualities, which affect our Senses do subsist, by supposing a Substance wherein Thinking, Knowing, Doubting, and a Power of Moving do subsist, we have as clear a Notion of the Nature, or Substance of Spirit as we have of Body; the One being supposed to be (without knowing what it is) the Substratum to those simple Ideas which we have from without; and the other supposed (with a like Ignorance of what it is) to be the Substratum of those Operations which we experiment in our selves within: It's plain then, that the Idea of corporeal Substance in Matter, is as remote from our Conceptions and Apprehensions as that of spiritual Substance; and therefore from our not having any Notion of the Substance of Spirit, we can no more conclude its Non-existence, than we can for the same Reason deny the Existence of Body; it being as rational to affirm there is no Body, because we cannot know it's Essence as it's called, or have the Idea of the Substance of Matter; as to say there is no Spirit, because we know not it's Essence, or have no Idea of a spiritual Substance.'

Mr. Lock also comparing our Idea of Spirit with our Idea of Body, thinks there may seem rather lest Obscurity in the Former, than in the Latter. Our Idea of Body he takes to be an extended solid Substance, capable of Communicating Motion by

Impulse; and our Idea of Soul is a Substance that thinks, and hath a Power of exciting Motion in Body, by Will or Thought. Now some perhaps will say, they cannot comprehend a thinking Thing, which perhaps is true; but he says, if they consider it well, they can no more comprehend an extended Thing: And if they say, they know not what it is that thinks in them, they mean, they know not what the Substance is of that thinking Thing; no more, says he, do they know what the Substance is of that solid Thing: And if they say they know not how they think, he says, neither do they know how they are extended, how the solid Parts of Body are united to make Extension, &c.

And consonant to what is here delivered by Mr. Lock, Monsieur Le Clerc, in his Coronis, thus argues; says he, 'When we contemplate the corporeal Nature, we can see nothing in it but Extension, Divisibility, Mobility, and various Determinations of Quantity or Figures; which being so, it were a rash Thing, and contrary to the Laws of right Reasoning, to affirm other Things of Bodies; and consequently from meer Body, nothing can be deduced by us, which is not joined in a necessary Connection with the said Properties: Therefore those who have thought the Properties of perceiving by Sense, of Understanding, of Willing, Imagining, Remembring, and others the like, which have no Affinity with corporeal Things, to have risen from the Body, have greatly transgressed in the Method of right, Reasoning and Philosophizing, which hath been done by Epicurus, and those who have thought as he did, having affirmed our Minds to be composed of corporeal Atoms. But whence shall we say they have had their Rife? Truly, they do not owe their Rise to Matter, which is wholly destitute of Sense and Thought; nor are they spontaneously sprung up of nothing; it being a received Maxim of most evident Truth, that Nothing sprung from nothing.'

Therefore the Learned Dr. Cudworth, in his Intellectual System of the World, seeing nothing in Matter but what we have mentioned, and considering the abovementioned Maxim; passed from the Consideration of Bodies, to the Contemplation of a much more excellent Nature, by which he as well as other

Physiologers, understood that Human Minds, and all other intelligent Minds were created; therefore the Consideration of the corporeal Nature, joyned with the Knowledge of the Properties of the Mind lead Men the direct Way to the two Tenets of the greatest Moment, viz. The Existence of a supreme Deity, and the Creation of a Man's Soul, by God, whence also is deduced it's Immortality: To which we may add, that though the Authority of divine Revelation, be worthy of Credit by it self; yet it is not a little confirmed in our Minds, when we fee Revelation and Reason both conspire to confirm our Faith.

The above-mentioned Monsieur Le Clerc hath delivered several Things concerning Spirits and their Operations, of which we shall subjoyn the following Heads, being of Use to direct our Judgment in the Consideration of their Natures. '

First, Those who affirm, or deny that Spirits can be, without any corporeal Property, go farther than they ought; for we cannot gather from the Nature of Spirits, whether they are without all corporeal Property, or have a subtle Body. Sect. 2. c. I.

Secondly, As for Apparitions of Spirits, he says, we cannot by any Reason, shew from the Nature of the Thing it self, that it is not possible for Spirits to be joyned with a subtle Body; nor is it likely that so many Nations, and so remote in Places and Opinions agreed in a Lye, as to all they have said concerning the Apparitions of Spirits. It's much more likely, that the Ground of the Lyes invented about this Matter, was some true Apparition, to which, as it is usual, a World of other Relations of the like Kind have been feigned.

Thirdly, We are so far from determining what is the Nature of an Angel's Intellection, that we do not comprehend what is the Nature of our own Intellection.

Fourthly, In what the Gentiles say of Dæmons, and the Hebrews, of Angels, there is nothing contrary to any certain Knowledge we have; therefore what they say may be true, if the Thing be considered in it self.

Fifthly, As it cannot be doubted but there may be many Errors in what is related concerning the strange Performances of

Witches, upon a Contract with Dæmons; so it would be Rashness to charge them all with Falshood, especially since the Scriptures relate some Things like them; and truly the Thing it self is not so known to us, that we may gather from the Nature of Dæmons, which may not consist at least with many Things that are related of them; if any Man, (because both good and evil Angels are believed to be thinking Substances,) should contend that they have no Power on Bodies, because naked Thought hath no Power on Bodies: Before this were granted he ought to shew, and that evidently, First, That there is nothing in Angels besides Thought; Secondly, That there is no Tye instituted by God betwixt their Wills, and some Changes of Bodies; for if either of these may be admitted without Absurdity, they may be also thought able to act on Bodies without Absurdity.

Sixthly, Some say no true Miracles, but Cheats are performed by Dæmons; but to understand what this means, we must define the Words that are here used; a Portent, a Miracle, or a Prodigy, are here the same Things; and they denote an Effect; First, Above human Power; Secondly, Besides the constant Course of Nature; Thirdly, That it's done at Man's Pleasure, or at the Moment he will. Now who can make out by certain Arguments, that nothing can be done by evil Dæmons, above human Power, besides the usual Concourse of Nature, at the Moment the Magician pleases, since the Bounds of Angelick Power are unknown? We can here assert nothing but from Experience.

Seventhly, Those that deny some wonderful Facts, for the most Part contend they are Præstigia; but besides that they affirm what they know not; this Word may be taken in a twofold Sense; Præstigia, by some, are so understood, as though Dæmons present to the Senses, a Thing thing that is not, as if it were; as that an House, for instance, may seem to be there where there is none; but to do this, either they move the Brain of the Spectator, as it is wont to be affected when a House is before them, or they present a certain Sort of an Appearance of a House in the Air, which strikes the Eyes of the Spectators; but chuse either of these, it must be shewn how this is no Miracle, for both are done above human Power, and besides the Order of Nature, and at the Time the Magician pleases.

Eightly, Those Opinions or Diseases of the Brain which Witches have, who think they go to Feasts and Dancings, upon their Talking of it to others that are of a timorous Disposition and weak Brains, bring others into the same Fits of Fury, and like a Contagion spread far and near, infecting many Heads; though it is observable, those Diseases are more frequent amongst the Inhabitants of Mountains and solitary Places, than amongst those that live in Cities, or amongst a Concourse of People, &c.--to which he adds--whoever weighs these Things, will not wonder if Opinions of Witches are accounted melancholly Diseases.

Yet though these Things may be so, I will not affirm that those Things which Witches relate, have never happened,-- &c.'

From whence it sufficiently appears, that according to the Opinion of the most learned and greatest Philosophers, as well as the Testimony of Divine Revelation, there may be such Things as Spirits, which may produce Effects above the Power of Human Nature.

If it should be asked what Definition we give of Spirits, we may offer on this Occasion what Monsieur Le Clerc says in his Preface to his Pneumatologia, viz. 'We call all Things endowed with an Understanding and a Will, Spirits; as we consider them as spiritual Substances, he says, he hath shewn in his Logick, that the inward Nature of any Substances whatever, as well as that of Spirit is unknown to us; wherefore Men ought not to expect an absolute compleat Description of Spirits.'

From what we have offered, we doubt not but sufficient Arguments may be be drawn to confirm the Belief and Existence of Spirits, as well as from the Testimony of Holy Writ, which may be confirmed by the Examples recited in the following Histories: For as Reason and Revelation serve to confirm our Belief, and make Way for our Credit and assent to Historical Truths; so Historical Truths confirm, as well as lay a Foundation for Moral Demonstration, nothing presuming a stronger Pretence to Truth, than Histories attested by good Authority and sufficient Witnesses.

We might add a great many Arguments to prove the Existence of Spirits, and to demonstrate the Possibility of producing such Effects and Operations; but as in this History we have taken Notice of none but what seem to be authentick; so we have rather chose to produce the Opinions and Arguments of approved and noted Writers to prove their Possibility, than to offer any of our own, which might be less valid as of less Authority, though Reason, of what Authority soever, ought to be prevalent, as far as it carries the Probability of Truth along with it.

All that we shall add on this Occasion, by Way of Preface, is, That since the Design of this Work, is to shew what Power the Devil hath to torment, as well as deceive Mankind, when God Almighty pleases to permit him, and what evil Instruments he often makes use of to their own Destruction, as well as the Disadvantage of those that are tormented by them; if it answers the Design proposed, and may contribute to put us in Mind, how much we owe our Safety to an Almighty Providence, and how much we ought to reverence and adore our Great Protector, as well as to detest and abominate the Works of the Devil; we shall be not a little satisfied, that these Ends may render our Endeavours both acceptable and useful to the Publick.

A COMPLEAT HISTORY
OF WITCHCRAFT, SORCERY,
and all Magical Performances;
Together with
Relations of APPARITIONS, SPIRITS, and other reternatural Appearances, &c.

The INTRODUCTION.

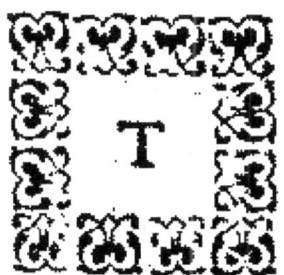

THE Diabolical Art of Witchcraft, Sorcery, and other Magical Performances, have been practised thro' so many Ages, and in so many Countries, with such dreadful and surprizing Effects; and have been attested by the Authority and Testimony of so many Writers of undoubted Repute and Credit, that it would be as absurd and unreasonable to deny the Truth of such Relations, as to dispute the Existence of that Diabolical Power by which they were performed, or of those pernicious Instruments the Devil makes use of to put them in Practice.

Nor are the Relations of Apparitions, Spirits, and other preternatural Appearances, less indisputable; since the Truth of such are testify'd by the unquestionable Testimony of a great many Eye-witnesses of Probity and Verity, who have been struck with Terror and Amazement at the Appearance of such

Spectacles, as well as by the dreadful Examples of such wicked Persons as have suffer'd by the Insults of those wicked Spirits.

Since then the Truth of such Things is indisputable, being confirmed by the Testimony of Eye-witnesses, and the undoubted Authority of both ancient and modern Authors, we shall not here trouble the Reader with a tedious Recital of Arguments, to prove the Possibility of such Things, since that sufficiently appears from the History of those wicked Practices, attested both by Sacred and other Writers; and is also confirmed by the severe Punishments inflicted on such as have practis'd such unlawful Arts, and the dreadful Effects produced by their unwarrantable Proceedings: Nor need we make use of stronger or more convincing Arguments, to prove the Possibility of Spectres and Apparitions, than the ocular Demonstration and Testimony of the Senses of those who have seen such Things, and have been terrify'd with such unwelcome Appearances.

Since then Historical Proofs of these unlawful Practices, and such preternatural Appearances, are the most convincing Arguments of the Truth of what we are about to treat of, we shall in the following Sheets consult the most authentick and learned Historians, both ancient and modern, who have wrote upon these Subjects, making use of the best Authority to prove the Practice of such Diabolical Arts; and shall, as briefly as we can, collect the most attested Relations of those Authors, to prove the Truth of Apparitions, Spirits, and preternatural Appearances.

And that this History may be the more compleat and methodical, we shall make use of the following Method, viz. First we shall begin with the most ancient and noted Historians of this kind, and shall continue that History down to the Moderns, collecting the most remarkable Relations and Passages contained in those Writers, according to the Time they were wrote in, whether they relate to Witchcraft, Sorcery, Magick, &c. or contain the most remarkable Relations of Apparitions, Spirits, or preternatural Appearances, comprising all Things that have been deliver'd, worthy our Notice, for above a Hundred Years.

But tho' the Testimony of Historians, and the undoubted and indisputable Relations of Matters of Fact, may be sufficient, and the best Arguments, to prove the Truth of such wicked Practices and Arts as have been made use of by Witches, Sorcerers, Necromancers, Magicians, &c. and to prove the Truth of such frightful and amazing Appearances of Dæmons, Spectres, Spirits, and other Apparitions; yet, that the Reader may have a clearer Apprehension of the Manner and Method of such unlawful Practices, and of the Nature of those Apparitions which are so frightful and surprizing, before we proceed to such Historical Relations above-mention'd, and to pursue the Method propos'd, to illustrate this History, we shall first consider what those unlawful Arts are in themselves, and how the Devil comes to delude Men to the Practice of them; what Contract the Devil makes with them, with the Difference between God's Miracles and the Devil's: We shall also prove from Scripture, the Possibility of such wicked Practices, and shew after what Manner wicked Men engage themselves in such Practices. We shall also consider the Nature of Witches Actions, and the Manner of their coming together, and what Adoration they pay to their Master the Devil. We shall also take Notice of the Methods Witches make use of to transport themselves from Places far distant from one another. We shall also consider their Actions, particularly in respect of those Persons they act upon, and why Women frequently practise that Art more than Men; what is the Extent of their Power, and what is the properest Method to remedy the Mischief done by them; what sort of Persons are more subject to be damaged by Witchcraft; and for what Reasons, and to what End, the Devil often appears to them, and assumes different Shapes and Forms. We shall also consider the different kinds of Spirits which troubles either Men or Women, and then proceed to the Method above-propos'd.

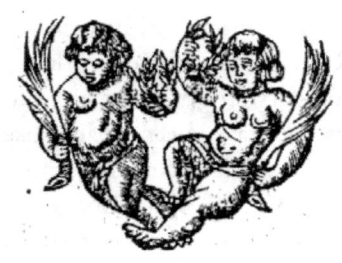

Chapter I

CHAP. I. Containing a brief Account of the Diabolical Arts of Witchcraft, Sorcery, and other Magical Practices, and how the Devil comes to delude Men to the Practice of them; what Contract the Devil makes with them, with the Difference betwixt God's Miracles and the Devil's; with the Manner how Men engage themselves in such Practices: As also the Actions of Witches, and their Manner of Meeting together, and what Adoration they pay the Devil their Master; as also how they transport themselves from Place to Place; what are their Actions in respect of the Persons they work upon, with the Extent of their Power, and what Methods are proper to remedy the Mischief done by them: What sort of Persons are most subject to be affected by them; why the Devil appears to them in different Shapes, as also the different Kinds of Spirits that disturb Men or Women.

THAT the Art of Witchcraft hath been practised in former Ages plainly appears from sacred History: For when Saul was troubled in Spirit, and his heinous Offences troubled his Conscience, he presently applied himself to a Woman who dealt with a familiar Spirit; I Sam. 28. who at his Desire raised up an unclean Spirit, which, according to the Text, Saul knew to be Samuel, it appearing in his Likeness so exactly, that Saul took it to be the Spirit of Samuel; the Devil being able to transform himself, and to appear in different Shapes, as 2 Cor. xi. 14. Satan is said to transform himself into an Angel of Light; and that God permits the Devil thus, upon some Occasions, to represent the Spirits of Men, and to foretel things to come, is not only apparent in this Case, but the like is plain from Michaiahs's Prophetick Discourse to King Ahab; I King 22. And that there is such an evil Practice as Witchcraft, and Witches, is apparent from several other Places in Scripture, it being plainly prohibited by the Law of God; Exod. 22. and the Truth of this appears further from the Power of Pharaoh's Wisemen, Exod. 5 and 8. who imitated a great many of the Miracles performed by Moses, which hardened that wicked Tyrant's Heart. And further, I Sam. 15. Samuel said to Saul, that Disobedience is as the Sin of Witchcraft. And that there were others of the same Craft, is manifest from the Story of Simon Magus, Acts 8. and the Woman that had the Spirit of Python, Acts 16. not to mention several other Places in Scripture which mention the Practice of Witchcraft, and such Diabolical Arts.

As for the Means by which the Devil allures Men to these wicked Practices, since he is the common Enemy of Man's Salvation, he is industrous to prompt them to such Vices as are most agreeable to their Tempers and Dispositions, the most heinous Impieties, being the most pleasant and delightful to such who have forsaken God, and are given over into the Hands of the Devil, whom he endeavours to lead so far into his Snares, that it is impossible for them to get out again. The chief and principle Motives by which Men are often led into these Snares, are Curiosity in some Men, who to please their Fansie, sell their Souls and Bodies to the Devil; others are moved to it, by an inordinate Thirst after Revenge, for some Injuries they have suffered, or through too greedy an Appetite of Gain.

And as there are three Inducements to allure Men to such unwarrantable Practices, so there are two Sort of Persons that may be enticed to the Pursuit of this Art, viz. learned and unlearned; and two Methods also of exciting them to this forbidden Curiosity, viz the Devil's School and his Rudiments. The Devil's School is a too eager Desire and Pursuit of Knowledge and natural Causes, where, when Men begin to find themselves Proficients in some Measure, and that they can account for several things by natural Causes, they are apt to advance too high; and where lawful Arts and Sciences fail of giving them Satisfaction, they are apt to apply themselves to the black and unlawful Science of Magick; and finding that several kinds of Circles, and Conjurations added to them, will raise several kinds of Spirits to resolve their Doubts, attributing these Effects to the Power inherently inseparable from the Circles, and several Words of God. confusedly wrapped together, they flatter themselves that they are Masters, and can command the Devil; though at the same time they enter themselves as his Slaves, and lose Paradise, as Adam did, by eating of forbidden Fruits. The Rudiments of the Devil are such unlawful Charms, which old Women often make use of to produce Effects without natural Causes; as Charms to prevent evil Eyes, &c. by knatting round Trees several kinds of Herbs; also curing of Worms, or stopping of Blood, by healing of Horse-crooks, or turning the Riddle, or meerly by Words, without the Application of Medicines: For though by such Practices they often do what they pretend to; yet it is not through any inherent Virtue in the thing done, but by the Power of the Devil, by which he deceives Men; and thus he allures them to seek Reputation by this deceitful Art, or entices them to it through Ambition, or the hopes of Gain; and makes a firm Contract with them upon that Account.

Of this kind of unlawful and unwarrantable Proceedings, is that Part of Astrology which pretends, by the Influence of the Stars, to foretel what Kingdoms will flourish or decay; what Persons will be fortunate or unfortunate; what Side shall gain the Victory in Battle; who shall overcome in single Combats; how, or at what Age Men shall die; what Horse shall win the Race, which Cardanus and Cornelius Agrippa have written at large. Of the same kind are those other Arts of Chyromancie, Physiognomie; and Fortune-telling, &c. which are unfit to be practised amongst Christians; the Prophet Jeremy plainly forbidding us to believe or give ear to Prophesies, and such as foretel by the Course of the Planets and Stars; Jerem. 10.

But the Art of Magick is not only unlawful but dangerous, which soon makes the Magicians weary of that Art which they at first Practise, and willing to agree with the Devil at an easie, Rats, and less Hazard; for as in practising the Magical Art, not only certain Seasons, Days and Hours, are to be made use of, but likewise Circles are to be made triangular, quadrangular, round, double or single, according to the Form of the Apparition that is desired: So besides the different Forms of the Circles, the innumerable Characters and Crosses, both within and without, and through the same; and the divers Forms of Apparitions that the Devil deceives them with, when once the conjured Spirit appears, if the Magician hath missed one of the least of all the Rights and Ceremonies, or if frightned with the Apparition, he slides over the Circle, he forfeits both Soul and Body, and is presently carried away with that Spirit, and the Devil directly pays himself that Debt which otherwise he must have stayed longer for.

But to proceed to the Manner of the Contract the Devil makes with them, it consists either in Forms of Effects; by Forms I mean in what Shape he is to appear to them in, when they call for him; by Effects I mean what Services he obliges himself to be subject to them in; which Forms and Effects are greater, according to the Skill and Art of the Magician: Some he obliges himself to appear to in the Form of a Dog, a Cat, an Ape, &c. or only to answer them by a Voice; and obliges himself to be serviceable to them in the Cure of Diseases, or some other base thing required of him. To oblige the most Curious, he often obliges himself to enter into dead Bodies, and out of them to answer Questions, in relation to future Events, as the success of Battles, or other Matters in respect of the Affairs of Kingdoms or Commonwealths; some he constantly pays his Attendance to in the Form of a Page: Sometimes he suffers himself to be conjured into the Form of a Tablet or Ring, which the Person he hath contracted with may constantly carry about with him; some he empowers to sell such Goods, which will be dearer or better cheap, as the Spirit conjured in them Lyes, or shall speak Truth.

And though all Devils are according to their Nature, Lyars; yet they deceive their wretched Slaves, and make them believe, that when Lucifer fell, some Spirits fell into the Air, some in the Water, some in the Fire, and some on the Land, and continue still in those Elements; and conclude, that such as fell in the Fire or Air, are truer than those that fell in the Water, or on the Land: And though by falling from the Grace of God, they are all of the same Quality, and wander through the Earth to execute what God permits them; and when those Executors of God's Wrath have finished their Work upon Earth, they are at the last Day to be enclosed in Hell along with those they have deceiv'd; yet they endeavour to perswade Men, that there are Princes, Dukes, and Kings amongst them, which command less or greater Legions, and have Empire and Power in several Arts, and different Quarters of the Earth.

But to proceed; as the Forms which the Devil obliges himself to appear in to the most curious Magicians, are wonderful, so the Effects are proportionable; he obliging himself to teach them Arts and Sciences; to carry them News from any Part of the World; to reveal to them any Persons Secrets, if once spoken: Nay, further he teaches his Scholars how to insinuate themselves into the Favour of Princes, by informing them of several great things, some of which prove to be true, and some false. He can also enable them to please Princes with dainty Entertainments, supplying them with such in a little time from the remotest Parts of all the World. Sometimes he pretends to guard his Scholars with the Appearance only of Armies of Horse and Foot, as well as with Castles and Sorts, which are only such in Appearance, formed by a Spirit making such Impressions on some Substances in the Air. He likewise teaches them several jugling Tricks with Cards or Dice, to enable them to deceive Mens Senses, and other such like false Practises, as we are inform'd by those who are acquainted with the Italian called Scoto. Thus the Devil enables them to deceive Mens Senses, as the Magicians did Pharaoh with their false Miracles which counterfeited those wrought by Moses. Thus the difference betwixt the Miracles wrought by God, and those perform'd by the Devil, is, that God, as the Creator, makes his Miracles appear in Effect, as Moses's Rod was turn'd into a real Serpent; whereas the Magicians Wands were only counterfeited by the Devil, and appear'd so only to deceive Mens Senses. One thing which we are here to observe further is, that when the Devil makes his Agreement with Magicians, it is either written with the Magician's own Blood, or else Touches; or else he touches them in some Part, without any visible Mark remaining, which are always perceivable in Witches.

Thus far we have consider'd the Nature and dangerous Practice of Magicians chiefly; we shall in the next place proceed to shew, that the Law of God, as plainly proves the evil Practices of Witchcraft, since it condemns and prohibits all such as consult with Devils, as Magicians, Diviners, Enchanters, Sorcerers and Witches: And that the Woman who had the Spirit of Python was a Witch seems evident, since he entered into her Body by her own Consent, and spoke with her Tongue; she being tormented with him, as those Demoniacks are, who are said to be possessed with an evil Spirit against their Will.

But to proceed: As the Being of Witches is undeniable from their ill Practices, and the Mischief they do, so it is not amiss, if we observe, that they are of two kinds, viz. either rich or wealthy, or poor and of low Degree; which Difference answers to the different Passions of the Mind, by which he entices them to follow such Practices; such as are in Misery and Poverty he allures to it by fair Promises of great Riches and worldly Gain. Those that are revengeful he promises the Satisfaction of obtaining the Ends they desire; yet the Devil is so crafty, that he pretends not to allure any Body, though possess'd with the above-mentioned Passions, except encouraged by their small Degree of Sense, or the ill Course of their Life, or their Carelessness and Contempt of God; and when he finds them in Despair, for any of these Causes, then he thinks it a proper time to attack them, and to discover himself to them; and then either as they walk solitarily in the Fields, or in their Beds, and without Company, he either by a Voice only, or in the Shape of a Man, enquires of them, what it is that troubles them, and promises them a certain Remedy, provided they follow his Advice, and what he requires of them; to which they are too ready to comply with, their Minds being before-hand prepared to admit of his Temptations. Having thus gained his End, he presently appoints another Meeting; and before he makes any further Proposals, he first perswades them to give themselves up to his Service, and then discovers to them what he is, obliges them to renounce their God and Baptism directly, and fixes his Mark upon some secret Part of their Body, which continues soar and unheal'd 'till their next Meeting, and ever after unsensible, though never so much nipped or pricked, which is proved by daily Trials, to let them know, that as he could both hurt and heal them, so all their future Evils or Happiness must depend on him. And besides, that the intolerable Pain which they felt in that Place where he marked them, serves to make them, and hinders them from resting 'till their next Meeting, lest in the mean time they should forget him, being not as yet confirmed sufficiently in their new Folly; or lest remembering the horrid Promise they made him at their last Meeting, they should repent of their Bargain, and endeavour to call it back. At their third Meeting he endeavours to make them sensible, how careful he is to observe his Promise, either by teaching them how to revenge themselves of any Injury; or how by unlawful ways they may obtain Riches and worldly Wealth.

As for their Actions they are of two kinds, viz. either in respect of themselves or other Persons. In respect of their own Actions, that they may perform such Services as the Devil employs them in, he counterfeits in his Servants the like Service that God requires of those that serve him: For as the Servants of God meet together to serve him, so these Servants of the Devil meet together in great Numbers to serve him, though not publickly; and as the Ministers of God teach his Servants how to serve him in Verity and Truth, so the Devil at these Meetings teaches his Servants how to act all manner of Mischief, and demands an Account of all their horrible Proceedings past for the Advancement of his Service. And as God formerly had Churches sanctify'd to his Service with Altars, Priests, Sacrifices and Prayers, the Devil had the like polluted to his Service: And as God gave answers by Urim and Thummim, so did the Devil by the Intrails of Beasts, the Singing of Fowls, and their Actions in the Air; and as God by Visions, Dreams and Extasies, revealed what was to come, and what was his Will, so the Devil used the like Methods to forewarn his Slaves of things to come. And as God loved Cleanness, expressed his Hatred to Vice and Impurity, and inflicted Punishments for the same; so the Devil dissembled with his Priests, appointing them to keep their Bodies clean and undefiled before they asked Questions of him; that by seeming to avoid less Crimes, he might lead them into greater: And even the Witches confess, that the Devil often, in defiance of God, appoints his Meetings in the Churches, and himself makes use of the Pulpit; and that in the Form of Adoration they are oblig'd to kiss his hinder Parts: And this, though ridiculous, seems probable, since we read in Calicute, appearing in the Likeness of a He-Goat, he had this Homage publickly paid him; his Ambition being so great, that he coveted to imitate God in this; it being said, Exod. 33 that Moses could only see the hinder Parts of God, for the Brightness of his Glory.

As to the Manner of their Meeting together thus, they say they have several Methods, either to adore their Master, or to execute any of his Commands, as by rideing, going, or sailing, whith are natural Ways, which they do upon their first Notice from their Master. Another Way is, by being carried through the Air, either over Land or Water, very swiftly, by the Force of the Spirit. Thus the Devil imitates God, Habbakkuk being carried by the Angel to the Den where Daniel lay. And one thing worthy our Notice is, that when they are thus transported, they are invisible to every Body, except themselves, which is very probable, since the Devil hath Power to make such Impressions on the Air, so as to form the Representations of Castles, Sorts, &c. Another way which they say they come together, is, by being transformed into the Likeness of a Beast or Fowl, in which Form they can pass through any House or Church, or any Place where the Air hath free Passage. Some say that when their Bodies lie still, and are in an Extasy, their Spirits may be ravished out of their Bodies, and carried to such Places, which appears both from the Testimony of those who have seen their Bodies lie sensless in the mean time, and also from the Designs they have formed at such Meetings; and in this Form they pass, when they are transported from one Country to another.

Thus much being said in respect of their Actions towards themselves, we shall next take Notice of their Actions in respect of others, in which we are to consider, First, The Manner of their Consultations; Secondly, What is done on their Part, as Instruments; and what the Devil does who puts such things in Execution.

As for their Consultations, those are most commonly made in Churches when they meet together to adore; when their Master asking each of them what they would be doing, every one proposes the mischievous Purpose they are inclined to, either for obtaining Riches, or to revenge themselves for some Injury, or on any Person they are maliciously inclin'd against, who presently puts them in the way to accomplish any Design that is evil. To accomplish some small Designs which they aim at, he teaches them how to dis-joynt dead Bodies, and powdering them to mix some other things with them which he furnishes them with.

As for the Reason why Women are more frequently concerned in this Craft than Men; it is partly occasion'd by their Frailty, as Eve was thought the fitter Subject for the Devil to work upon, and partly because they are more inclined to revenge.

But to proceed to the Arts which the Devil contrives to deceive his Scholars with. He teaches some to make Pictures of Wax or Clay; that by roasting of them, the Persons whose Names they bear, may be continually wasted and consumed by Sickness. Some he furnishes with such Stones or Powders, as will assist them to occasion Diseases, or to cure them. Others he instructs how to give uncommon Poysons, which are not easily remedied by Medicines; the Devil better knowing the Nature and Properties of Medicines than Men, and consequently how to evade the Power of those Medicines they make use of. Thus, as God opened the Eyes of the Blind with Clay and Spittle, which could not have that Effect, by their own Natures; so the Devil endeavours to delude his Servants, by making use of external Means, which have no Virtue to perform what is propos'd, but is brought about some other way: And by such like Means, these Servants of the Devil pretend to make Men and Women love or hate; the Devil himself disposing the corrupted Affections of those God permits him to work upon, which way he will. Thus, by God's Permission, he inflicted Sickness upon Job; for as the Devil is a subtle Spirit, and knows what Humours prevails in us, so he can alter the Temper of them, and make them of a vicious Temper, when God will permit him.

And further, That they can take away the Life of Men or Women, by roasting of Pictures, is very likely; for though the Instrument of Wax hath no Vertue to produce such Effects, yet the Devil being a subtle Spirit can dissolve the Form of the Spirits, and thus prevent the Concurrence of Spirits to promote Digestion, and supply the Body with fresh Nourishment, whilst the other is dispersed and consumed. But further, they can raise Storms or Tempests in the Air, either by Sea or Land, if God permits them, though not universal, but only in some particular Places, which are different from others, being sudden and violent, but not so lasting as those which naturally happen; which is very possible for the Devil to do, since he is a Spirit, and of near Affinity with the Air, which may easily be moved by a Spirit; and we read that the Scripture it self gives the Devil the Title of Prince of the Air.

Another thing which is said to be in their Power is, to make People phrensical and mad; which being but natural Sicknesses, the Devil may as well occasion as any other Sickness. They can likewise occasion Spirits to follow and trouble Persons, or to haunt certain Houses, and frighten the Inhabitants, which we have often known the Witches do. They likewise can cause some to be possessed with Spirits, as Dæmoniacks.

As for the Persons whom God permits to be afflicted thus, and to be under the Power of Witchcraft, they are of three kinds, viz. either such as God thinks fit should be punished for their horrid Sins; or sometimes the Godly, to awaken them out of some great Sins or Infirmities, or to try their Patience as Job's was, it being in God's Power to suffer any Punishments to be inflicted as he pleases. And as God may permit some Persons to be more under their Power than others, so those often are most subject to the Power of Witchcraft, that are of a weak and infirm Mind, being weak in Faith, whereas those who through Faith in God defie their Power, he will not suffer the Devil their Master to hurt them that trust in him.

But though Witches have the Power we have observed, to transport themselves from one Place to another, and to bring about such things as the Devil their Master can help them out in; yet when God Almighty thinks fit to bring them to Justice, and they are imprisoned and confined by the Laws of God, the Devil hath no Power any further to help them, being not able to wrest them out of his Hands: Yet when they are imprisoned, and like to be punished for their Offences, the Devil is still ready to deceive them; and if they flatter themselves with vain Hopes, he is ready to promote their vain Expectations; or of he find them in Despair, he is as ready to augment it, and urges them to use some extraordinary Means to endeavour to rescue themselves.

As to the Forms the Devil appears in on such Occasions, it is either according to their Agreement, or the Nature of their Circles and Conjurations they make; yet to some he appears as he pleases, or as he thinks it will suit with their Humours; so that at the same time he makes himself appear in different Forms to several Persons, as he thinks will best suit his Ends. And though he be an airy Body, yet he will sometimes so delude the Senses, as to appear to them like a Substance; or assumes a dead Body, which he makes use of as long as he thinks fit.

Thus much being said of Magick and Witchcraft, we shall, in the next place, proceed to consider the Nature of those

Spirits which appear and trouble both Men and Women, frequently affrightening them with their dreadful Appearances.

These Spirits then which fright and disturb Men frequently by their amazing Effects they produce, or by their dismal and astonishing Appearances, may be divided into four different kinds; the First are those which trouble Houses and solitary Places; the Second are such as haunt and follow several Persons, and are often troublesome to them; the Third are such as enter into Persons and possess them; the fourth Sort are such as are commonly called Fayries.

How these Spirits have been troublesome to Persons by the Power of Witchcraft, hath been shewn already. We shall in the next place say something of their natural Appearance, without the Power of Witchcraft; though no doubt but they are one kind of Spirits, which only differ in their Form of Appearance, and the Manner of their Actions.

As for the first kind of these Spirits, which haunt Houses, and appear in several horrible Forms, making a great Noise, they are called Lemures or Spectra, which sometimes appear in the Form of dead Persons, and are called by different Names, according to the Difference of their Actions. That there are such Appearances of Spirits, we are assured by the Holy Scriptures, where the Prophet Esay, 13. and 34. threatning the Destruction of Jerusalem, declares, That it shall not only be sacked, but become so great a Solitude, that it shall be the Habitation of Howlets, and of Ziim and Jim, which are Hebrew Names for these Spirits. They haunt solitary Places, that they may the better terrify and shake the Faith of such Persons as frequent Places of that kind; and when they haunt Houses, it shews either a great deal of Ignorance, or they are suffered to disturb the Neighbours for their gross and slanderous Sins.

As for the Manner of their entering such Houses, it is different, according to the Form they are in at that Time. If they have assumed a dead Body, they can easily open a Door or a Window without any Noise; and if they enter as a Spirit only, any Place where the Air can pass thro', is sufficient for their Passage.

If it be asked whether the Devil hath equal Power to enter the Bodies of just, as well as those of wicked Men; I answer, That his Entrance into their Bodies when the Soul is absent, cannot defile them, and therefore in that there can be no Inconveniency in respect of the Person that the Body belong'd to; nor can it be any greater Dishonour to them than the hanging, heading, or other shameful Deaths good Men frequently suffer, the Bodies of both the Faithful and Unfaithful being equally free from Corruption, and worthy of Honour, till the last Day, when those of the Just shall be purged and purified.

But though these Spirits actually haunt such Places, yet are they not to be seen by all Persons, but only such as God Almighty shall think fit: And as for their appearing in the Form and Shape of a Person who is dead, or is to die, as the Devil formerly thus appeared to amuse the Gentiles, and mislead them, by foretelling the Death of a Person, the Will of the Dead, or the Manner of their Death, so he now appears to some ignorant Christians to delude and mislead them, since it is not possible the Souls of the Defunct should return, or that Angels should put on such Forms.

As for the other two kinds of Spirits, which outwardly haunt and trouble some Persons, or otherwise inwardly possesses them; these, for the Likeliness of their Appearance and Actions, may be both esteemed of one kind, as well as the Persons they are permitted to trouble.

As for the Persons that are usually troubled with these kind of Spirits they are of two kinds, viz. either such as are guilty of great Offences, or such as God permits to be tempted for a Trial of their Patience, or the admonishing of the Beholders, or that others may have Reason to praise God that they are not corrected in the same dreadful Manner. The Intent and Design of the Devil tormenting Persons after this Manner is, either to provoke them to mistrust and blaspheme God, either for the Intolerableness of their Torments, as he endeavour'd to do with Job, or that they might make him some Promises, to perswade him to leave off troubling of them. And though these fort of

Spirits not only molest and torment some Persons, but sometimes forewarn them of what Dangers may happen to them; yet this is only to deceive Men, that they might think themselves safe, and confide in him who appear'd willing to do them what Service he could, though all the while he was outwardly seeming to do good, his Intentions were evil, he endeavouring to perswade them that God's Enemy was their Friend.

There were other sorts of Spirits, called Incubi and Succubi, according to the Difference of the Sexes they conversed with. Sometimes he made use of the Semen taken out of a dead Body, which he deceived several with, who were not able to feel any thing, but that which was so contrary to Nature in that Part: And sometimes he made use of a dead Body to abuse Men, though the Deceit might be discovered by the Coldness of the Semen, perceived easily by the Person abused. This hath been confessed by some Witches who have been perswaded by the Devil to suffer him to abuse them after this Manner, that he might secure them the faster in his Snares. And here it may not be amiss to take Notice, that the Mare, which is called Incubus, ab incumbendo, is much different from this kind, that depending on a Distemper and Disorder of the Body.

As for those who are possess'd with these kind of Spirits, tho' they may be thought by some only to be sick of a Phrensy or some other Distemper, yet those who are truly possess'd, may easily be distinguish'd from such Persons, by several Symptoms, especially three; not to mention the vain Signs which the Papists assign for the Difference, as their raging at Holy Water, flying back from the Cross, &c. The first of the true Signs, is the incredible Strength of the possess'd Creature, being six times greater than the Strength of other Men who are not thus possess'd. The second is, the violent lifting up of the Person's Breast and Belly with violent Motions and Agitations within, the Sinews being extended and stretched out as hard as Iron it self. The third is, their speaking of divers Languages, such as the Person is known never to have learned, and that too with a strange and hollow Voice, having, all the Time of speaking, a greater Motion in the Breast than Mouth. But such as are possess'd with a dumb and blind Spirit, have not this last Sign; such a one our Saviour relieved in the 12th of Mathew.

As for the Manner of casting out these Devils when Persons are possess'd with them: That our Saviour gave his Disciples Power to do it, is evident from Scripture; and that those who are not true Disciples may have this Power, is evident, since Judas had that Power as well as any of the rest, the Method of doing it being by Fasting and Prayer, and calling upon the Name of God; and our Saviour tells us of the Power false Prophets may have to cast out Devils. But to proceed to the last kind of Spirits, which were called Fairies: These were most frequent in the Time of Papistry here in England; and though it was esteemed odious to prophesy by the Name of the Devil, yet those that these kind of Spirits carry'd away, and informed, were thought to be the best Tort of Persons. Of these we are told that there was a King and Queen, who had a noble Court and Train; that they had a Duty of all sorts of Goods; also how they naturally rode and went about, eat and drank, and exercised all other Actions natural to Men and Women, the Devil deluding the Senses of People so much, that these Spirits appeared to them actually to do such Things.

But tho' the Devil deludes his Scholars with the Appearance of such Things, yet it appears from those that have been carried along with these Fairies, that they never saw the Appearance of any in that Court, except of those who were Brothers and Sisters of the Art of Witchcraft. This hath been proved by the Relation of a young Woman, who was troubled with Spirits, thro the Power of Witchcraft; who, though she saw the Shapes of several Men and Women disturbing her, and could name the Persons whom these Shadows represented, yet most of those have been try'd and found guilty, and confessed the same.

To conclude: The surest way to discover such as practise this odious Craft, besides their evil Lives and Conversations, is, first, by their Mark, which is insensible; and, secondly, by their swimming upon the Water, God having ordained, that such as had cast off the Water of Baptism should not be received into Water, but swim upon it.

CHAP. II.

Of Ghosts and Spirits walking by Night, and of strange Noises, Cracks, and Things that happen before the Death of Men, great Slaughters, and Alterations of Kingdoms.

Having in the foregoing Chapter given the Reader a general Notion or Scheme of the Art of Magick and Witchcraft, and also of the Actions of Magicians and Witches, both in respect of themselves and others; and having also shewn briefly the Nature of Spirits, and their Difference, which are concerned in Spectres, Apparitions, and other preternatural Appearances, we shall in this Chapter proceed to Particulars, and give an Historical Account of Witchcraft, Magick, Apparitions, Ghosts, &c. according to the Time and Places they occur in, in the Method above-propos'd.

And, first, though a great many melancholy, mad, fearful, and Men of weak Sense, frequently imagine Things to be that really are not, and are oftentimes deceived by Men or brute Beasts, and sometimes mistake those Things which proceed from natural Causes, to be Bugbears and Spirits; yet it is most certain, and beyond Dispute, that those Things which appear to Men and fright them, do not always proceed from natural Causes, but that Spirits do often appear, producing very strange and wonderful Effects, such Things being attested by ancient Historians of very good Credit, who have delivered their Histories upon the Testimony of such Persons as have seen them both in the Day-time as well as by Night.

Suetonius tells us, that when Julius Cæsar marched out of France into Italy with his Army, and came to the River Rubicon, which parts Italy from South France, staying there a while, and considering with himself how great an Enterprize he had taken in Hand, and being doubtful whether he should pass the River or not, there suddenly appeared to him a Man of excellent Stature, and well shaped, who sat hard by him, piping upon a Reed. This drew together a great many Shepherds and Soldiers from the Camp, and also a great many Trumpeters, who flocked together to hear him. Having by this Means collected a great Number together, he suddenly snatched a Trumpet from one of them and leaped into the River, and, with a strong Breath blowing up the Alarum, went over to the other Side. Upon which, says Cæsar, Good Luck attends us, let us go where the Gods give us Encouragement, and where the Iniquity of the People calls us. The Dice are thrown; and, upon this, he immediately passed over the River.

To this we shall add what Plutarch relates in the Life of Theseus, viz. That many who were in the Battle of Marathonia against the Medians, affirm'd that they saw the Soul of Theseus armed, (who died a long time before by a Fall) before the Vanguard of the Grecians, running before and encouraging the barbarous Medians; which caused the Athenians afterwards to honour him as a Demi-God.

Pausanias writeth in Atticis, That in the Field of Maratho, Four hundred Years after the Battle was fought, they distinctly heard the neighing of Horses, and the encountering of Soldiers, as if they were engaged in Battle every Night. And what was very remarkable was, that those that came there on purpose to hear these Things, could hear nothing; whereas those that came that Way by Chance, heard these Things very sensibly.

And Plutarch writes, in the Life of Cimon, That when the Citizens of Cheronesus had entreated their Captain Damon with fair Words to return home, who fled from the City for several Murthers he had committed, and had afterwards killed him barbarously in a hot House, as he was bathing himself; after that Time there were several strange Sights seen in the same Place, and oftentimes most grievous Groanings were heard, so that ever after they were obliged to shut up the Hot-house Doors.

He also tells us, in the Life of Dion, That the same Dion being a stout and courageous Man, and not subject to Fear, saw a very strange and wonderful, as well as horrible Sight: For sitting alone in the Entry of his House, in the Evening and meditating and discoursing of several Things with himself, being suddenly surprized with a great Noise, he rose and looked back towards the other Side of the Gallery, where he saw a monstrous great Woman, whose Countenance and Apparel made her appear like a Tragical Fury, sweeping the House with a Broom. Being very much amazed and frighten'd with this astonishing Sight, he called his Friends and Acquaintance to him, declaring to them what he had seen, and desiring their Company all that Night; for being extreamly amazed at the Appaparition, he feared it might appear to him again if he were alone, though it never did: But a few Days after his Son threw himself headlong from the Top of the House, and died; and he himself, being stabbed through the Body, ended his miserable Life.

The same Author tells us, in the Life of Decius Brutus, That when Brutus determin'd to transport his Army out of Asia into Europe, being in his Tent about Midnight, and the Candle burning dimly, and the whole Army being quiet and silent, as he was considering with himself, he fancy'd he heard one entering into his Tent, and, Looking back towards the Door, he saw the Form of a terrible and monstrous Body, much exceeding the common Stature of Men, which stood close by him, without speaking a Word; which frightful Apparition, tho' it made him not a little afraid, he even ventur'd to ask this Question: What art thou? a God, or a Man? And for what camest thou to me? To which the Apparition answerd; I am, O Brutus, thy evil Ghost, at Philippus thou shalt see me. Then says Brutus, recovering his Surprize, I will see thee. When this Sight was vanished, he called his Servants, who told him, that they neither saw any such Thing, neither heard any Voice at all. All that Night Brutus could not sleep at all, but in the Morning went to Cassius, and told him the whole Story of this strange Vision; but Cassius contemned and despised all such Things, attributing them to natural Causes: But afterward Brutus, being overcome in the Field by Augustus and Anthony at Philippi, slew himself, rather than to be deliver'd into the Hands of his Enemies.

To this we shall add, that Valerius Maximus tells us, that Caius Cassius saw Julius Cæsar in the Battle at Philippi, appearing in much more Majestick Shape than could belong to any Man, setting Spurs to his Horse, and running on with a terrible threatning Countenance; upon the Sight of which Cassius turned his Back to the Enemy, and fled, and soon after murther'd himself.

Dio Cassius Nicæus, in his Roman History, tells us of Drusus, that having ravaged and over-run Germany on every Side, he came to the River Abbis, which being not able to get over, he there erected Memories of his Victories, and returned back again; for he there met a Woman exceeding the rest of mortal Creatures in Majesty, who said to him; Drusus, who can set no Limits to thy boundless Ambition, whither goest thou? It is not lawful for thee to go any further, therefore get thee hence, for the the End both of thy Life and worthy Actions are now at hand. Drusus hearing this, presently altered his Course; and, as he was on his Journey, before he came to the River of Rein, fell sick and died. The same Author mentions several other Things which foretold his Death, tho' he did not regard them; for two young Men appeared upon the Ramparts on Horse-back; and the Shrieking of Women were also heard, with several such-like Omens.

Plinius Secundus, a Citizen of Novocomensis, writ an Epistle of the Appearance of Spirits to his Friend Sura, which we shall in the next Place take Notice of. He tells us, That Curtius Rufus, who was then Companion to the Pro-consul of Africa, being both poor and of small Reputation, walking one Day in a Gallery, towards the Evening, he met with an Apparition in the Shape of a Woman, greater and more beautiful than any living Creature. He being amaz'd at the Sight, she told him that she was Africa, and was come to acquaint him before-hand with the News of future good Fortunes: First, that he should go to Rome, and there be promoted to great Honour; and that afterwards he should return into the same Province with great Power and Authority, and there end his Days: All which came to pass. The same Figure met with him again by the Sea-side, as he landed out of a Ship, and came towards Carthage to take Charge and Command of a Regiment. Afterwards falling sick, when no Man despaired of his Recovery, conjecturing what would come to pass for the future, by what had already happen'd, and comparing his Adversity with his former Prosperity, he utterly laid aside all Hopes of Recovery.

But what is much more terrible and wonderful, is the following Relation. There was in Athens a goodly and very large House, but reported to be very unlucky and unfortunate; for about Midnight there was heard the strange Noise of Iron, and, if well observ'd, the rattleing of Chains, which at first seemed to be afar off, but by degrees approached nearer and nearer. In a little time, there appeared the Image of an old Man, who, to Sight, was lean and loathsome, with a long Beard and staring Hair: He had Fetters on his Legs, and carry'd Chains in his Hands, which he always rattled together. Those that lived in the House, being terrify'd with these Things, spent many a dismal Night in watching, after which they were afflicted with Sickness, and in a little time, their Fear encreasing, it ended in Death; for in the Day-time, tho' the Apparition was vanished, yet the Remembrance of it was still before their Eyes, so that their Fear continued longer than the Cause. Upon this, the House stood empty, desart, and solitary, being only possessed by the Monster that haunted it, notwithstanding it was proposed to be sold, if any Body who was ignorant of its being haunted, would have bought it or lived in it. Athenodorus, by Chance coming to Athens, read the Writing over the Door, and when he understood the Price, thinking it a good Bargain, he enquired further, and hearing the Truth of the Matter, he was the more forwards to hire the House. When Night came on, he commanded his Servants to make his Bed in the outward Part of the House; and, having fixed his Writing-Table, and other Things, in Order, he sent all his Servants into the inner Part of the House. Having done this, he composed his Mind, and fixing his Eyes upon what was before him, he was very intent upon his writing, lest his Mind, being unemploy'd, should be apt to imagine strange Things, which might create groundless Fears. In the Beginning of the Night there was Silence, as in all other Places, but not long after the Iron began to ring, and the Chains to move; but not withstanding all that, he would not look up, but continued his writing, and stopped both his Ears. Upon that the Noise encreased, and drew nearer, sometimes seeming to be without the Porch, and sometimes within; upon which he looked back, and saw the same Things which he had been told of before. The Apparition stood still and beckon'd with his Fingers, as if he called him: The Philosopher, on the other side, moved his Hand, to signify that he should stay a while, and fell to writing again: Upon that the Image shook his Chains over his Head, as he was writing. He looked about, and saw him beckoning, as before; therefore he rose up directly, and, taking the Candle in his Hand, followed the Apparition, who walked softly before, as if he was heavy loaden with Chains; but as soon as he had turned aside into the Court of the House, he suddenly vanished away, leaving the Philosopher alone; who gathering Herbs and Leaves together, left them upon the Place. The next Day he went to the Governours of the City, and desired them to command the Place to be dug up, which accordingly was done, where they found Bones wrapped up, and bound in Chains, which continued in Bonds, tho' the Body was rotted and putrify'd with lying long in the Earth. These Bones being gathered together, were solemnly bury'd; and the House, after they were decently laid in the Ground, was ever after clear from such Ghosts.

    The same Author who relates this Story, delivers the following upon his own Knowledge, after this manner. Says he, I have one with me, who was some time my Slave, but now at Liberty and free, a Man not altogether unlearned. who lay in the same Bed with my younger Brother: He imagined he saw a certain Person sitting on the Bed-side where he lay, putting Knives to his Head, and by that Means pulling off his Hair. In the Day-time the Hairs were found upon the Ground, and the Loss of them was plainly discernable about the Crown of his Head. In a little Time after the same Thing happen'd again, which confirmed the first Report: The Boy, among the rest of his School-Fellows, happen'd to sleep in the School; and when he was asleep, some coming in at the Windows, cloathed in white Garments, and shaving the Hair off his Head as he lay, they went out again the same Way they came in. The Hair that was shaved off his Head, as well as those scatter'd Hairs before-mention'd, were found when it was Day light. No remarkable Accident happened after these Things, except that I was not accus'd of Treason, as I should have been, if Domitianus had lived longer, who dy'd about this Time, there being a Libel found amongst his Writings against me, given him by Master Carus. Whence it may be conjectured, since those that were accused used to wear their Hair long, that the cutting off my Friend's Hair was an eminent Token of my escaping that great Danger which hung over my Head.

The like History may be found in a Collection of John Manlius's common Places, who tells us, That Theodorus Gaza having a Lordship or Manour in Campania given him by Nicholas, Pope of Rome; one of the Farmers having digged up a Coffin with dead Men's Bones in it, in that Manour, a Spirit suddenly appeared to him, commanding him to bury the Coffin again, otherwise his Son should die in a little Time after; which the Farmer refusing to do, his Son was soon after slain in the Night. In a few Days after the Spirit appeared again to the Husbandman, threatning him, that if he did not bury the aforesaid Bones, he would kill his other Son. The Man being surprized at this, and finding his other Son sick, related the whole Matter to Master Theodorus; which as soon as he had heard, he went along with the Man, and, digging a Grave just by the Place where the Coffin was dug up, they bury'd the Coffin and Bones in it; upon which the Husbandman's Son immediately recovered his Health.

Dion tells us, That the Emperor Trajanus was lead out of the House where had taken up his Inn, in the Time of an Earthquake, into a safer Place. And Julius Capitolinus, writing of the Roman Emperors, reports, That Pertinax, for three Days Space before he was killed by a Stab, saw a Shadow in one of his Fish-Ponds, which, with a Sword ready drawn, threatened to kill him; which was no small Trouble and Occasion of Uneasiness to him.

Flavius Vopiscus says, That Tacitus Father's Grave open'd it self, the Sides falling down of their own Accord; and that his Mother's Soul appear'd both to him and Florinus Day and Night, as if she had been living; which was a Sign that he should die soon after. And Ammianus Marcellinus, writing of the Signs and Prognostications of Constantius's Death, says, that he was troubled and terrify'd in the Night with Shapes and Figures. And the same Author affirms, that a little before Julianus dy'd, as he was writing in the Tents, after the the Example of Julius Cæsar, he saw the Image of the publick Genius or God of the Place, which used to be painted with Amalthæas's Horn in his Hand, departing from him, more deformed and ill-favoured, than when it began to mount up towards the Top of the Tent. And Lucan, who was both an excellent Historian, and a learned Poet, reckons up as many of such Fore-warnings in his Book of the Battle of Pharsalia, which happened before the great Conflict between Julius Cæsar and the great Pompey.

And if we read over the Ecclesiastical Histories, we shall find many of these Examples.

Sozomenus, in his Ecclesiastical History, tells us of one Apelles a Blacksmith (whose Name was very famous at that Time through Ægypt, for the Gift of working Miracles, which he was endowed with) who, one Night as he was hard at work, was surprized with the Appearance of a Vision, which was the Devil in the Likeness and Attire of a very beautiful Woman, endeavouring to move and entice him to the Vice of Lechery: Whereupon he suddenly snatched the Iron which he worked with, glowing hot, out of the Fire, and thrust it in the Devil's Face, and scorched his Vizard; which being done, he fretted, and cry'd out, and fled away.

In another place, writing of the Sedition rais'd at Antioch, upon the immoderate Exaction and Tribute, which Theodosius laid on the City in the Time of the Wars, in which the People being offended, overthrew the Images of the Emperor and his Wife, and dragged them in Ropes about the City, using all the villanous Expressions they could, and shewing what Spite they could against them, says, that the Night before, as soon as the Rebellion begun, immediately at break of Day, there was a strange Sight seen, a Woman of a huge Stature appearing, with most horrible Looks, running up and down the City through the Streets in the Air, whisking and beating the Air with a Whip, and making a fearful Noise: So that as Men usually provoke wild Beasts to Anger, which serve for publick Spectacles, so ic appeared, that some evil Angel, by the Craft of the Devil, stirred up that Commotion amongst the People.

Theodorus Lector, in his Collections of the Ecclesiastical History, writes, that as Gennadius, Patriarch of Constantinople, came down to the high Altar to pray, a certain Vision or Spirit appeared to him, in a most horrible Shape and Figure; which as soon as he had sharply rebuked, he heard a Voice crying out aloud, that as long as he lived he would withdraw and cease; but as soon as he was dead, he would certainly ransack and spoil the Church; which the good Father hearing, he earnestly prayed for the Preservation of the Church, and soon after departed this Life.

St. Ambrose, in his 90th Sermon, tells us of a noble Virgin, named Agnes, who was crowned with Martyrdom for professing the Christian Religion; who when she was buried, her Parents watching one Night by her Grave, they saw, about Midnight, a great Company of Virgins cloathed in Golden Vails, amongst whom was their Daughter adorn'd like the rest, who desiring the other Virgins to stay a while, and turning towards her Parents, she desired them that they would by no means bewail her as if she were dead, but rather to rejoyce, because she had obtained of God eternal Life; which as soon as she had spoke, she immediately vanished out of sight. And St. Augustin reports, that when the City of Nold was besieged by the Barbarians, the Citizens saw Felix the Martyr plainly appearing to them. And in the Life of Chrysostom, it is said, that Basiliscus, Bishop of Comanè, (who suffered as a Martyr with Lucianus the Priest of Antioch, under Maimianus the Emperor) appeared to St. Chrysostom, when he was in Exile, and said. Brother John, be of good Comfort, for to Morrow we shall be together. But first he appeared to the Priest of that Church, and said to him, prepare a Place for our dear Brother John, who will shortly come hither: Which things proved true in the Event.

To these Relations we shall add several Histories of the Appearance of Spirits from very credible Authors.

Alexanderab Alexandria, an excellent Lawyer, born at Naples, writes, that a certain Friend of his, of good Credit, having celebrated the Funeral of one of his Acquaintance, as he returned towards Rome, being benighted, he went to an Inn by the Way, and there layed himself down to rest; where as he lay there alone, and broad awake, suddenly the Image of his Friend lately deceas'd came before him, very pale and lean, just as he saw him last on his Death-bed. When he beheld this Spectacle, being almost out of his Wits with the Fright, he demanded of him, who he was? But the Ghost making no Answer, slip'd off his Cloaths, and lay'd down in the same Bed, drawing nearer to him, as if he would have embraced him: The other gave way to him, and endeavouring to keep him off from him, by chance touched his Face, which seemed to be extremely cold, and much colder than Ice: Whereupon the other looking upon him very lowringly, took up his Cloaths again, and rose out of the Bed, and was never afterwards seen.

Baptista Fulgosus, Duke of Genoa, in a Book of the worthy Sayings and Actions of Princes, Emperors, &c. concerning strange and monstrous things, writes, that in the Court of Mattheus, Great Sheriff of the City, in the Evening, after Sun-set, there was seen a Man far exceeding the common Stature, sitting on a Horse, in compleat Armour; who, when he had continued there, and was seen by many, for the Space of an Hour, vanished away to the great Terrour of those that beheld him. About three Days after, two Men on Horseback, of the same Stature, were seen in the same Place, about three Hours after it was Night, fighting together a long time, and at last vanished as the other did before. Not long after Henry the Seventh, Emperor, departed this Life, which proved the utter Ruin of all Sheriffs.

To which History he adds the following: Ludovicus, Father to Alodisius Ruler of Immola, not long after he died, appeared to a Secretary, whom Ludovicus had sent to Ferraria, as he was on his Journey, riding upon a Horse with a Hawk on his Hand, as he used to do when he was living, and desired the Secretary, who was much afraid, to bid his Son come to the same Place the next Day, having Matters of great Importance to declare to him. When he heard this, partly because he could not believe it, and partly lest some Body should lie in wait for him, he sent another to answer for him in his Room; with whom the same Soul meeting, as it did before, much lamented that his Son was not come thither; for if he had, he said he would have discovered several other things to him: However he desired one Messenger to tell him, that after twenty-two Years, one Month and one Day, he should lose the Rule and Government he now possessed. As soon as the time foretold by the Ghost was expired, though he was very circumspect and careful, yet the same Night the Soldiers belonging to Philip Duke of Millan, with whom he was in League, and therefore stood in no fear of him, came over the Ditches hard frozen with Ice to the Walls, and raising up Ladders, took both the City and Prince together.

Philip Malancthon writes himself, that he hath seen four Spirits, and that he hath known many Men of good Credit, who vouched, that they had seen Ghosts themselves, and talked with them a great while. And in his Examen Theologicum he relates the following History; which was, that he had an Aunt, who sitting very sorrowfully by the Fire, after her Husband was dead, two Men came into her House, one of which being very like, said he was her Husband deceased, and the other being very tall, appeared like a Franciscan Fryar. That which seemed to be the Husband came near the Chimney, saluting his sorrowful Wife, and bidding her not to be afraid, for he came to command her to do several things: Then he bid the long Monk to go aside a while into the Stove hard by, and then began his Discourse; and after many Words, at last he earnestly beseeched her, and desired her to have a Priest to say Mass for his Soul; and then being ready to depart, he bid her give him her right Hand, which she was very unwilling to do; but upon his Promise that she should come by no Harm, she gave it him; which, notwithstanding it had no hurt, it seemed to be so scorched, that ever after it remained black.

Ludevicus Vives says, that in that Part of the World which was then lately found out, that nothing is more common than for Spirits, not only in the Night-time but at Noon-day, to appear, both in the City and in the Fields, which speak, command, forbid, assault and strike Men, as well as make them afraid. And Olaus Magnus tells us, that in Iseland Spirits appear in the Figure and Likeness of such as Men are acquainted with, whom the Inhabitants take by the Hand instead of their Acquaintance, before they have heard a Word of their Death, whose Likeness those Spirits take upon them; nor do they understand that they are deceived before they shrink and vanish away.

Sometimes men walking alone in their Houses, have been surprized with the dismal Appearance of Spirits in our own Country, which even the Dogs have perceived, and fell down at their Masters Feet, and would by no means depart from them: Others lying down in their Beds to rest, have been pinched, or had the Cloaths pulled off them; and sometimes the Spirit hath sat upon them, or lain down in the same Bed, or would walk up and down in the Chamber. They have often also appeared, walking on Foot, or rideing on Horse-back with a fierce Countenance, and in such Shapes as were known to Men, and of such as died not long before. Others who have been slain in the Wars, or who have died in their Beds, have appeared to their Acquaintance, and have been known by their Voice.

And very frequently in the Night-time Spirits have been heard, either going softly, spitting or groaning; and being asked what they were, answered that they were the Souls of particular Men, and that they suffered extreme Torments. Sometimes the People of the House have thought, that some Body in the House had over-set Pots, Platters, Tables and Trenchers, and trumbled them down the Stairs, though when Day-light appeared, they have found things set in their Places again. Sometimes Spirits have thrown own Doors off the Hooks, and set all things in he House out of order, and never set them in their Places again, and have strangely disturbed People with rumbling and making a great Noise. Sometimes a great Noise hath been heard in Abbies and other solitary Places, as if Cowpers were hooping and stopping up Wine-casks, or other Tradesmen were about their Labour, whilst all the People have been in their Houses and at rest. When Houses have been building likewise, the the Neighbours have heard Carpenters and Masons handling their Tools, as if they had been at work in the Day-time: Also Pioneers, or those that dig for Metals, affirm, that several times in the Mines, Spirits have appeared in strange Shapes, or dressed like other Labourers, which wandering up and down in Mines, employ themselves in all sorts of Work, as to dig after the Vein, to carry together the Oar, to put it into Baskets, and to turn the Wheel to draw it up; yet they seldom hurt the Labourers, except provoked by laughing or railing at them.

A very godly and learned Man gives an Account, that in a Silver Mine at Derosium in the Alps, there was a Devil of the Mountain, who every Friday, when the Labourers were filling their Baskets, would be very busie putting the Mettal-out of one Basket into another, which also would go down into the Pit, and come up again, without doing any Body any harm: But once, whilst this Spirit was very busie about every thing, one of the Miners being much offended, began to rail and curse at him, and bid him begone in the Devil's Name; upon which the Spirit caught him by the Head, and twisted his Neck till his Face stood behind his Back, yet he lived a long time after, being well known to his familiar Friends.

It often happens, that when Persons are sick of any mortal Disease, something is heard to walk about the Room, as the sick Person used to do when in Health, which the sick Person often hears himself, which puts him in mind of his End. And sometimes just before they die, or sometime after, something is seen much like the same Person in Shape, or in the Fashion of other Men. And sometimes when their Acquaintance lie a dying, or their Friends, though several Miles off, some strange Noises are heard: And sometimes the whole House seems likely to fall, or a great noise is heard, as if some weighty substance fell quite through the House, which, as it appears after wards, happened at the same time that our Friends departed this Life. And in some Families, before any of them dies, there are particular Signs and Tokens, either the Doors and Windows opening and shutting; or something runs up Stairs, or walketh up and down the House.

Cardanus tell us of a noble Family of Parma in Italy, out of which, as often as one died an old Woman was seen in the Chimney-Corner: Once she appear'd when a Maid of the same Family lay sick, which made them despair of her Life, but she afterwards recovered, but another in the Family presently fell sick and died.

There was a certain Parish Priest, a very honest and godly Man, who in the Plague-time could tell when any of his Parish should die; for in the Night-time he heard a great Noise over his Bed, as if one had thrown down a Sack of Corn from his Shoulders; upon which he would say, now another bids me farewell; and the next Day he used to enquire who died that Night, or who was taken with the Plague, that he might comfort them.

It hath been often observed in Guildhalls, where Aldermen fit, that when one of them hath been near Death, either a Rattling hath been heard about his Seat, or some other Sign of Death: And the same thing happens about rows or Stalls in Churches, or in other Places where Men have been used to follow their Labour. In Country Villages, before the Death of some Persons, either in the Evening, or in the Night, they hear a Grave diging in the Church-Yard, and the next Day they have found the Grave diged. Likewise in the Night, when the Moon hath shone, they have seen some solemnly going with a Corps, according to the Custom of the People, or standing before the Doors as if some Body was to be carried to Church to be buried. Oftentimes in Prisons, when Prisoners lie in Chains under the Sentence of

Death, in the Night there is heard a great Noise and Rumbling, as if some Body was breaking into the Prison to rescue them; which the Prisoners knew nothing of, nor can any Signs of such things, being offered, be perceived: And some Executioners or Hangmen say, that most commonly they can tell before-hand, when any Man is to be deilvered into their Hands to suffer, for their Swords will move of their own accord; and others say, they can tell before-hand what Deaths they shall die. Plato tells us in the Books of his Laws; that the Souls of those that are slain, often cruelly trouble and molest the Souls of them that slew them.

Before the Alterations and Changes of Kingdoms, and in the Time of Wars, Seditions, and other dangerous Times, most commonly very strange things happen in the Air, the Earth, and amongst Jiving Creatures, quite contrary to the Course of Nature, which are called Wonders, Signs, Monsters, and Forewarnings of things to come. There are often seen in the Air, Swords and Spears, and whole Armies of Men encountering with one another, or seen or heard in the Air, or upon the Land, where one Part is obliged to fly; and then there are heard most horrid Cries, and Clattering of Armour, Guns, Launces and Halberts, and other kind of Weapons also, often move in Armories of their own accord. It is also said, that Horses will be very sad and heavy, and will scarce suffer their Masters to sit on their Backs before they go to a Battle where they are like to be overcome; but when they are couragious and hostile, it often betokens Victory. It is reported by Suetonius, that the Horses which Julius Cæsar let run at Liberty, never to be put to Labour again, wept when Cæsar was slain.

When Miltiades addressed his People against the Persians, terrible Noises were heard before the Battle: And before the Lacedemonians were overthrown in the Battle of Leuctris, the Armour moved and made a great Noise in the Temple of Hector. At the same time the Doors of Hercules's Temple at Thebes, being fast shut with Bars, opened suddenly of their own accord; and the Weapons and Armour which hung fast on the Wall, were found lying on the Ground. In the second Wars of Carthage the

Standard-bearer of the first Battalia of Pikemen, could not remove his Ensign out of its Place, nor could he do it when a great many came to help him; and though Caius Flaminius the Consul did not regard it, yet soon after his Army was routed, and he himself slain. In the Beginning of the Wars waged with the People called Marsi, out of secret Places there were heard certain Voices, and the Noise of Harness, which foretold the Danger of the Wars to come. And Pliny tells us, that in the War with the Danes, and many times before, there was heard the Clashing of Armour, and the Sound of Trumpets out of Heaven. And Appianus relates what Signs and Wonders happened before the Civil Wars at Rome; what miserable Cries of Men, Clashing of Armour, and Running of Horses were heard, though Men could see nothing.

Valerius Maximus writing of strange Wonders, tells us how Gnæius Pompeius was forewarned not to fight with Julius Cæsar; for as he launced off at Dirrachium his Shouldiers were seized with a sudden Fear, and in the Night before the Battle, they were seized with Fear, and their Hearts failed them. And Cæsar himself, in his Book of Civil War says, that the same Day that he fought the fortunate Battle, the Crying of the Army, and the Sound of Trumpets, was heard at Antioch in Syria so plainly, that the whole City ran in Armour to defend their Walls: And the same happened in Ptolemais.

Josephus in his History of the Wars in Jury, reports what strange Signs happened before the Destruction of Jerusalem, which were, that a Brazen Gate, made fast with Iron Bars, opened in the Night-time of its own accord; and that before the Sun set, there were seen Charriots in the Alt, and Armies of Men round the City; and that at Whitsontide, as the Priests went into the Temple to celebrate Divine Service, they heard a great Noise, and by and by a Voice, crying, Let us depart hence. And the same Night that Leo of Constantinople was slain in the Temple, Travellers by the Sea-side heard the Voice of Leo at that Distance.

Felix Malleolus, Doctor of Law, Master of Sclodor, and Canon of Tigurum, a Man of great Reading, tells us, that in the History of Rodolphus King of the Romans; the said Rodolphus, having vanquished Othotaras King of Bohemia, continuing in the Place all Night where the Battle was fought, about Midnight certain Spirits or Devils, making a horrible Noise and Tumult, troubled and disordered his whole Army: And that those were Spirits walking by Night was certain, since they suddenly vanished a way like Smoak.

And the same Author tells us, that in the Year of our Lord 1280, as one of the Plebans belonging to the Church of Tigurum, preached to the People, the Grave-stone of the Sepulchre of the two Martyrs, Fælix and Regula, Patrons of the same Place, violently broke asunder, no Man moving or touching it, making a horrible Noise like Thunder; so that the People were as much astonished and afraid, as if the Roof of the Church had broken down. And he says, that the same Year, the third Day of October, the greater Part of the City of Tigurum was burnt down; and moreover, that Sedition was moved amongst the People, upon the Account of certain Ecclesiastical Disciplines, and the Imperial Bann. And in the Year of our Lord 1440, the Twelfth Day of December, at the Dedication of the above-mentioned Church, about Midnight, the like Noise was heard, and immediately after followed Civil Wars, which the Tigurins made with uncertain Success against the other Helvetians, for the Space of seven Years and more.

The same Author likewise asserts, that in the Year of our Lord 1444, before that valiant Battle, which a small Number of the Helvetians fought against an innumerable Company, belonging to Lewis Dauphin of France, under the Wall of Basill, in the Time of the General Council, there were heard several Nights about those Places, the Alarms of Souldiers clattering of Harnesses, and the Noise of Men encountering together.

We are told also of a grave and wise Man who was a Magistrate in the Territories of Tigurum, who affirmed, that as he and his Servants went early in the Morning through the

Pasture Lands, he espied one whom he knew very well, wickedly difiling himself with a Mare; being amazed at which, he returned back again and knocked at his House, whom he supposed he had seen, where he was assured that he went not one. Step out of his Chamber that Morning: So that if he had not diligently enquired into the Matter, the honest Man had certainly been cast into Prison, and been put upon the Rack.

Chunegunda, Wife to Henry, the second Emperour of that Name, was very much suspected of Adultery, and Rumours were spread about that she was too familiar with a certain young Man in the Court; for the Devil was often seen to come out of the Empress's Chamber in the Likeness of this young Man; but she afterwards discovered her Innocency, by treading upon hot glowing Plowshares, according to the Custom of those Times, without burning her Feet, as Hebbertus Cranzius witnesseth.

St. Hierom tells us, that St. Anthony being in a stony Valley, a Spirit appeared to him in the Form of a Dwarf of a small Stature, having a crooked Nose, and his Forehead rough with Horns, the hinder Part of his Body and his Feet like a Goat. Anthony not at all amazed at the Sight, but being armed with Faith, this Creature presented him with Dates, to refresh him in his Journey, as Tokens of Peace and Friendship; upon which Anthony enquired of him what he was; who answered, I am a Mortal Creature, and one of the Inhabitants of this Desert, whom the Gentiles, deceived with many Errors, worship; calling us Finns, Satyrs, and Night-Mares; and I am sent as Ambassador from our Company, who earnestly beseech thee, that thou wilt pray unto the God of all Creatures for us, whom we acknowledge to be come into the World to save the same.

Plutarch tells a Story, related to him by Epitherces his Country-man, Father to Æmilianus, which was, that once designing to sail into Italy, and carrying along with him, not only good Store of Passengers, but also of Merchants Goods; in the Evening, when they were about the Islands Echinadæ, the Wind quite ceased; and whilst the Ship was driving at Sea, 'till at last they were near Paxe, several being awake, and others drinking after Supper, they suddenly heard the Voice of one calling Thamus, to the great Wonder and Astonishment of them all. Thamus was a Pilot born in Ægypt, unknown to a great many that were in the Ship, who though twice called held his Peace, but the third Time he answered; upon which the other, with a loud Voice, commanded him that when he came to Palades, he should tell them that the great God Pan was departed. Upon this every one was struck with Fear and Amazement, as Epitherces told us, and consulting whether they should comply with these Commands, or not. Upon which Thamus gave his Opinion, that if the Wind blowed, they must pass by silent; but if it was calm, he must declare what he had heard. When therefore they came to Palades, it being calm, and neither Wind nor Waves stirring, Thamus looking towards the Land, cried out, as he was told by the Voice, that the great God Pan was dead He had scarce said these Words, before a great Groaning of a Multitude, mixed with Admiration, was heard. The same of which being spread abroad, Thamus was presently sent for by Tiberius the Emperour, to give him an Account of this Relation.

To these we might add several others of the like kind, as also of the Chasing or Hunting of Devils, and the Dancing of dead Men. These walking Spirits sometimes stop the Way as Men are upon their Journies, and leading them out of their Way, put them in so much Fear, that some have become Gray-headed in one Night. Of this an Acquaintance of Lewes Evaterus, one John Welling was an Example; who not many Years ago meeting with a walking Spirit in the Night, was so much altered, that when he came home his Daughters did not know him. To these we shall add the following Relation, viz. A certain Magistrate within the Liberties of Tigurine, entertaining several Friends at Breakfast, before he took a Journey; whilst they were thus attending him, they supposed they heard a Knife fall from the upper Part of the Room, yet could see nothing. Whilst they were talking together of it, they thought they heard it again; at which time in came the Magistrate, whom they acquainted with what had happened; but before they had finished the Story, they heard it fall again, the Magistrate, who could scarce believe it, being a Witness of it himself; upon which he began to exhort them, that since a great Marriage was to be celebrated in a few Days in the same Place, they should endeavour to preserve the Peace, and keep themselves sober, lest by Quarrelling Murder should happen, and make it a bloody Marriage. After this he took his Journey, and dispatching his Business in a few Days, as he returned towards his Castle, his Horse falling into a River, which was suddenly increased with Rain, after he had long strove to get out of the Water he died miserably.

From hence it appears, that it is no hard Matter for the Devil to appear in divers Shapes, not only of those who are alive, but also of dead Men, or in the Form of Beasts and Birds, he sometimes appearing in the Likeness of a black Dog, a Horse, an Owl; and by these and several other Methods brings several things to pass; since he, by long and great Experience, understands the Effects and Force of natural things, and by that means brings wonderful things to pass; And as he is a subtle and quick Spirit, and can readily take things in Hand, so by his Quickness and Knowledge in natural things, he may easily deceive the Eye-Sight, and Mens Senses, and hide those things which are before our Faces, and convey other things into their Room. Thus Simon Magus bewitch'd the Samaritans with his unlawful Arts: Egisippus writing of the Destruction of Jerusalem says, that he came to Rome, and there set himself against Peter, boasting that he could flie up into Heaven; and coming at the Day appointed to the Mount Capitoline, and leaping from the Rock, he flew a great while to the Wonder and Admiration of the People, who began to give Credit to his Words; but suddenly fell down and broke his Leg, and being afterwards carried into Aritia there died.

Johannes Tritenhemius tells us, that one of the Sons of Simon a Monk, who ruled over the Bulgarians, whose Name was Baianus, was seen to exercise the Art of Necromancy, transforming himself into a Wolf as often as he pleased, or into the Likeness of another Beast, or could make himself invisible to any Man. And the same Author tells us, that in the Year 876 a certain Jew named Sedechias, sometime Physician and Phylosopher to Lewes the Emperour, was so skilful in Sorcery, that he could visibly devour an armed Man and his Horse with all his Harness, or a Cart loaden with Hay, together with the Horse and Carter. He likewise cut off Men Heads, with their Hands and Feet, which he set in a Bason before the Spectators, with the Blood manifestly running about the Bason, which he would presently fix upon their proper Places again, without any Hurt to the Persons. He would like Exercise, Hunting, and Running in the Air and Clouds, as Men are used to do upon Earth.

In the Year 1313 when Frederick Duke of Austrick was chosen Emperour, and was overcome in a great Battle against Lewis, between Ottinga and Moindorfus, and delivered into the Hands of Lewsi, who sent him into a strange Castle to be secured; it chanced, that a Conjurer going to his Brother Lupoldus in Austricke told him, that in an Hour's time, by the Help of a Spirit, he would deliver his Brother Frederick out of Captivity, if he would promise him a good Reward for his Pains: The Duke answered, that if he would perform his Promise he should have a good Reward. Upon which the Conjurer, along with the Duke, entering into his Circle of Conjuration in an Hour most convenient, called the Spirit that was accustomed to obey his Commands, who appearing in the Likeness of a Man, he commanded him, by Virtue of his Conjurations, that he should speedily bring unto him into Austricke, Duke Frederick safely delivered out of Prison; unto whom the Spirit answered, If the Duke will come with me, I will obey thy Commands. Then the Spirit flew away, and taking upon him the Form of a Pilgrim, he entered into the Prison, where the Duke was kept Prisoner, and told him, If thou wilt be delivered out of Captivity, presently mount upon this Horse, and I will bring thee safe and sound without any Hurt into Austricke unto Duke Lupoldus thy Brother; to whom the Duke said, who art thou? To whom the Spirit answered, ask not who I am, that being nothing to the purpose, but get thee up upon the Horse, and I will bring thee safe into Austricke: Upon which the Duke being seiz'd with

Horror and Fear, blessed himself with the Sign of the Cross, and the Spirit immediately vanished away with the black Horse, and returned empty to him that sent him, and told him the Reason why he did not bring him. Duke Fredcrick being at the last delivered out of Prison, confessed what happened in the Time of his Imprisonment the same Day they mentioned: This History is to be seen in the Chronicles of the Helvetians.

Chapter 3

CHAP. III. Containing the most strange and admirable Discovery of the Three Witches of Warboyse, arraigned, convicted, and executed at an Assizes at Huntington, for Bewitching of Five Daughters of Robert Throckmorton, Esq; and divers other Persons, with sundry devilish and grievous Torments; and also the Bewitching to Death the Lady Cromwell; the like hath not been heard of in that Age.

HAVING in the former Chapter given the Reader an Account, according to the Method proposed of the Appearance of Ghosts, Spirits, and Apparitions; we shall in the next Place give an Historical Account of true and particular Observations of a notable Piece of Witchcraft, practised by John Samuel the Father, Alice Samuel the Mother, and Agnes Samuel the Daughter, of Warboyse in the County of Huntington, upon five Daughters of Robert Throckmorton, of the same Town and County, Esq; and other Maid-Servants, amounting to the Number of Twelve, all belonging to one House, in November 1589. About the Tenth of November, in the Year 1589, Mistriss Jane, one of the Daughters of Mr. Throckmorton, being near ten Years of Age, was suddenly seized with a strange sort of Sickness, and Indisposition of Body, viz. sometimes she would screek very loud and often, for the space of half an Hour together, and presently like one in a Trance, would swoon and lie quietly down all along; soon after she would begin to swell and lift her Belly up, so that no Body was able to bend her, or to keep her down: Sometimes she would shake one Leg, and no other Part of her, as if the Palsie had been in it, and sometimes the other; presently she would shake one of her Aims, and the other, and soon after her Head, as if she had been affected with a running Palsie, continuing in this Condition two or three Days. Amongst other Neighbours in the Town, Alite Samuel came into Mr. Throckmorton's House to visit the Child, who lived next Door on the North Side. The Child, when the old Woman came into the House, was held in another Woman's

Arms by the Fire side; so she went into the Chimney-Corner and sate down hard by the Child, the Grandmother of the Child and the Mother being both present: She had not been there long before the Child grew something worse than at her coming, and suddenly cried, pointing to the said Mother Samuel, Did you ever see one more like a Witch than she is? Take off her black thrumb'd Cap, for I cannot abide to look at her.

The Mother of the Child little suspecting any such Matter, was very angry with her Child, and reproved her for saying so, thinking it might proceed from some Lightness in the Child's Brain, seized with such a violent Sneezing and wanting Rest, and therefore took her and laid her down upon a Bed, and hanged Curtains against the Windows, hoping, by that means, she might be inclined to rest; but it was not without great difficulty she could pacifie the Child.

The old Woman hearing this sate still, without saying a Word, yet looked very dismally, as those that saw her remembered very well. The Child continuing still after the same manner, rather worse than better, the Parents within two Days after sent the Child's Urine to Cambridge to Dr. Barrow, a very skilful Physician, who return'd this Answer, viz. That he could perceive no Distemper, only he thought she might be troubled with Worms, and sent Medicines accordingly, but the Child was no better. In two Days time they sent to the same Man again, describing her Sickness more at large; he then told them, that the Urine they then brought shewed no such kind of Disquiet to be in her Body, and that he would warrant her clear of the falling Sickness, which her Parents suspected; upon which he sent other Medicines proper to purge her, which had not the expected Effects; upon which they sent to him a third Time, and told him, that the Medicines had no Effect, and that the Child was no better. The Doctor then looking again upon the Urine, and perceiving the Child's Body to be in good Temper, which appeared for any thing he saw to the contrary, asked if there was no Sorcery or Witchcraft suspected in the Child, to which they answered, No. Upon which he declared it was impossible it should be occasioned by any natural Cause, without any Signs appearing in the Urine: Nevertheless he desired they would send to any other skilful Man in the Town for their Satisfaction. Upon which the Messenger went to Mr. Butler, who considering the Urine, and hearing the manner of the Child's Distemper, said, he thought it might be the Worms, which nevertheless he did not perceive by the Urine, and thought it strange they should occasion such Symptoms, ordering the same Medicines before described, which were not used: Dr. Barrow having before advised them not to make use of any more Medicines, suspecting that the Distemper was occasion'd by Witchcraft. Yet tho' Mr. Throckmorton and his Wife resolved to trust to God Almighty's Will, they neither suspected any such thing as Witchcraft, till about a Month after, two others of his Daughters, about two or three Years older, fell into the same Extremities with the other, and cry'd out upon Mother Samuel, Take her away, look where she standeth there before us in a black thrumb'd Cap; (which she commonly wore, tho' not then,) it's she that hath bewitched us, and she will kill us if you don't take her away. This moved their Parents to suspect Witchcraft, yet could not imagine why it should be wrought upon them or their Children, being come to Town but the Michaelmas before, and having given no Occasion of Malice to any Body About a Month after, another Sister, younger than the rest, being about nine Years old, was seized with the like Malady, and cried out of Mother Samuel, as the others had done.

Soon after, Mrs. Joan, the eldest Daughter, about Fifteen Years of Age, was in the same Condition, but handled more severely than the rest; for she being stronger than the others, and striving more with the Spirit, and not able to overcome it, was more grievously tormented; for it caused her to sneeze, shriek, and groan, most fearfully; sometimes it would heave up her Belly, and bounce up her Body with so much Violence, that if she had not been kept upon her Bed, she must have been extreamly bruised: And several times, when she had her Fit in a Chair, with starting and heaving, she would almost break the Chair she sate in. Yet the more they strove to help them and to keep them down, the more violently they were handled, being deprived of the Use of their Senses during the Fit, being neither able to see, hear, or feel any Body, only cry'd out of Mother Samuel, desiring her to be taken away from them; who never came after she perceived her self to be suspected.

These Fits would hold them sometimes longer, and sometimes a less while; sometimes an Hour or two, and sometimes half a Day, or a whole Day; and sometimes they would have six or seven Fits in an Hour: Yet when they were cut of them, they neither knew what they had said, nor what they had suffered. When Mrs. Joan had been thus handled a while, the Spirit would sound something in her Ear, which she could declare in her Fit; and once particularly it shewed her, that twelve of them should be bewitched in that House, naming them to her, being all Women and Servants in the House, her self and Sisters being five of the Number: Which afterwards proved very true, for all of them had their several Afflictions, in the same manner with those five Sisters.

The Servants, when they first fell into Fits, all cry'd out of Mother Samuel, as the Children did, saying, Take her away, Mistress; for God's Sake, take her away, and burn her, for she will kill us all if you les her alone, undergoing the same Miseries and Extremities the others did: And when they were out of their Fits, they knew no more what they said or did than the Children; and, as soon as they left Mrs. Throckmorton's House, they were all presently well, as before, and so continued, without any further Suspicion of such Vexations: And those Servants which came in their Places, were afflicted much after the same Manner for near two Years.

On Friday the Thirteenth of February, being St. Valentine's Eve, Gilbert Pickering, of Tickmerch Grove, in the County of Northampton, Esquire, Uncle to the said Children, hearing how strangely they were troubled, went to Warboyse, as well to see them as to visit their Parents; and coming to the House where they lived, found them as well as any Children could be; and about half an Hour after, Mr. Pickering was informed, that Mrs. Hadley, and Mr. Whittle of St. Ives, and others, were gone to Mother Samuel's House, to perswade her to come and see and visit the Children: But she staying long, Mr. Pickering concluded that she would not come, though she had promised that she would come and see them whenever their Parents should send for her; and that she would venture up to her Chin in the Water, and lose some of her best Blood, to do them Service: But now her Mind, it seemed, was altered, because, as she said, that all the Children cry'd out of her, and said that she had bewitched them; and she also feared that the common Practice of Scratching would be used upon her; which, indeed, was intended; for both the Parents and Mr. Pickering had taken Advice of good Divines of the Unlawfulness of it: Wherefore Mr. Pickering went to Mother Samuel's House, both to see her, and to perswade her, that if she was any Cause of the Children's Trouble, to amend it. When he came to the House, he found there Mr. Whittle, Mrs. Audley, and others, endeavouring to perswade her, but she refused it; whereupon Mr. Pickering told her that he had Authority to bring her, and if she would not go willingly, he would compel her, which accordingly he did, along with her Daughter Agnes, and one Cicily Burder, who were are all suspected to be Witches, or in Confederacy with Mother Samuel.

As they were going to Mr. Throckmorton's House, Mr. Whittle and Mrs. Audley, and others, going before; Mother Samuel, Agnes Samuel, and Cicily Burder, in the middle; and Mr. Pickering behind; Mr. Pickering perceived that Mother Samuel would fain have talked with her Daughter Agnes, if he had not followed so close that they could have no Opportunity; and when they came to Mr. Throckmorton's Door, Mother Samuel made a Curtesy to Mr. Pickering, offering him to go in before her, that she might have had an Opportunity to confer with her Daughter in the Entry, but he refus'd; where she thrust her Head as near as she could to her Daughter's Head, and said these Words; I charge thee, do not confess any thing. Mr. Pickering being behind them, and perceiving it, thrust his Head as near as he could betwixt theirs, whilst the Words were speaking, and hearing them presently, reply'd to old Mother Samuel, Dost thou charge thy Daughter not to confess? To which she answer'd, I said not so, but charged her to hasten Home to get her Father his Dinner. Whilst these Words were speaking, Mr. Whittle, Mrs. Audley. and the rest, went into the House, and three of the Children stood in the Hall by the Fire, perfectly well; but no sooner Mother Samuel enter'd the Hall, but these three Children fell down, at one Moment, on the Ground, strangely tormented, so that if they had been let alone, they would have leap'd and sprung about like a Fish newly taken out of the Water their Bellies lifting up, and their Head and Heels still remaining on the Ground; and would have drawn their Head and their Heels backwards, throwing out their Arms, with great Groans, which were terrible and troublesome to those that beheld them. But Mr. Whittle soon took up one of the Children, which was Jane Throckmorton, and carry'd her to an inward Chamber, and laid it upon a Bed, and though as strong a Man as most in England, and the Child but nine Years old, yet he could not hold her down to the Bed, but she would lift up her Belly as high as a Woman big with Child, and ready to be deliver'd, and very hard; and thus it would rise and fall an hundred times in an Hour, her Eyes being closed, and her Arms spread abroad so stiff and strong, that a Man could not, with all his Strength, bring them to her Body. Then Mr. Pickering went into the Chamber where the Child was, and, going on the other Side of the Bed, he perceived that she presently stretched out her Right-Hand that Way, and, scratching the Covering of the Bed, said, O! that I had her! O! that I had her! Which Mr. Pickering wonder'd at, he thinking that Scratching was altogether unlawful: Yet he put his own Hand to the Child's, whilst she was speaking those Words; but the Child feeling his Hand, would not scratch it, but let it go, and continued to scratch the Bed, her Face being turned the other way from Mr. Pickering, her Eyes shut, and Mr. Whittle lying with almost his whole Weight upon her, to hold down her Belly, being afraid otherwise she would have broke her Back.

Notwithstanding this Offer being made by the Child, or the Spirit within-her, to discover some Secret by which Witches might be discover'd, Mr. Pickering went into the Hall, and took Mother Samuel by the Hand, who went much against her Will, and brought her to the further Side of the Bed from the Child, who still lay scraping upon the Bed-Cloaths, and crying, O! that I had her! Then Mr. Pickering, very softly, that the Child should not hear, desired Mother Samuel to put her Hand to the Child's, which she refus'd; upon which Mr. Pickering put his Hand to the Child's, and so did Mrs. Audley, and others, but ths Child would scratch none of-them; upon that Mr. Pickering took Mother Samuel's Hand, and thrust it to the Child's Hand, and as soon as she felt it, she scratched with so much Vehemence, that she splinter'd her Nails, with her eager Desire of Revenge. Whilst the Child was thus scratching, Mr. Pickering cover'd Mother Samuel's Hand with his own, to try what the Child would do in this extream Passion; but it would not scratch his, but felt too and fro for that which it missed, and if it could but come with one Finger to Mother Samuel's Hand, she would scratch that Hand, and no other; nay, sometimes when Mr. Pickering cover'd Mother Samuel's Hand, the Child would put one of her Fingers between his, and scratch Mother Samuel's Hand with that Finger, the rest of her Fingers lying upon his Hand unmov'd.

And if at any time Mother Samuel's Hand was moved from the Child, she would mourn, and shew evident Tokens of Dislike. And this is a Truth to be noted as most certain, Mr. Pickering giving it in Evidence at the Assizes at Huntington the Child's Eyes being shut that she could see nothing; and had her Eyes been open, her Face was turned the other way, and covered so much by Mr. Whittle, that it was impossible for her to see any Body on the other Side of the Bed.

When this was done, Mr. Pickering went out of this into another Parlour, where a Woman was holding one of the other Children; which Child, as Mr. Pickering passed by, was scraping the Woman's Apron that held her, drying out, O! that I had her! O! that I had her! Then Mr. Pickering went to the Hall, and brought Cicily Burder, and served her as he did Mother Samuel with the other; and as the first Child acted in respect of Mother Samuel, so did this to Cicily Burder in every Respect.

The third Child being in the Hall, spoke the same Words; but the Father of the Children, and Dr. Dorrington, Parson of the Parish, would not admit the same to be practised upon the other.

The same Night, after Supper, the Children being then out of their Fits, and well, Dr. Dorrington moved to have Prayers before the Company departed; and the Company kneeling down, he began to pray; but as soon as he began, all the Children fell into their Fits, with such terrible Shrieks and strange Sneezings, and so strangely tormented, as if they would have been torn in Pieces; upon which, Dr. Dorrington stopped in the middle of his Prayers, and said, Had we best go any further? But he no sooner left off praying, but the Children were quiet, yet still in their Fits: Then he began to pray again, and at the same time the Fits returned with the same Violence, the wicked Spirit being moved within them. And this was often try'd, for as soon as he left off praying they were quiet, and whenever he began to pray they began to shriek.

The next Day, being Valentine's Day, Mr. Pickering brought Elizabeth Throckmorton home to his own House at Tichmerch Grove; who, as the first, was in her Fit, but she was no sooner on Horseback, and out of Warboyse Town, but she was well, and continued so till she came to Mr. Pickering's House, where she no sooner was come, but the was suddenly seized with a Fit, and taken gasping, and not able to speak, the Fit beginning after the following manner; First, she pitched her self backwards, all the Joints of her Back being contracted together, and thrusting out her Belly so violently, that no Body could bend her back again, being very strong and heavy, shaking her Limbs, and oftentimes her Head, but especially her Arms, like those that are convulsive before Death, being both dumb, deaf, and blind, her Eyes being closed up. This Fit held her not above a Quarter of an

Hour before (with a Gasp) she came to her self, stroaking her Eyes as if she had been asleep.

Sometimes in the Fit the is only deaf; when she can speak, but rather, as we think, the Spirit, in her, yet it is very vainly; and though she can see, yet it is but with a Glimmering, so that if you were to look upon her, you would think she could not see at all.

Sometimes she can hear only; yet not every Body, but one that she likes best. Sometimes she can see only, but as plainly as any Body, and can neither hear nor speak, her Teeth being set in her Head. Sometimes she can both hear and see, but cannot speak at all.

Above all Things, she delights in Play, chusing some particular Person to play at Cards with her, yet but one only, neither hearing, seeing, or speaking to any other; and when awake, she remembers not what she did, heard, or spoke, affirming that he was not sick, but asleep.

She continued well till Night, and before Supper, at Thanksgiving, was strangely troubled at the very Word of Grace, which held her no longer than Grace was saying. She sat well at Table, but had no sooner put up her Knife, but it pitched her backwards; and then being taken from the Table, she was well till Thanksgiving, at which Time she was very much tormented, and no longer. After she was very quiet, till they moved to go to Prayers; all which Time she seemed as if she would be torn in Pieces, with such Shrieking and Outcries, and violent Sneezing, that she terrify'd the whole Company; but when Prayers was ended, she continued quiet.

Mr. Pickering, and others, observing this, said, that if they should read the Bible, or any other Godly Book, it would put her in a Rage as before, as long as they read; to try which, one took a Bible and read the first Chapter of St. John, and the first Verse: At the reading of which, she was as one distracted in Mind, but was quiet when they left off; and when they read again, was again tormented; which ceased several times, when they ceased to read.

Nay, at the Motion of any good Word, as God, or Pray God bless her, or when any thing was named that tended to God or Godliness, she raged all one as if one read or prayed by her, and was carry'd to Bed, still continuing in her Fit.

On Sabbath-Day Morning she came down into the Hall about Prayer-time; and being asked whether she would stay in Prayer-time or not, she answer'd, that she would do as they would have her: And being asked whether she could read, she answered, That she could once, but had almost forgot now: And being asked whether she had prayed that Day, she answer'd, It would not suffer her: And being asked further, whether she used to pray at home, she answered, That it would not give her so much Time: Upon which one said, Since it will not let you pray, or any other for you, pray to your self secretly in your Heart and Spirit; and beginning to tell her, that God understood the inward Sighs and Groans of the Heart, as well as the loudest Cries of the Mouth, she suddenly fell into her Fit, being more violently and strangely tormented than ever; and being carry'd away, her Fit continued and encreased all Prayer-time, though out of Hearing, with such vehement Cries, Screetching, and continual Sneezing, that several times they were obliged to leave off Prayers for some Time, the whole Company being amazed: When Prayers were ended, she came to her self, with a Gasp, wiping her Eyes, being presently as well as any Body, and as it she had not been disorder'd.

She came' down to Dinner, and, whilst Grace was saying, it seized her again; yet she could better bear any Body else to say Grace than her self, but no Body well. At Dinner-time she was tolerably well; and sometimes she hath merrry Fits, putting her Hands beside her Meat, and her Meat beside of her Mouth, mocking her, and making her miss her Mouth; at which she would sometimes smile, and sometimes laugh exceedingly: And, what was remarkable was, that in her Fit she looked much more sweetly and cheerfully than when awake; and, tho' violently tormented, yet out of her Fit she was as well as any Body. At last Mr. Pickering remembring what was done at Warboyse, viz. That if a Child, in the Time of the Fit, was carry'd into the Church yard, it would presently be out of it; but as soon as they were brought into the House again, the Fit would presently return; but, upon their being brought out again, they presently recovered; To try the same with this Child, he carry'd her out of the House, and she presently recover'd; but upon her Return into the House, the Fit returned as before. But the Success of this Experiment lasted not above three Days.

We rejoyc'd however at these welcome Intervals, and concluded, that as the Devil was but a Vassal for the wicked Purpose of her that detain'd him, so the wicked Spirit had no Power to torment her abroad; for as the Angel of God said to Lot, I can do nothing till thou come hither, much less can the Devils go beyond their Commission. But this Experiment presently failed, for after that Time, when she was carry'd abroad, you would have thought that she would have been torn in Pieces, to the Surprize and Amazement of those that savv her.

From the Sixteenth Day of February, to the 26th Day, she vvas taken most commonly five or fix times a Day; sometimes ten times, and sometimes but once or tvvice, and not till Night. On the Seventeenth of February, she could not refrain from gasping and gaping; and being asked the Reason, she ansvvered, that it vvould not let her forbear. Being perswaded to strive against it, and to shut her Mouth, or stop it, yet it was some Time before she could overcome it, and not before she heard the Standers-by say, that they thought it was the Spirit of the Air, entering and departing by a Breath, since it was a Token of the Fit leaving her, when she stretched her Arms, and gaped frequently and long, with a little rubbing of her Eyes, and then this continual Gaping ceased.

On the 26th of February, she read and sung Psalms, being well all the Day till Evening, when the Fit seizing her, she cry'd out of Mother Samuel, fearing, as she cry'd, that she would put a Mouse into her Mouth; sometimes a Cat or a Frog, and sometimes a Toad, clapping her Hands before her Mouth. Being suddenly seized with this Fear, she would start out of the Hands of them that held her, and run away out of Doors into another

Room, where suddenly her Legs failed her, and she was catched by one that followed her, still crying, Away with your Mouse, Mother Samuel, I will have none of your Mouse: After which Time she imagined she had a Mouse in her Belly.

The 27th of February she was pretty well, yet in her Fit all the Day long, and, tho' awake, she nodded at every second Word, as if she were drowsy, often with Meat in her Mouth; or whatever she did she gave a Nod with her Head, very low, and every Minute. This Drowsy Fit continued near two Days.

The 28th Whereas before she bended backwards, she now bended forwards, coveting to touch the Ground, as if she would have stood upon her Head, turning her Hands backwards; and if any moved her contrary to her bending, the would cry out all the while, being in danger of tearing her Limbs; nor was any Body able to bend her straight.

The First Day of March, after Dinner she was seized with such a violent Sneezing forty times together, and faster than one could well count them, so that Blood issued out of her Nose and Mouth; but all Night, being in Bed, she fell into the most sorrowful Fit of all, weeping with most sorrowful Sobs and Sighs, crying out so that no Body could appease her, that now the Witches would kill her Father, and destroy her and all her Sisters; which continued above two Hours: After, in a Sleep, she fell into a sad Bleeding, losing at least a Pint at both Nostrils and Mouth; but in the Morning remember'd nothing of her Fit or bleeding.

The Second of March, all her Fits were merry, full of exceeding Laughter, and so hearty and excessive, that if they had been awake they would have been ashamed of being so full of trifling Toys, and some merry Jests of her own making, which would occasion her self, as well as the Standers-by, to laugh at them. In this Fit, she chose one of her Uncles to go to Cards with her; and, desiring to see the End of it, they play'd together. Soon after, there was a Book brought and lay'd before her; upon which she threw her self backwards: but that being taken away, she pesently recover'd, and play'd again: Which was often try'd, and found true. As she thus play'd at Cards, her Eyes were almost shut, so that she saw the Cards, and nothing else; knew her Uncle, and no Body else; she heard and answer'd him, and no other Person; she perceived when he play'd foul or stole from her, either Counters or Cards, but another might steal them out of her Hands, without her seeing or feeling of them. Sometimes she would chuse another whom she did see and hear; sometimes a little Child; but never above one in a Fit.

The Fifth of March she fell into a Fit in the Morning and longed to go home to her Father's. The Sixth, one of her Father's Men came over to Tichmerch-Grove, whom she had often call'd in her Fit, to carry her to Warboyse, to her Father's, saying, If she were but half way the knew that she should be well. To try this, she carry'd her towards Warboyse on Horse-back; and being scarce gone a Bow-shot, by a Pond-side, she awaked, wondering where she was, not knowing any thing; but no sooner the Horse's Head was turned back, but she fell into her Fit again; and for three Days after, and no longer, as often as she was carry'd to the Pond, she awaked, and was well; but as soon as she turned back again, her Fit returned.

The Eighth Day of March she had a new antick Trick; for she could go well enough two Steps, but the third she down-right halted, giving a Beck with her Head as low as her Knees; and as she was sitting by the Fire, she would suddenly start up, saying she would go to Warboyse; but she was stopped at the Door, where going out, with a Nod, she hit her Forehead against the Latch, which raised a Lump as big as a Walnut; and being carry'd to the Pond, and there awaking, she asked how she came to be hurt. There she continued all Day well, playing with other Children at Bowls, or some other Sport, for the foolisher Sport she made use of, the less she was tormented with the Spirit; but as soon as any Motion was made of coming into the House, the Fit presently took her; so that for Twelve Days she was never out of her Pit within Doors, eating and drinking in it, but neither seeing, hearing, nor understanding; and without Memory or Speaking.

The Ninth of March she could not go, but hop, the one Leg being drawn up, so that it would not touch the Ground by a Foot; and then being carry'd to the Pond, she did not awake, yet her Leg was restored. This continued three other Days, yet she could go but upon one Leg in the House.

The Tenth, after eating some Milk, she listen'd and hearken'd, as she us'd to do, asking if no Body heard the Spirit in her Belly lapping the Milk she had eaten. Then she began to dislike all bad Things, and delighted in reading, saying, the Spirit loved no Goodness; therefore she burned all the Cards she could come at, and she would read when you would not have thought that she could have seen the Book; but sometimes her Eyes were quite clos'd up; sometimes her Tongue was ty'd; sometimes her Teeth were set; sometimes she would fling away the Book, especially at any good Word: If she could catch the Book, and hold it, with striving to do so, she would clap it to her Face till she could see; for sometimes, as she was reading, it would fling her backwards, and swell her Belly after so strange a manner, that two strong Men were not able to hold her down.

On the Eleventh, one asked her if she loved the Word of God; whereupon she was much troubled and tormented. When they asked, Love you witchcraft? she was content. Love you the Bible? it shaked her. Love you Papistry? the Devil within her was quiet. Love you Prayer? it raged. Love you the Mass? it was still. Love you the Gospel? it heaved up her Belly: So that every good thing it disliked; but whatever concerned Popish Idolatry, it was pleased with.

The Twelfth Day she was carry'd to the Pond, yet halted still. The Thirteenth, Fourteenth, and Fifteenth Days, she was troubled with a severe Fit; and on the Sixteenth in the Afternoon she started up suddenly, and ran out of the Place she was in, and awaked in the Way; but at Five a Clock it seized her again, till next Day at Three a Clock; and at Five a Clock it took her again, and so it did the third Day: Yet as she sat at Supper she awaked; whereupon, one said, Thanks be to God; at which World she fell backwards into her Fit again.

And here we are to observe, that all the while this Elizabeth Throckmorton stay'd at Tichmerch-Grove, every Month, from March to July, she was troubled with some Disorder of Body, called Fits, being never free from he first Visitation; tho' in some Months she had only one Fit.

The 29th of July, she had a Fit from Noon till Night, sleeping most of the Time. The 30th she had three several Fits in the Afternoon, going to bed each Fit; yet all of them were mild, and without violent Plunges, or excessive Sneezing, as in her former Fits.

The Second of August, she fell very suddenly, after Dinner, into her usual Fits, having not so much Time as to say, It comes; which Words she used to express suddenly before the Approach of a Fit, which was very strong and troublesome at this Time; yet towards the End she fell into a Sleep, and continued in it till Supper-time, when awaking, she was very sick, and complain'd that she was grip'd at her Stomach and Belly; but the next Day Morning all her Pain ceased, and then she fell to eat her Meat chearfully, and was very well, as at any other Time. But the same Night, before she went to bed, she had two grievous Fits, which brought a great many Tears from her Eyes, as well as those of the Standersby, and she was brought to Bed. The next Morning she was found to be in her Fit, which continued the whole Day, she lying in her Bed, as in a drowsy Sleep, eating and drinking in her Fit, and speaking very little; but sometimes she would say that she would go to Warboyse, for there her Sisters were well, and named some of them; whereas, out of her Fit, she was loth to go to any Place from Tichmerch-Grove.

The next Day, being the Thirteenth of August, she was taken up in her Fit, and made ready; but when she came to move her self, one of her Legs was drawn close to her Body, almost a Foot from the Ground; so she sat in a Chair all the Day, and eat her Meat, at due Times when it was brought her; yet she never moved her Countenance, appearing like one in a Trance, void of Sense and Motion, and no other Signs of Life but breathing; yet would lift up her Hand, in Token of Thanksgiving, after Meat, which was comfortable to the Beholders.

The Fourteenh of August, the was carry'd abroad into the open Air, but it made no Alteration in her: But now she began to complain of that Side on which the Leg was drawn up; and if any Body touch'd her on that Side, she would whimper and groan as if it were sore, without any Appearance of outward Hurt. If you touched her on the other Side, she would laugh after a jesting manner, and look of a merry Countenance, yet without speaking a Word all the Day, from this Time till the Eighth of September, this drowsy Fit continuing a whole Month. Several Things happen'd worthy Notice; for sometimes she would sow all the Day long, and mourn if her Work were taken away from her; sometimes she would wind Yarn or knit, but never cast up her Eyes or Countenance: Some Days she would be merry and lightsome, finding many Things wherein she would take Delight, as playing with her Cousins at light and childish Sports, like Children.

Sometimes she would be so heavy and drooping, that she could not sit in her Chair, but would cast her self on the Ground, and lie with a Pillow or Cushion under her Head half the Day. Sometimes she would take a Book, and read. Chapters or Prayers very well; but whenever she miscall'd a Word, or slipped any thing, she could not hear any that corrected her, though he spoke never so loud; yet if he pointed to the Place with his Finger, or gave some other Sign, she would turn back, and read it over again, sometimes reading it true, and sometimes not. When the came to the Word Satan, or the Devil, she had much ado to pass it over quietly, or to keep the Book in her Hands; for it would shake her Arms, and strain her Body so much, that she would often say, Wilt thou not suffer me to say my Prayers? Wilt thou not suffer me to read? To which she would answer, I will say them, I will read, with frequent and vehement Repetitions; and would by no means forsake her Book, except by great Force and Violence the Spirit cast it out of her Hands; yet would she receive it again when brought to her, and many times fetch it her self; and, at last, with much Contention and striving, she would read quietly. And thus she was used most commonly when she went to bed, and in Time of Prayer.

Further, for two or three Days, if Satan or the Devil had been named to her, it would have troubled her; and as often as those names had been used, she would have so many Twitches; which was very strange to the Beholders: And at the naming of Mother Samuel, it would shake her by the Shoulders and Arms, as if it would shiver her in Pieces, giving Tokens of great Disgust at it: And sometimes her very Name would cast her into her Fit, in the midst of which she would say, Could not you have held your Tongue? I was well enough before you named her.

She continued long in this drowsy Condition' speaking very little all the Time; but sometimes she would say she could not be well till she came to Warboyse, or a Mile upon the Way. Once she asked if any Body in the House had slept so long as she had done, saying, it had been a long Night with her, having then continued so Five Days; and if every Body had slept so long as she had done, says she, I wonder how all the Work could be done.

The last of August, she had a very sudden and violent Fit presently after Dinner, crying out very grievously, that Mother Samuel stood, before her in a white Sheet, with a black Child sitting upon her Shoulders, saying. Look where she is, look where she is; away with your Child, Mother Samuel; I will have none of your Child; and trembling every Joint of her, and sweating extreamly, calling upon her Uncle Pickering, and others, to save her from Mother Samuel's Child, with very lamentable Expressions, because no Body would relieve her. When this Fit was ended, her Teeth were set in her Head, so that she lost her Speech; after which, she mourned inwardly, and shed a great many Tears, often puting her Hand to her Mouth, and shaking her Head. The closing of her Month very much frighten'd us all, it hindering her from taking her Food; which, by putting her Hands to her Mouth, and lifting up her Head, she endeavour'd to let us know she stood in need of, having a hungry Desire for Meat and Drink.

Towards Night we observed that the Child wanted a Tooth, so that by the Help of a Quill, she sucked up some Milk, and the same Way received her Drink. Upon which she shewed great outward Signs of rejoycing tho she could not speak, but clapping her Hands on her Breast and Belly, for Joy she had found a Way to deceive her Enemy. For though the Children were foyl'd for a time, yet when it pleased God to give them a little Ease, they would greatly triumph in Words, as I defie thee thou wicked Spirit; do what thou canst, thou canst do me no hurt; thou seest God is stronger than thee; thou hadst as good let me alone; I am glad in my Heart that thou canst not overcome me; yet at the same time the Enemy seemed to check and torment them for it, either by straining their Bodies, checking their Speech, as if they could not speak, and then they would rejoyce in Countenance and outward Signs; and thus they all of them triumphed after the Fit was over.

But to return to this Child who was carried to Bed in her Fit, and in the time of her Prayers, as she inwardly mourned in her Mind, and was tormented, yet she would not cease 'till she had ended them; for though her Torments increasing might interrupt her Prayers, yet as soon as she had a little Advantage of her Enemy, she went on with them 'till she had ended them.

The next Morning, which was the first of September, she was taken up in the same manner as she lay down, her Teeth still remaining fast together, yet she could receive Milk by a Quill as before: After Dinner she had a little struggling with her Fit, in which her Teeth were got one over the other, whereas before they were but one against another; the Devil being so malicious, that now she could not receive any Nourishment by the Quill. Seeing therefore that it was impossible to preserve her Life without a Supply of Nourishment, and that she often said, she should not be well till she came to Warboyse, or a Mile on her Way, we resolved to try what this would do; and therefore, in Company with Mrs. Pickering, she was set on Horseback; at which she presently rejoyced, making Signs with her Hands for them to go forwards.

As soon as she was got about a Mile on the Way, though not the direct Road to Warboyse, yet the same Way she came to Tichmerch Grove, as it happened; she began to be more chearful, and her Teeth were untied, and she presently spoke, and said, I am not yet gone a Mile, I shall soon, and then I shall be well. Presently after she rubbed her Eyes, and came to her self, yet wondered how she came thither, and why; as also at the Company and the Strangers that were there: Afterwards alighting from the Horse her Leg was restored to her, which she had had no use of for three Weeks before, and desired her Aunt to pray God to bless her. Thus she walked on perfectly, and Meat being brought to her, she eat and drank chearfully: Then she took a Prayer-Book and read a good while, but when she came to the Word Satan, it shaked and wrung her Shoulders; and the Devil was so malicious, that no sooner Mention was made of their going home, but she was presently taken with a shakeing of her Shoulders, Arms and Body, as if it would have shuffled her together; a little after she arose, and as soon as she turned her Face homewards, her Eyes were shut, her Legs taken from her, and her Teeth fast set in her Head, and her Belly began to heave and swell, as when she was first seized with the Fits. But as long as she was going towards Warboyse, without mentioning going back, she was chearful and well; but if you stand still and talk of going home, she presently sinks in your Arms as in a Swoon, struggling betwixt Life and Death; but as soon as you turn her Face the other way, she presently recovers, and is restored to her Health. This was several times proved, both on Foot and on Horseback; so that at last we were obliged to bring her back the same way she came; a dead Child to look upon for Sense or Motion, but of a very lovely and amiable Complexion, that being not at all altered. At Night it pleased God she received Milk by the help of a Quill, as before; yet not without some Difficulty, the Place being closer shut than at the first, so that within Doors she was fed with Milk like a Suckling; and if Meat was brought her, she pointed to go towards the Place where she was used to awake.

The next Day, therefore, after Dinner, she was carried out again; and when she came to the same Place, she began to rub her Eyes, and was awake again; and gasping once or twice, she stretched forth her Arms, and eat her Meat with a good Appetite as before: But when she was about to return Thanks, the Devil appeared again in his Likeness, and endeavoured to hinder that good Office, by hindering her from speaking, twisting and winding her Body also, so that she could not bring out one good Word; and the better the Word, the more difficult it was to express it.

After this it was thought convenient to put a little Stick into her Mouth, to keep her Teeth open, which was tried,; so that when she was turned about she held the Stick fast in her Mouth, which kept her Teeth open; but she her self was in a dead Sleep, small Signs of Strength or Life appearing in her, and so she continued 'till she was turned about again, which at that time was not soon done, being willing to see the Event of it. A little time after she strove with her Hands to pull the Stick out of her Mouth, lamenting inwardly as if it was a great Trouble to her; but she held it so fast with her Teeth, that it could not be pulled out without great Force, which appeared by the Dents her Teeth had made in it when she recovered: This we durst not venture to do a second time, because she complained her Mouth was very cold, the Stick keeping it open. And now we told her of the Quill she made use of at home; she asking whether she did not eat Meat at other any Place, which she much wondered at, not believing that she could do it.

After this she was carried back out of the Fields into the Grove, and continued in the same State as usual, taking all her Nourishment through the Quill; only sometimes she would take some buttered Meat, minced small, and rubbed against the Outside of her Teeth, and so suck in the Juice and Moisture.

From this Day, which was the Third of September, 'till Tuesday, which was the Eighth, she was carried every Day abroad into the Fields to eat her Meat, she always awaking at the same Place; and though she was carried a Mile or two another way towards Warboyse, yet it had no such Effect, she notwithstanding continuing in the same Condition as before.

This Tuesday she was carried from Tichmarch Grove to her Father's House at Warboyse, and at the Corner of a Hedge she made the usual Signs; and it being the same Place we used to carry her too, she awaked and came to her self, being very hearty and well; her only Grief being that she had left Tichmarch Grove, though she was glad to go to Warboyse.

By what hath been related of this, you may guess what might happen to the rest of the Sisters, who were no less tormented than her, and some in a more grievous Manner; but to relate the Particulars of all their Misfortunes would be too long and tedious.

About a Month after Mr. Pickering had carried this Child to his House, the Lady Cromwell. Wife of Sir Henry Cromwell, Kt. (who then lay in Ramsey a Town two Miles from Warboyse, came to Master Throckmorton's House, with her Daughter-in-Law, Mistriss Cromwell, to visit the Children, and to comfort their Parents; but before she had been long there, the Children all fell into their Fits, and were so grievously tormented, that it moved the good Lady's Heart with Pity to see them, so that she could not forbear Tears, and caused old Mother Samuel to be sent for, who durst not deny to come, because her Husband was Tenant to Sir Henry Cromwell; but after she was come, the Children grew worse than they were before: Then my Lady Cromwell took Mother Samuel aside, and charged her strictly with this Witchcraft, using threatening Words to her, but she stifly denied all, and said, that Mr. Throckmorton and his Wife did her a great deal of Wrong, to blame her without Cause, to which the Lady answered, that neither Mr. Throckmorton nor his Wife accused her, but the Children themselves in their Fits, or rather the Spirit within them. Mrs. Joan, who was then in her Fit, hearing the old Woman thus clearing her self, though she heard not the Lady, nor any Body besides, said, that it was she that caused all this, and that something told her so just then, and asked if no Body heard it but her self, affirming that it squeaked so loud in her Ear, that she wondered they could not hear it, and desired the old Woman to listen if she could not hear it; but Mother Samuel still continued to deny it. Then the Lady Cromwell would have taken her up into a Chamber to examined her more strictly, Dr. Hall a Divine being present; but she would by no means go with them, but made several Excuses to go home: When the Lady found that neither she nor any Body else could prevail, and that she wanted to be gone, she suddenly pulled off her Kircher, and with a Pair of Scissors cut off a Lock of her Hair, and gave it privately to Mrs. Throckmorton with her Hairlace, desiring her to burn them.

Mother Samuel finding her self so served spoke thus to the Lady, Madam, Why do you use me thus? I never did you any harm as yet: These Words were afterwards remembred, though not taken notice of at that time; towards Night the Lady went away, leaving the Children much as she found them.

That Night my Lady Cromwell left Warboyse, she was mightily troubled in a Dream about Mother Samuel; and as she imagined was mightily disturbed in her Sleep by a Cat which Mother Samuel had sent her, which offered to pluck off the Skin and Flesh off her Bones and Arms. The Strugling betwixt the Cat and the Lady was so great in her Bed that Night, and she made so terrible a Noise, that she waked her Bed-fellow Mrs. Cromwell, Wife to the Worshipful Mr. Oliver Cromwell, Son and Heir to Sir Henry Cromwell, who that Night was from Home.

Mrs. Cromwell perceiving the Lady thus disquieted, awaked her, whom the Lady thanked for so doing, and told her how much she had been troubled with Mother Samuel and her Cat, with many other Circumstances; which made her so uneasy, that she could not rest all that Night for fear of the same Soon after the Lady fell very sick, and continued so till her dying Day, which was four Years and a Quarter after her being at Warboyse. The Manner of her Firts was much like those of the Children, only she retained her perfect Senses all the while; sometimes Pain would be in one Arm, and sometimes in another, sometimes in one Leg, and would thence remove into the other, and was oftentimes in her Head. Sometimes it would seize only one Finger or two, and always shake the Part affected, as if it had been the Palsie. And that Saying of Mother Samuel's at Warboyse, Madam, I never hurt you yet, would never be out of her Mind: And thus leaving this good Lady in Heaven with God, we shall return to the Children.

About Christmas after 1590, Mr. Henry Pickering being then a Scholar in Cambridge, went to Mr. Throckmorton's House, and staid there three of four Days, being desirous to speak to Mother Samuel, and taking a convenient time, he desired two or three other Scholars of his Acquaintance to go along with him, who consenting, they went without the Knowledge of any belonging to Master Throckmorton's House. As they were going, she came out of her own House, and crossed the Street before them; so they rather chose to follow her where she went, than to stay for her Return, because her Husband was a cross Man, and would not suffer her to talk with any Body, if he knew it: She went to a Neighbour's House for Barm or Yest, where the Scholars immediately followed her, where they proposed some Questions to her, but she was very impatient, and loath to stay, not suffering any to speak but her self; they desired her to be more silent, but she answered, she was born in a Mill, begot in a Kiln, and must have her Will, and could speak no softiler: The greatest Part of her Discourse was Railing against Mr. Throckmorton and his Children, saying, he misused her, in suffering his Children to accuse her, and bring her Name in Question, and that their Distemper proceeded from their Wantonness, and that if they were her Children she would punish them for it: Then they asked her about her Service of God, and her Faith, to which she answered, that her God would deliver her, defend her, and revenge her of her Enemies. Then one of them asked her if she served the same God that others did, to which she answered, Yes; but had much adoe to bring her from the Phrase of her God, to name the GOD of Heaven and Earth: At last she told them, that if she stayed her Husband would beat her. Then Mr. Pickering told her, the Vengence of God would surely wait on her, however she might deceive the World and her self, and that the only way to prevent God's Vengence was Confession and Repentance, if she had worked that Wickedness upon the Children; and that if she did not, he hoped, one Day, to see her burn at a Stake, and that he would bring Wood and Faggots, and the Children should blow the Coals; she answered, she had rather see him doused over Head in the Pond, and so went away.

But to proceed, the Eldest of Mr. Throckmorton's Daughters was then in her Fit, sitting at home in a Parlour, her Father and Grandmother, and some of her Sisters in their Fits along with her, who suddenly said, now my Uncle and two others, whom the named, are going to Mother Samuel, we shall hear News by and by. See, says she, where Mother Samuel goes trotting in the Streets before them, with her wooden Tankard, and her Apron tucked up before her, naming the House where they went, and all the Passages mentioned above which passed betwixt them. Mr. Throckmorton hearing this, and further, that his Daughter said, now Mr. Pickering and Mother Samuel are parted; he enquired after Mr. Pickering, and finding he was gone out, supposed he was at Mother Samuel's; therefore going out of Doors to look for him, he met him in the Church-Yard, and told him what had passed: Mr. Pickering upon that coming into the Parlour where they were, discoursed with them, they being able to hear no Body but him, and found that they could repeat every Word and Passage exactly that passed betwixt him and Mother Samuel, but that there was so much Wind, that they had much adoe to hear what was said, though at the same time there was no Wind at all.

After this the Spirit would several times appear to them in the Form of a Dun Chicken, and would talk familiarly with them, saying, it came from Mother Samuel, whom it called Dame, and was sent by her to the Children to torment and vex them after that manner. It would likewise declare to the Children concerning Mother Samuel so much, that for a long Time she could do nothing at home, but the Spirit would disclose it, if the Children desired it, in their Fits; as what she was then doing at home; in what Part of the House; or the Spirit would tell where she was: Which was proved true by a Messenger sent on purpose to discover it.

And now the Spirit began to accuse Mother Samuel to the Children in their Fits, telling them it was she that had bewitched them, and all the Servants in the House; and also that whenever they were in their Fits, and carried to Mother Samuel's House, or she was caused to come to them, they should be well. This was often proved, and never once failed; for if the Children, in their Fits, were carry'd to Mother Samuel's House, as soon as they came to the Door, they would rub their Eyes, and say they were well, Why do you carry me? set me down; as if they were ashamed to be carried in the Streets, not knowing in what Condition they had been in. As long as they continued in the House they were well, but once thinking of going away, and offering to go out of the Doors, they fell down on the Ground, and were brought away in the same Condition they were carried thither; and when Mother Samuel went to Mr. Throckmorton's House, though in the greatest Extremity, as soon as she came into the Parlour or Hall where they were, the Children would presently start upon their Feet, and be as well as any in the House, and continue so as long as she stay'd, but when she was about to go, they would fall down like a Stone on the Ground. If she turned about, and came towards them, they would be well again; which was try'd twenty times in an Hour: And when she went away, she left them in the same Condition she found them.

After this, Master Throckmorton resolved to disperse his Children, and send them abroad amongst his Friends, to see how they would then be dealt with, yet always kept some of them at home with him.

It would be too tedious to relate all that happen'd to them whilst abroad; but this was remarkable, that tho' they were eight, ten, or eleven Miles distant, they could tell what happen'd to each other in the Time of their Fits; as they would say, Now is my Sister sore handled, as she her self was at that Time; which was proved to be true, by the Computation of Time, and other Circumstances.

Whilst they were abroad, they were never all clear and free from their Fits, though some of them had not their Fits once in a Month, or half a Year, and one of them was clear of them for a whole Year. But some of them were scarce three Days without them, except since last Lent Assizes, when those Witches were executed.

But to pass by what happen'd for near a Year and a half, we shall proceed to those latter Times, when the Spirits either moved by their own Malice or those that sent them, or their Parents Impatience, it pleased God to grant them the Liberty to exercise their Malice against these Children: However, it was in these latter Times they were more tormented in Body and Mind than formerly. At which Time four of them were at their Father's House at Warboyse, and the other, which was the eldest, at Mr. Pickering's at Tichmersh-Grove.

About this Time, which was in the Year 1592, the youngest but one, being about Fourteen Years of Age, was in a very strange Fit. Every Day, for about three Weeks, she had a senseless Fit, one time of the Day or other, and sometimes many times in one Day. But in this Fit she could neither hear, see, nor speak to any Body: Besides her inward Grief, she would heave, and start, and swell up her Body, which was very troublesome to her for the time. When she was out of these Fits, she would go up and down the House very well, eat and drink, and sometimes be very pleasant with her Sisters, and would do any thing which by any Sign she could understand ought to Be done, and would pay her Respects as she passed by, to those to whom it was due, so that those who were ignorant of her Condition could not perceive that she was out of order, yet she could neither speak to, nor hear any Body speak to her, except sometimes she would prattle to an Infant that was new born, which she took a great deal of delight in.

In the Beginning of these Fits, an Aunt of hers was delivered of a Child in the House, and several of their Friends stay'd there for a Week or Ten Days; all which Time this Child was in these Fits, when Mother Samuel came to the House as well as the rest, and was brought up to the Gentlewoman's Chamber, where commonly most of the Company was: As soon as she came in, this Child, being there, 'spy'd her, and bid her welcome, saying, she was a great Stranger there, and fetched her up both Meat and Drink, and would do any thing she desired her. At last she asked Mother Samuel whose little Child that was she had in her Arms; which she told, and its Name: At which the Child wonder'd, and said, She was glad her Aunt was brought to bed. Why then said she, several of my Aunts and Uncles said they would be here; who were then in the House, and some of them in the Room. Mother Samuel told her, that those she asked for were present; but the Girl said, She saw no-body but her and the little Child in her Arms, tho' she looked full in their Faces. As soon as the old Woman departed, the Child lost all her Senses, and was in the same Condition as before she came.

Continuing in this Condition three Weeks, she came out of her Aunt's Chamber into the Hall, where, in a little time, she fell into a very troublesome Fit; but it lasted not long. Her Mother being in the Hall, she asked her Blessing; and enquiring about several Things, she asked how her Aunt did, from whom she just came; nor could she tell any thing that had been done for the three Weeks past.

But both her's and the rest of her Sisters Troubles grew more severe, as the Year grew nearer an end, their Fits every Day growing more painful, and after a strange Manner.

Towards Hollantide the Spirits grew very familiar with the Children, and, when the Fits were almost at end, would talk with them for half an Hour or more, about the Manner of the Fits they should have, and concerning Mother Samuel, whose Pleasure it was they should be used after that Manner; but they said several times they would bring her to Shame for it at the last. The Spirits likewise would have told them how long their Fits would last, and when they should have another, as likewise the Manner of them, or whether more or less grievous; which was set down in Writing as the Children spoke it, and proved exactly true.

The Times and Signs which the Spirits appointed for the beginning or ending of their Fits were, That in the Morning they should happen, either as soon as they offered to rise out of their Beds; or as soon as they were up or ready; as soon as they asked their Father or their Mother, or their Grandmother, Blessing; as soon as they took a Book in their Hand to pray, or when they had ended their Prayers; as soon as they went to Breakfast, or Dinner was set upon the Table; or as soon as themselves were set down to Dinner, or when the Meat was first put into their Mouths; when Dinner was ended, or when they had put up their Knives after Dinner, observing the same Circumstances at Supper: Or if it were on the Sabbath-day, or when their Bellies were to be twisted, as soon as the first, second, or third Peal was rung, or was ended, with many other such Signs of their Fits beginning or ending.

When they had continued in this Condition above a Month, whether the Devil was weary of it (for he often told the Children in their Fits, that he was weary of his Dame Mother Samuel,) or whether, through God's Providence, the Spitits found they could not kill the Children as they desired, they told them, that in a little Time they would either bring their Dame to a Confession or Confusion. And now they began to accuse Mother Samuel openly to her Face, and tell her that they would not be well in any Place but in her House, or she was confined to continue with them; and if one of these Things was not brought to pass, their Fits would be more violent than over.

Mr. Throckmorton still thinking the Spirits might lie, was resolved to try the utmost for three Weeks together, all which Time the Children had very severe Fits; so that when Night came, not one of them was able to go to bed alone, their Legs being very full of Pains and Sores, besides other Grievances not usual. One of them, for all that Time, never had the Use of her Legs, except an Hour or two in a Day, whilst Mother Samuel was in the House, her Legs otherwise being thrust up to her Body as if they had been ty'd with Strings, so that where you sat her down she was oblig'd to to stay, except she crept away.

Mr. Throckmorton then perceiving that it could not be avoided, offered Ten Pounds a Year for the best Servant in Huntington to do her Work, that she might stay with the Children; but old John Samuel would not consent to it: So that there was no way to preserve the Health of his Children, but to carry them thither; which, as soon as he did, they no sooner came into his House, but they were well: Upon which, he said his. Children should live there, and he would provide what they wanted. The old Man seeing that, put out the Fire, the Weather being cold, and said he would starve them then, several other ill Words coming from him and his Daughter at the same time.

All that Day they continued there well, both eating and drinking, and very merry. At Night, when the old Man perceived that they should lodge there, and that they would be very troublesome to him, promised that his Wife should come next Morning to Mr. Throckmorton's House and continue with him; upon which he took his Children home, who were in their Fits as soon as they came out of the door, and continued so all Night.

Next Morning Mr. Throckmorton went for the old Woman, but she was gone no Body knew whither, upon which he sent for his Children, who as soon as they came into the House were well. Towards Night the old Woman came in, who said she had been two or three Miles out of Town, her Husband knowing of her going, that she might not come to Mr. Throckmorton's; but the Husband forswore the Matter, and presently fell upon his Wife, and beat her severely with a Cudgel, before she could be rescued from him. The Man finding Mr. Throckmorton in the same Mind, consented that his Wife should go along with him that Night, they being all very well, and so they continued eight or nine Days. This made their Parents use the Woman as a welcome Guest. The next Day, the old Woman entreated Mrs. Throckmorton to let her go Home, to fetch something she wanted; which she was loath to grant, offering rather to fetch what she wanted, than to let her go out of the House; but the old

Woman telling her no Body could come at it but her self, and that she would return, she granted her Request.

Soon after she was gone, some of the Children fell into their Fits again, and then the Spirit talked with them, and told them, that then Mother Samuel' was feeding her Spirits, and making a new League with them, which was, That tho' she came again to the House, they should be never the better, but the worse, for her being there, she not being willing to tarry there any longer; which accordingly proved true, for when she came again, those that were in their Fits continued so, and those that were not, fell into them, after her coming, and cry'd out, Now Mother Samuel hath made a new Composition with her Spirits, and that now they should be never the better, but the worse.

Mr. Throckmorton coming Home, and perceiving the Matter, could not chuse but be concerned; yet leaving all to God Almighty, would not suffer the old Woman to leave his House, since his Children, when in their Fits, could neither hear, see, nor speak to any Body but her; and some of them could take nothing but what she gave or touched with her Hands.

Mother Samuel remaining thus in the House, could do or say nothing in any Part of it, but the Children, in their Fits, would reveal it, especially when feeding her Spirits, for then the Children would say, Now Mother Samuel is in such a Place feeding her Spirits; and when they went to look they found her there, but what she was doing they could not discover.

And as often as she sat talking to these Children in their Fits, they would say to her, Look Mother Samuel, do you see this Thing that sits here by us? To which she would answer, No, not she: To this they would answer, That they wonder'd she could not see it leap, skip, and play up and down, pointing with their Fingers. Sometimes they would say, Hark Mother Samuel, don't you hear it? Hark how loud it is, I wonder you cannot hear it; nay, you cannot but hear it. She would deny it, and bid them ask their Father, or some Body else that stood by, whether they heard it or no. The Children would answer, that They saw no Body, though they stood by. Then they would tell Mother Samuel, that it told them she both heard it, saw it, and sent it. Mr. Throckmorton, desirous to make an Experiment of this Matter, one Night desired Mother Samuel to name how many Fits the Children would have next Day, and what kind of Fits they should have, when they should begin, and how long they should continue. Mother Samuel was loath to consent to it; but at last, he saying she should do it, she said, one of them, naming the Child, shall have three Fits, and after such a Manner, appointing the Time for their Beginning and Ending; the other shall have two, likewise appointing the Time; and the third shall have none, but be well all the Day. All which came to pass.

Not long after, Mother Samuel sitting by the Children in their Fits, as before, Mr. Throckmorton, and some others who were along with him, told Mother Samuel, that they had heard that those that were acquainted with these Spirits, and had them at their Command to do what they desired, used to reward them with something, and commonly with some of their Blood every Day; now confess openly, and shame the Devil, whether you do so or not. She utterly deny'd it, with many bitter Words and Curses, desiring the Lord from Heaven might shew some Token upon her, that she was no such Woman as they suspected, or had any Spirits, or rewarded them, or knew any thing of such Matters, or what they were.

Soon after, Mr. Throckmorton and Mr. Henry Pickering, then present, hearing such Protestations, being half terrified at it, that she should thus violently pull down God's Judgments upon her own Head, went out of Doors, and before they were gone ten Paces, Mr. John Lawrence, a Relation of theirs, came to them, and told them that Mother Samuel's Chin bled; whereupon they returned again into the Parlour, and saw eight or ten Drops of Blood upon a Napkin, which she had wiped off her Chin. Then they looked upon her Chin, and could see no Marks of any thing, all being clean and smooth, except some little red Spots, like Flea-bitings. Then Mr. Throckmorton asked her if her Chin used to bleed so or not; to which she answered, Very often: He then asked her, who could witness it; and she said no Body, for it always bled when she was alone, and she never told any Body of it.

After she was condemned, she confessed, that then Mr. Throckmorton demanded the Question of her, that then the Spirits were sucking, and that when she wiped them off with her Hand it bled so, but never had bled above one Drop at a time before, and sometimes not at all.

What we have here related, was proved upon Evidence at the Assizes at Huntington; and those which were not proved there, have been attested by several honest and worthy Gentlemen.

Not long after, the Spirits told the Children, that if their Father did not presently go to John Samuel's House, his Daughter Agnes Samuel, who was concerned in these Matters, and not yet brought in Question, would hide her self, and not be seen by him: Upon which, he being told of it, went presently to try how it would be. When he went to the House, Agnes Samuel, whether she suspected the Matter or not, went up into the Chamber, the Stairs being in the Room where her Father was, and a Trap-door at the Top of the Stairs, upon which she set Sacks of Corn and Tubs to keep it down. Mr. Throckmorton suspecting some such Matter, by the Noise in the House, continued knocking at the Door. In a little time John Samuel asked who was there, and what he wanted, &c. and at last knowing who he was, would not let him in. Then Mr. Throckmorton went on the other Side of the House, and finding the Back-door open, he went in; where he found the old Man in his Bed, it being about Eight a-Clock in the Morning. Mr. Throckmorton asked where his Daughter Agnes Samuel was; to which he answered with his usual Oath (which he commonly used, and continued the Use of it both at the Bench upon his Arraignment, and at his Execution, till the last Period) as God judge his Soul, he knew not where she was.

Mr. Throckmorton asked when he saw her; to which he answered, that she was in the House since the Evening, but where then she was he did not know. He asked, if she was not in the Chamber over him; he swore he could not tell, though it was certain he could not be ignorant of it. Mr. Throckmorton suspecting she was there, called three or four times, and desired her to answer if she was there, which was all he wanted; but she would not answer. Then he took a Candle, and said he would go and see, and finding the Trap-door fast, he knew she must needs be there; upon which he told them, that he would go into the Room before he went out of the House, and would break open the Trap-door or the Floor, and accordingly bid one of the Company fetch him a Crow or an Iron-bar. The Maid hearing him so resolute, answered, and taking the Things off the Door at his Desire, came down. Upon which he returned Home.

But to pass by such Things as these, and to proceed to the old Woman's Confession; Mother Samuel, by this time, began to be weary of Mr. Throckmorton's House, not only because she could do nothing in the House, but what the Children discovered in their Fits; but especially because the Children told her plainly to her Face, that she should confess these Things before Tuesday after Twelfth-day, and that the Spirits had told them that they would oblige her to confess in spite of her.

At this Time this Tuesday was not thought on to be the Sessions-Day at Huntington; yet they were often whispering with themselves about that Tuesday, which they longed mightily for, the Spirits telling them, that after that Day they should have no Fits. They further added, that if she confessed before that Tuesday, they should be well sooner.

The Children often desired her to confess, that they might be well; but she still denied it, saying, Why should she confess what was not true, and that she knew nothing of, nor consented to? The Children answered, They did not desire her to accuse her self falsely, and bid her look to that; yet in their Fits they gave her very good and divine Counsel concerning her Confession at several times.

The Speeches which they at several times made to her, were to this Purpose. They represented to her the Joys of Heaven she should lose, and the Torments of Hell which she should endure, if she were guilty, and did not confess; and what Advantages she might reap on the contrary, if she confessed and was sorry for what she had done. They put her in mind of her ill way of living, and of her cursing every thing that displeased her, especially their Parents and themselves. They put her in mind of her Neglect of the Church, and God's Service; which, she said she would begin to mend: Also her lewd bringing up her Daughter, and her suffering her to controul and beat her: They told her also how she said their Fits were but Wantonness, and desired to know if she thought so now; she answer'd, No. They concluded with their hearty Prayers to God for her, and said if she would confess, that they might be well, they would forgive her from the Bottom of their Hearts, and would entreat their Parents and Friends to forgive what was past. All the while they thus talked to her, it was with Tears, which moved all that stood by to Tears, except the old Woman, who was little or nothing concerned.

This Behaviour of the Children passed not till near Christmass, without moving the old Woman, who almost every Day had a Fit of bleeding at the Nose in considerable Quantities, which made her grow faint and pale, so that Mr. Throckmorton and his Wife were very careful of her, lest any Harm should come to her in their House, letting her want nothing she desired; so that she confessed to all that came to her, that she was very well used, and thought her self much obliged to him, if she had no other Cause; for she did nothing but her own Work, eat with him or his Children, and lay in his Chamber, and commonly with one of his Children.

One Day Mrs. Elizabeth Throckmorton was very uneasy, and could not eat any Meat; yet at Night, when Supper was ready, she thought to make her self amends; but when she was ready to sit at Table, she fell into a Fit, her Mouth being closed up, that she could neither eat, drink, nor speak, as it was usual, their Mouths being shut up, especially about Meal-times, and sometimes shut and open about half a dozen times at Dinner; but she went to bed, sorrowful and weeping. Next Day she was sick and ill, and ear little or nothing at all; yet at Night she found her self better, and very hungry; and being advised to eat then, she deferred it till Supper, but when the Meat was set upon the Table, she fell into the same Condition as before.

Mr. Throckmorton perceiving this, said, Mother Samuel, I believe you have a mind to starve that Wench; to which she answered, No, she was rather sorry to see it. Well, says he, you shall neither eat nor drink, till she does both, use the Matter as you will. Thus they continued both fasting till the Supper was almost ended, and the Company ready to rise. The old Woman seeing he was in good earnest, and that the Meat was carry'd out of the Parlour, the Child suddenly fetched a great Sigh, and said, If I had some Meat now I could eat. Upon which Mrs. Throckmorton ordered Meat to be given to them both, the Company not taking Notice of it to Mother Samuel; so they both began to eat very heartily, especially the old Woman, who was then very hungry: And from that Time, whilst the old Woman was in the House, none of the Children had their Mouths closed up when they had Occasion to eat, and if they were, they did not continue long so, which before commonly happen'd.

When all this was over, and the Time drew nearer, Mother Samuel complained every Day of some new Grief that befell her; sometimes she would cry out of her Back, being so full of Pain, that she was not able to stir her self in Bed all the Day, nor to rest at Night; sometimes she would complain of her Head or her Stomach, yet she would eat her Meat, saying, She had a gnawing at her Heart. The next Day after, it would be at her Knee, or lower, so that she would go halting up and down the House: And, indeed, one would have thought that something troubled her, for she would groan all the Night, and moan her self, one time complaining of one Part, and then of another; so that she rested very little her self, and disturbed every Body in the Chamber.

One Night she cried out so much of her Belly, that she awaken'd Mr. Throckmorton and his Wife, who lay by her. In God's Name, says he, what is the Matter with you, Mother Samuel, and what makes you groan so? Says she, I have great Pain in my Belly, and cannot imagine the Cause of it. He asked her what was the Matter in it: She answered, She felt something stir in it, and imagined it to be as big as a Penny-Loaf, and put her to a great deal of Pain. Mrs. Throckmorton got out of her Bed, and felt her Belly, and found something in it as she had complained, but did not feel it stir, not staying long, for the Weather was very cold: And, doubtless, she was then breeding the Child she pleaded under Sentence of Condemnation. But she still complained of her Belly, and said to Mr. Throckmorton, That she had often been told some evil Spirit haunted his House, which tormented his Children. This, he told her, he did believe. Then saith she, I believe one of them is got into my Belly. That, says Mr. Throckmorton, may be true. So she said it was an evil House, and haunted with evil Spirits, and wished she had never come into it. He told her, If any evil Spirits haunted the House, they were of her sending; and so granted all she said. In the Morning she complained much, but said the Swelling in her Belly was gone, and could not tell where the greatest Pain was, it was in so many Places, but her Stomach was the best of any Part; and after this, she always complain'd of one Part of her Body or other, whilst she stay'd in the House.

A little while after, one of the Children fell into a violent Fit, Mother Samuel standing by, which was the worst that ever any of them had; her sneezing was very terrible and strong, as if it would-have caused her Eyes to fly out of her Head. This surprized Mother Samuel, for she thought the Child would have died that Minute; and this brought her to Prayers, desiring the Lord to help her and preserve her in that Danger, and she hoped never to see her in the like again. But the more she prayed, the worse it was; and when she named God, or Jesus Christ, the Fit grew more violent. When she had continued thus about two Hours, the Spirit spoke to the Child, and say'd, There was a worse Fit than this to come yet. The Child answered, She cared not for him nor his Dame, but bid them do their worst, for she hoped God would deliver her; and soon after she was very well. But that Fit was so terrible to Mother Samuel, that she prayed after she might never see the like again.

The Children all continued crying upon Mother Samuel to confess, for she must do it at the last, and if she would let them be well before Christmass, they should think themselves obliged to her; but if she did not, they should soon be well, for Christmass was near, and they hoped to keep a merry one. She said she would do them all the Good she could, but would not confess to a Thing she knew not of, nor ever consented to.

Mr. Throckmorton hearing what was said, went in, and told Mother Samuel, Since you hear what the Children say, and that they shall be well if you confess, and that you must before it be long; and since you know that they never tell Lies in their Fits; In the Name of God, if there be any such Matter, confess it; it is never too late to repent, and ask Mercy: But she deny'd it, as before. But, says he, what say you to that grievous Fit the Spirit threaten'd my Daughter Jane with. Says she, I hope never to see any of them in such again. But says he, You know the Spirit never uses to fail of what he promises. I trust in God, says she very confidently, I shall never see it. Then says Mr. Throckmorton, Charge the Spirit in the Name of God, that she may escape this Fit: Upon which she said, I charge thee, Spirit, in the Name of God, that Mrs. Jane may never have this fit. The Child said, sitting by, The Thing said, I thank God that I shall never have this Fit that was threaten'd; then says he, Thank God that is well. Then says he again, Go on, Mother Samuel, and charge the Spirit in the Name of God, and speak from your Heart, that neither she, nor any of the rest, shall have their Fits any more: Which she did very heartily. The same Child said again, Truly I shall never have it any more, after the Tuesday following Twelfth day. It's well, thank God, says Mr. Throckmorton, charge the Spirit again in the Name of God, and speak from your Heart, and be not afraid, that he depart from them all now at this present, and that he never return to them again; which Words she expressed very loud and boldly. As soon as she had ended, the three Children, then in their Fits, and who had continued so three Weeks, wiped their Eyes, and presently thrust back the Stools they sat on, and stood upon their Legs, being as well as ever they were in their Lives.

Mr. Throckmorton's Face was then towards the Children, and his Back to the old Woman, and seeing them start up at once, said, Thanks be to God. In the mean time the old Woman fell down on her Knees behind him, and said, Good Master, forgive me. He turning about, and seeing her down, said, Why, Mother Samuel, what is the Matter? O Sir, said she, I have been the Cause of all this Trouble to your Children. Have you, Mother Samuel? says he: And why? What Cause did I ever give you to use me and my Children thus? None at all, said she. Then says he, you have done me the more wrong. Good Master, said she, forgive me. God forgive you, said he, and I do; but tell me how you came to be such a Woman? Master, said she, I have forsaken my Maker, and given my Soul to the Devil.

Then the Grandmother and Mother of the Children, who were in the Hall, hearing them so loud in the Parlour, came in, whom Mother Samuel asked Pardon of likewise. Mrs. Throckmorton, the Mother, presently forgave her with all her Heart, but could not well tell what was the Matter. Then Mother Samuel asked the three Children that were there, and the rest, Forgiveness, and kissed them, the Children easily forgiving her.

Mr. Throckmorton and his Wife perceiving the old Woman so penitent, and cast down, she weeping and lamenting all the time, did all they could to comfort her, and told her, They would freely forgive her from their Hearts, provided their Children were no more troubled. She said, She trusted in God they would never be troubled again; yet could not be comforted. Mr. Throckmorton then sent for Dr. Dorrington, Minister of the Town, and told him all the Circumstances; and all of them endeavoured to make her easy, but nevertheless the wept all that Night.

The next Day, being Christmas Even, and the Sabbath, Dr. Dorrington chose his Text of Repentance out of the Psalms, and communicating her Confession to the Assembly, directed his Discourse chiefly to that Purpose, to comfort a penitent Heart, that it might affect her. All the Sermon-time, Mother Samuel wept and lamented, and was frequently so loud in her Passions, that she drew the Eyes of all the Congregation upon her.

But Mr. Throckmorton reflecting on Mother Samuel's Inconstancy formerly, and that there were no Witnesses of her Confession, except himself and the Doctor, and those of his own Houshold, lest they should be thought partial, desired, after Prayers, that she should come into the Body of the Church, and there demanded that she would declare, whether the Confession she made before him and the Doctor, was forced from her, or whether she made it freely, and of her own Accord, She answered, That it came from her freely, before them all, and desired that her Neighbours would pray to God for her, and forgive her.

Towards Evening, Mr. Dorrington understanding she still continued in this sorrowful Condition, came to Mr. Throckmorton's House, and desired him in Pity to let her go Home to her Husband, and he would endeavour to reconcile them; to which the old Woman was much enclined; and to which Mr. Throckmorton readily consented, endeavouring to promote the same, little suspecting that any ill Consequence might happen upon it. The Man hearing of it, spoke bluntly, as usual, and said she might come Home if she would.

But, without doubt, she had a cold Welcome from both the Husband and the Daughter, for confessing this Matter; which we heard from her afterwards, both of them setting upon her, who prevailed with her to deny all she had said, and that it was not so. The next Day, being Christmass-day, she absolutely deny'd all she had said; which soon came to Mr. Throckmorton's Hearing, that this new Convert was revolted; though he was well satisfy'd with her open Confession in the Church, and could scarce believe what was reported of her.

The same Day Dr. Dorrington and Mr. Throckmorton went to Mother Samuel's House, and at the Door heard the old Man and Woman and her Daughter talking about it, and heard the Daughter saying, Believe them not, believe them not, for all their fair Speeches. Upon which, they went in, and charged them with it; but they all deny'd what was said: And the old Woman being charg'd with the Denial of her Confession, she said, She would deny that she was a Witch, or the Cause of his Children's Illness. Why, says he, did not you confess it. Says she, I did so indeed, but it is not so. Then, reply'd he, I must not shew you the Favour I promised; I will certainly have you before Justices. He then asked her, why she confessed it, if not true? She said, For Joy that his Prayers and her's so soon prevailed, and that they were well so soon. Then says Mr. Throckmorton, Since the Thing is published, and you or I must bear the Shame, it shall not pass so.

The next Day, that the common People might not think that he had done this to bring the old Woman into farther Danger, Mr. Throckmorton consulting with Dr. Dorrington, they concluded to send for the old Woman to Church again; but she was more averse to confessing than ever. Then Mr. Throckmorton took her by the Hand, and told her, That that Day she and her Daughter should go along with him to the Bishop of Lincoln's: Upon which he sent for the Constables, and charged them with the Mother and Daughter.

When the old Woman found that Preparations were made for the Journey, she came to Mr. Throckmorton, and told him she would confess to him alone; upon which, he took her into the Parlour, and she confessed again all she did before: Upon which, he asking her why she deny'd it again; she told him, She would not, but for her Husband and Daughter, who had told her she had better lived and died as she was, than to confess her self a Witch, and be called so as long as she lived. Then Mr. Throckmorton told her, if she would confess freely, he would shew her all the Favour he could; but Dr. Dorrington coming in, in the mean time, she seemed shy in confessing unto him; upon which Mr. Throckmorton left them together, and then Dr. Dorrington wrote down what she confessed.

And as it was then Prayer-time, Mr. Throckmorton sent to the Church, and desired some of his Neighbours to come to him, whom he placed under the Parlour-Window; and giving Notice of it to the Doctor, he both spoke loud himself, and made some Excuse to make her do so, by which means they without could hear all that passed. Then Mr. Throckmorton went into the Parlour, and desired them to come out into the Hall, where all the Neighbours stood who had heard what had pass'd; and the Doctor read over her Confession before them all, but she would fain have denied all again; but the Neighbours told her it was too late then to deny it, since they all heard it, and told her the Place where they were.

When she found her self thus catch'd, she would have made the best of it, if it would have prevailed. In the mean time in came John Samuel, who was told by Mr. Throckmorton, that his Wife would not have deny'd her Confession, but for him and his Daughter; who understanding that, gave her some ill Language, and would have given her Blows, had not the Standers-by prevented him: Upon which, she pretended to fall in a Swoon, but presently recovered again. The same Day Mr. Throckmorton resolved to continue his Journey, and clear himself of that Matter, and caused the old Woman and her Daughter to be carried to the Bishop of Lincoln to be examin'd.

The Examination of Alice Samuel, of Warboyse in the County of Huntington, taken at Buckden, before the Right Reverend Father in God, William, by God's Permission, Bishop of Lincoln, the 26th of December, 1592.

BEing asked whether a Dun Chicken did ever suck on her Chin, and how often; the said Examinant says, That it sucked twice, and no more, since Christmass-Even last. Being asked whether it was a natural Chicken, because when it came to her Chin she did scarce feel it, but when she wiped it off, her Chin bled; she saith further, That the said Dun Chicken first came to her Chin and sucked, before it came to Mr. Throckmorton's House; and that the Evil and Trouble that came to Mr. Throckmorton's Children, came by means of the Dun Chicken; which Chicken she knows is now both gone from them and from her: And further she saith, That Mr. Throckmorton and Dr. Dorrington shall bring further Information of such Things which as yet she hath not declared.

The Examination of Alice Samuel of Warboyse, taken at Buckden the 29th Day of December 1592, before the Reverend Father in God, William, by God's Permission, Bishop of Lincoln; Francis Cromwell and Richard Tryce, Esquires, Justices of Her Majesty's Peace, of the County aforesaid.

SHE faith she never did Hurt to any, except the Children in Question. Being asked how she knows the said Dun Chicken is gone from the said Children, she says, Because the said Dun Chicken, with the rest, is now come into her, and are now in the Bottom of her Belly, and make her so full, that she is like to burst; and this Morning they caused her to be so full, that she could scarce lace her Coat; and that on the Way as she came they weighed so heavy, that the Horse she rid on was not able to carry her. And further she confessed, That the upright Man she told Mr. Throckmorton of, told her he was a hard Man, and would trouble her much, and therefore he would give her free Spirits that should vex and torment his Children, and so he did; and that these Spirits sucked their Blood often, as a Reward for what they did, and always before she sent them any whither. She also confessed, That whatever the Children said of the Spirits was true, and that the Spirits were there when the Children saw them, and that she saw them; and that often she gave a private Beck with her Finger or Head, and then the Spirits stopped the Children's Mouths, that they could not speak till they came out again; and then the Children would wipe their Eyes, and be well again. Further she said, That it was taught her by a Man that came to the House, but what his Name was, or where he lived, she could not tell: That if she would call the said Spirits, they would come, and when she called them they appeared in the Form of Dun Chickens: Their Names were Pluck, Catch, and White; and the other three she called with her Mouth with three Smacks; two of which she sent to Mr. Throckmorton and his Wife, which returned and told her that God would not suffer them to prevail; upon which she sent them to his Children, which tormented them after that strange manner.

She further confessed, That what the Children said in her Hearing was true: And being asked what the upright Man's Name was that gave her the Devils, she said she could not tell; whereupon she was asked to go into another Chamber, and demand of her Spirits what his Name was, which she presently did, and there, with a loud Voice, three times said, O thou Devil, I charge thee, in the Name of the Father, the Son, and the Holy Ghost, that thou tell me the Name of the upright Man that gave me the Devils; and then returning, she said her Spirits told her his Name was Langland. Being asked where he lived, she said she could not tell; wherefore she was again desired to consult with her Spirits, which she presently did, and with a loud Voice cried three times, O Devil, I charge thee, in the Name of the Father, the Son, and the Holy Ghost, tell me where the said Langland dwelleth; and returning, said he had no Dwelling: And being desired to demand where he was at that present, she did as before, and returned, answering, That her Spirits told her he went the last Voyage beyond Seas. After these Confessions, Mother Samuel and her Daughter were committed to Huntington Goal, where she was suspected for the Death of one of the Goaler's Servants, whom she threaten'd, and of the extream Sickness of one of his Children, who presently mended after scratching of her.

After Dinner, Mr. Throckmorton desired the High Sheriff and Justices to accept of Bail for Agnes Samuel, that he might have her home to his House, and try whether the like Evidences of Guiltiness might appear in her as in the Mother, which they with much Difficulty granted.

The Report of Dr. Dorrington of what happened at Warboyse, on Tuesday the Sessions-Day at Huntington, the Ninth of January.

About Twelve a-Clock, Mary, Jane, and Grace, Daughters of Mr. Throckmorton of Warboyse, Esq; fell into their usual Fits of Lameness, Blindness, Deafness, and Want of Feeling; only their youngest Brother Robert, of Nineteen Years of Age, could speak to Jane, and she to Mary and Grace. After Dinner, Dr. Dorrington coming to see them, with a Cambridge Scholar, found them all in their Fits, each of them often repeating the following Words, I am glad, I am glad, none so glad as I. The Doctor desired their Brother to ask them why they were so glad: Jane answered, Within two Hours we shall have good News, the other Sister affirming the same. Mary and Jane whispered to each other, I wonder how she should know that Thing, I am sure none of this House told her, and therefore her Spirits must tell her. Robert was again desired to ask Jane, and Jane to ask Mary and Grace, when they should come out of this Fit; to which they answered, By and by, and then we shall be all of us well in the Hall, and then returning quickly here again, we shall have another slight Fit, and then the two Hours will be over; but when we have been told the News we expect, we shall have a severe Fit, but very shore: All which happened true, for they role presently from their Stools, and went out of the great Parlour into an inward Parlour, to see how their Mother did; and from thence into the Hall, to see their Sister Elizabeth, who was sitting by the Fire; and thence into the great Parlour, where they no sooner came, but they all fell into their Fits again; and being carried to their Stools, began to repeat again, I am glad, I am glad, none so glad as I: And being asked, Why? they answered, That Agnes Samuel should be brought from Huntington to their Father's House; but they should not hear Agnes Samuel, as they did her Mother, in their Fits, because her Father should ask her no Questions.

After they had all said these Words, they sell into extream Fits, bowing their Bodies so that their Heads and Feet almost met together, their Bellies being highest, with great groaning; but in a little Time, rubbing their Eyes twice or thrice, they awaked, and were very well again; upon which the Spirits saying We are gone, Mrs. Jane answered, Farewel and be hang'd. Being asked how they had been these two Hours; they said, They had been asleep. And though they had dined before their Fits, yet they had forgot it, yet had no Stomachs to eat.

When Agnes Samuel was brought to Mr. Throckmorton's House, the Children continued for three or four Days without Fits at all: But when it was hoped that all was over, they fell fresh into their Fits again, and were as much tormented as in the old Woman's Time; and then the Spirits began to accuse the Daugher, as much as ever they did the Mother, and told the Children, that the Mother had given her Spirits over to the Daughter, who had bewitched them over again, and would handle them worse than ever the Mother did. The Children shewed the same disposition towards the Daughter as they had to the Mother, saying they cared not for her or her Spirits, what they could do to them; they trusted in God, who would deliver them out of their hands.

Soon after Agnes Samuel was brought to Mr. Throckmortons House, Mrs. Jane the eldest Daughter, was brought home from Tichmarch Grove to Warboyse; but to omit what she suffered whilst she remained there, we shall particularly observe what happened at Warboyse.

On Friday the Ninth of Feb. 1592. Mrs. Jane fell into her fits as usual, complaining of great pain in her Legs, which had been sore nine or ten Weeks before, being most of the time she was at Titchmarch Grove. But now she grew much worse in her Legs, and for a fortnight before they were so full of pain, that she could neither walk nor fit, but only ly upon her Bed, or on Cushions by the Fire. Her Fit continuing all that Day, at Night the Spirit came to her, and talked as usual with it, asking whence it came, what News it brought, with a great deal of disdain. The Thing would not tell her whence it came, but that she should have very severe Fits for the future, worse than ever; being in perfect Memory, and retaining all her Senses. She answered, she neither cared nor feared him, for God was on her side, and would protect her; upon which the Thing departed, she continuing in her Fit most of that Night, till she went to Bed.

The Tenth in the Afternoon she lay groaning in her Fit by the Fire side, and suddenly was taken with a Bleeding at the Nose, which surprized her very much, fearing ill News after it. When she had bled much in her Handkercheif, she said it was a good deed to throw it in the Fire and burn the Witch. After she had talked thus, it appeared that the Spirit came to her; she smiling and looking about her, saying, What is this in God's Name, that comes tumbling to me? it tumbles like a Footbal, it looks like a Puppit-player, and appears much like its Dame's old thrumb Cap. What is your Name I pray you said she? the Thing answered, his Name was Blew. To which she answered Mr. Blew you are welcome, I never saw you before; I thought my Nose bled not for nothing, what News have you brought? What, says she, dost thou say I shall be worse handled than ever I was? Ha! what dost thou say? that I shall now have my Fits, when I shall both hear and see, and know every Body; that's a new Trick indeed. I think never any of my Sisters were so used, but I care not for you; do your worst, and when you have done, you will make an end.

After this she was silent a while, but listning to something that was said, presently called for Agnes Samuel, asking where she was, and saying, that the had too much Liberty, and that she must be more strictly looked too; for lately she was in the Kitchen Chamber talking with her Spirits, and intreated Mr. Blew not to let me have any such extream Fits when I spoke, heard, and knew every Body. But he says he will torment me more and not rest till Dame Agnes Samuel is brought to her End; so that now, says she, to Agnes Samuel, who was just come to her, it will be no better with us till you and your Mother are both hanged. The Maid confessed she was in the Kitchen Chamber and alone, but denied that she talked with Spirits, or knew any such. Mrs. Jane bid her not deny it, for the Spirits would not lye. Soon after she came out of this Fit, and complained of great pain in her

Leggs, and being asked where she had been, and what she had said, she answered, that she had been asleep, and said nothing she knew of, and wondered how her Hankerchief came to be so bloody, saying, some Body else had bloodyed it, and not she, for she was not used to bleed.

At Night when her Father and Mother rose from Supper, she fell into the Fit Mr. Blew threatned her with, being severely twisted in every Part; sometimes she would thrust out her Arms so strong and stiff, that it was impossible to bend them. Sometimes she would so twist them backwards, that no Body could do the like by their natural Strength, crying out very pitifully; sometimes she complained of her Stomach, saying she was very sick and offered to Vomit; sometimes of her Head, or her Belly, never a Part being free from extream Pain, she often calling upon God to think upon her, and to deliver her; sometimes it would stop her Breath, and so long, that when she fetched her Breath again, it would be with a deep and loud Groan; and being often asked how she did, she answered, very Sick, and full of Pain, saying, she heard and saw all that was present.

She continued in this Condition about half an Hour, and as she was complaining she fell into her severest Fit, having her Mouth also shut up, being deprived of all manner of Sense. And thus remaining quiet a while, she fetched a great Groan, and then her Mouth being opened, she said, Here is a Rule indeed, I find you are as good as your Word with me; whence came you, or what News do you bring I pray you? The Thing answered, that she must be worse handled than all this; she answered, God is above the Devil, and do what you can, you shall not be able to hurt me? But why do you punish me worse than all my Sisters, having my Fits when I know every Body? Because she told Tales of their Dame, they said, Who is your Dame said she, Nan Samuel replyed the Spirit. Thus in all their Talk, they would repeat the Spirits Answer, before they asked another Question; says she then, if Nan Samuel be your Dame, I will tell more Tales of her, and I hope to tell such a Tale of her one Day, that she will not be able to answer, nor you for her. The Thing answered, he would not punish her the more for it, she said she cared not for that. Then said the Spirit, when was Smack with you, another of the Spirits, she answered, I know no such fellow as Smack, you do says the Thing, and it is he that tells you all these things, but I will curse him for it; do your worst to me or him, I care not for you, says she. Farewel says the Thing, do you bid me farewel says she, farewel and be hanged, and come again when you are sent for.

Soon after she came out of her Fit, and was very sick, and her Legs sore. The next Day being Sabbath, she was pretty well all the Forenoon; soon after Dinner Mr. Throckmorton of Brampton came into the House, to see how the Children did, and staying in the Parlour a while, Mrs. Elizabeth just as she was coming in at the Door, fell into a Fit, which was a little strange to the Gentleman. Says Mr. Throckmorton to the Gentleman, will you see a Wonder, says he, can I see a greater than this: To which he replyed, You shall see this Child brought out of this Condition, at the pronouncing of certain Words by a Maid in this House; upon which he called for Agnes Samuel, and desired her to say these Words: I charge thee thou Devil, as I love thee, and have Authority over thee, and am a Witch, and guilty of this Matter, that thou suffer this Child to be well at this present. These Words were no sooner ended, but the Child wiped her Eyes, and was as well as any of them. Whilst the Gentleman admiring what passed, was talking with the Maid, and telling her she could tell a pretty Tale for her self; Mrs. Jane standing by fell presently into her Fit, and the same Experiment was tryed with her, as with the other, and this answered exactly whenever any of them were in their Fits, it being foretold by the Spirit a Fortnight before, that whenever Mrs. Agnes Samuel repeated these Words, they should be well.

But to return to Mrs. Jane who was Sick and full of Pain all that Day; when Night came, after Supper she fell into her Fit as the Night before, being able to see, hear, and understand every thing that was asked of her; and having continued in this Fit some time, she fell into her senseless Fit, and being silent a while, and her Mouth shut, she fetched a great Groan, and said, whence came you Mr. Smack, and what News do you bring? The Spirit answered, that he came from fighting, said she, with whom? The Spirit answered with Pluck, where did you fight, I pray you, said she? The Spirit answered, in old Dames back House, which stood in Mother Samuels Yard; and they fought with great Cowlstaves last Night, and who got the Mastery I pray you, said she? He answered, he broke Plucks Head, says she, I wish he had broke your Neck also; saith the Spirit, is that all the thanks I shall have for my Labour? What, says she, do you look for thanks not my Hands? I wish you were all hanged up against one another, for you are all naught, but God will defend me from you; so he departed, and bid her farewel. Being asked when he would come again, he said on Wednesday Night. He was no sooner gone, but presently came Pluck to her, to whom she said from whence come you Pluck, with your Head hanging down so? He answered just as Smack had told her. Then said the Spirit to her, when saw you Smack? She answered, that she knew no such Fellow, yes says he, but you do, but you will not be known of him. It seems, says, she, that you have met with your Match, and after such like Expressions, he went away, and presently she came out of her Fit, and complained of Pain in her Legs.

The next Day she was very sick all Day, it being Monday, and in the Afternoon fell into a very strange Fit, having lost all her Senses for about half an Hour; Agnes Samuel seeing the Extremity of which, seemed to pray earnestly for her along with the rest; and being asked whether it proceeded from Wantonness, as she used to say, she could not deny but it must proceed from some Supernatural Power. When the Fit was over she was well, except the Pain in her Legs.

After Supper, as soon as her Parents were risen, she fell into the same Fit again, as before, and then became senseless, and in a little Time opening her Mouth, she said, Will this hold for ever? I hope it will be better one Day. From whence came you now Catch, said she, limping? I hope you have met with your Match. Catch answered, That Smack and he had been fighting, and that Smack had broken his Leg. Said she, That Smack is a shrewd Fellow, methinks, I would I could see him. Pluck came last Night, said she, with his Head broke, and now you have broken your Leg; I hope, said she, he will break both your Necks before he hath done with you. Catch answered, that he would be even with him before he had done. Then said she, Put forth your other Leg, and let me see if I can break that, having a Stick in her Hand. The Spirit told her, that she could not hit him. Can I not hit you, said she? Let me try. Then the Spirit put out his Leg, and she lifted up the Stick easily, and suddenly struck on the Ground. You have not hurt me, said the Spirit. Have I not hurt you, said she? No, but I would if I could, and then I would make some of you come short Home. So she seemed divers times to strike at the Spirit, but he leaped over the Stick, as she said, like a Jack-an-Apes. So after many such Tricks the Spirit went away, and she came out of her Fit, continuing all that Night, and the next Day, very Sick, and full of Pain in her Legs.

    At Night, when Supper was ended, she fell into her sensible Fit again, which continued as usual, and then she grew senseless, and after a little time, as usual, fetching a great Groan, she said, Ha! Sirrah, are you come now with your Arm in a Sling, Mr. Blew? Who hath met with you I pray? The Spirit said, You know well enough. She answered, Do I know well enough? How should I know? Why, said the Spirit, Smack and I were fighting, and he hath broken my Arm. Said she, That Smack is a stout Fellow indeed, I hope he will break all your Necks, because you punish me without a Cause. I wish, said she, that I could be once acquainted with him. We will be even with him, said Blew, one Day. Why, said she, what will ye do? The Spirit said, they would all fall upon him and beat him. Saith she, Perhaps he cares not for you all, for he has broken Pluck's Head, Catch's Leg, and your Arm, now you have something to do, you may go and heal your Arm. Yes, saith the Spirit, when my Arm is well, we will beat Smack. So they parted, and she came out of her Fit, and complained of most Parts of her Body; so that she seemed easier, while the Spirit was talking with her, than when she came out of the Fit.

The next Day, which was Wednesday, she was very ill, and when Night came she first fell into her sensible Fit, and then into her senseless one, and after fetching a great Sigh, said she, whence came you Mr. Smack? He said he was come according to his Promise on Sunday Night. Said she, It is very likely you will keep your Promise, but I had rather you would keep away till you art sent for; but what News have you brought? Said he, I told you I had been fighting last Sunday Night, but I have had many Battles since. So it seems, said she, for here was both Pluck, Catch and Blew, and all came lame to me. Yes, said he, I have met with them all. But I wonder, said she, you could beat them, for they are very great, and you are but a little one. Said he, I am good enough for two of the best of them together. But, said she, I can tell you News. What's that, said he? They will all of them fall upon you at once, and beat you. He said he cared not for that, he would beat two of the best of them. And who shall beat the other two, said she, for there is one who hath been often spoke of, called Hardname, his Name standing upon eight Letters, and every Letter standeth for a Word, but what his Name is otherwise, we know not. The Spirit answered, That his Cousin Smacks would help him to beat the other two. There are also two other Smacks, as appears from the old Woman's Confession. What, said she, will your Cousin Smacks help you? Is there Kindred amongst Devils? I never heard of that before, God keep me from that Kindred.

A great deal of such foolish Talk passed amongst them, but at the last the Spirit said, You shall have no more such Fits as you have had. No, said she, that's well, but you can do nothing but lye. Why, said he, will you not believe me? No, said she, shall I believe the Father of Lyes? But you shall find it true, said he. She reply'd, If I do, I will believe you, but not before. I pray God it may be true, but whether it is or not, I care not a rush for you. No, says he, will you not thank me? Thank you, hang you and all your Fellows, for I will believe yo no further than I see you, not do I care for any of you all.

This Smack hath often endeavoured to deceive her with fair Promises, that he would do any thing for her, if she would but love him; but by the Assistance of God, she always resisted and defy'd his Temptations.

At last, said she, You have often told me, that I should scratch Agnes Samuel, when shall I scratch her? The Spirit told her that she should scratch her before the Assizes. What, said she, shall she stand before the Assizes with a scratched Face? Yes, said the Spirit, so it should be. She said she would set it on whensoever it should be; and, said she, look you be as good as your Word in this, for I would fain scratch her; for whatsoever the Mother is, I cannot abide her now, and am sick when I look upon her, and loath her Company. At parting the Spirit told her she should have no more Fits after the Assizes. No, said she, I am very glad of that. But, says the Spirit, if you have, Woe be to Agnes Samuel, for I will bring her to her End. Thus the Spirit left her, saying nothing of his return, and presently she came out of her Fit, and was better than commonly she used to be, and the next Day was able to go upon her Legs, which she could not use a Month before.

On Monday the Twentieth of February she began to talk again, after she had been an Hour in her Fit; having eaten her Supper in her Fit, on a sudden she said, What are you come now? I thought you would have come no more, but where have you been said she? He answered, That his Cousin Smack and he had been fighting with Pluck and Catch, and had beaten them both very much, so that they durst not come to her no more; but after a great deal of Talk, she asked when she should scratch Agnes Samuel? The Spirit answered, That if she should scratch her now, her Face would be well before the Assizes, which must not be; so she bid him look to his Promise, for she would keep her Nails for her. Yes, saith the Spirit, and she was also consenting to the Death of the Lady Cromwell. Like enough, I thought so, said she. Yes, says the Spirit, and to prove this to be true, whensoever any Stranger shall come into the House, you shall fall into a Fit, and if then Agnes Samuel shall come unto you and say, As I am a

Witch and consenting unto the Death of the Lady Cromwell, so I charge thee to depart, and let her come forth of her Fit, you shall be presently well. So Mrs. Jane repeated the same Words after the Spirit, which were then set down in Writing. If it be so, saith Mrs. Joane, then I hope she will be hanged at the Assizes as well as her Mother, and that Sir Henry Cromwell will look to the matter. At last the Spirit told her, that she should have her Fits upon the Assizes-Day, and all manner of Fits that she ever had, but after that Day she should have no more; but if she had, then Woe be to Agnes Samuel, for then I will make her pay for it.

On Friday following, as soon as Supper was ended, she fell into her Talking Fit again, and on a sudden she said, Smack, where have you been all this time? And how did it happen I talked not with you, having had so many Fits all this time? Saith Smack, I was not at Home, but now I bring you good News. What is that said she? You shall have no more Fits till this Day Seven Night, if you will rise betimes to Morrow Morning, but if you do not, you shall have your Fit in the Morning; which shall continue all the Day to your Trouble. Then, said she, if rising betimes will prevent it, God-willing, I will to Morrow Morning, which she did, and had no Fit that Day. Then she asked, Why she should have no more Fits that Week? The Spirit answered, That Agnes Samuel intreated she should have no more Fits this Week, as I loved her, but I love her not says the Spirit, yet you shall have no more Fits this Week, if you rise betimes in the Morning. And why, said she, must I have my Fits if Strangers come? The Spirit answered, To bring her to Shame. But when did you talk with her, said she? Just now, said the Spirit, in the Church Chamber. She will deny that, said Mrs. Jane, when she is asked about it. Yes, says the Spirit, so she is obliged, and you must have one whole Week of sick Fits before the Assizes. Must I, said she, for whose Soul? Agnes Samuel will have it so, says the Spirit. Let me know, says she, when that Day will be. You shall know, said the Spirit, this Day Seven Night, and what manner of Fits they shall be.

Before they parted, the Spirit asked how her Legs did. She said, Well, Thanks be to God, why do you ask? He said, Because he was glad of it. Be glad for your self, said she, and be not glad for me, for I thank not you for it, but God, who I trust will deliver me in spight of you. Upon which he went away, and she came out of her Fit, and continued well all the next Day, rising betimes in the Morning.

On Sunday following, being the 25th of February, Mr. Throckmorton, of Brampton, who was the first Stranger that came to the House, pay'd a Visit; and in half an Hour after his coming, Mrs. Jane fell into her Fit, and had not long continued so, before Smack came to her, to whom she said, How comes it I have my Fit now, and you promised I should have none before Friday next? He said, She knew well enough. She said, She did not. Then he told her, That Strangers were come, and she must have her Fit to prove Agnes Samuel a Witch. The Spirit likewise told her, That there was a sore sick Week of Sick Fits to come yet. She said, She hoped in God to deliver her.

As she sat thus in her Fit, talking with Smack, one of her Sisters sat by her, in a quiet Fit also, who suddenly said to her, Sister Jane, the Thing tells me you shall have a very sore Fit by-and-by. And immediately she fell into a very sick and troublesome Fit, swelling and heaving her Body, and groaning and crying out after the usual manner. Then Mr. Throckmorton her Father, called for Agnes Samuel, and desired her to hold the Child, for I think said he, you are fittest to have the Trouble of it. After the Child had been in her Arms a considerable time, strugling and very troublesome, her Sister, who was foretold of her sick Fit, said, Be of good Comfort, Sister Jane, for the Thing tells me the worst is past, and you shall be well by-and-by, for the Thing says, That Agnes Samuel is weary of holding you, and therefore you shall be well, which presently proved true, for her troublesome Fit ended, and she continued quiet as before. Upon this, Mr. Throckmorton her Father, told his Cousin what his Daughter Jane had said before, viz. That when any Stranger come she should fall into her Fit, and then if Agnes Samuel should say such

Words, she should come forth of it to prove her a Witch, which his Cousin desired him to try. Upon which the Child's Father bid Agnes Samuel say after him, Even as I am a Witch, and consented to the Death of the Lady Cromwell, so I charge the Spirit to depart, and let her be well. The Maid began, but either could not, or would not speak them plain, but would always say, Consenting to our Death of our Lady Cromwell, and would not with repeating the Words three or four Times over, speak them plain; so that she that was in her Fit, said, Here is something telleth me that she will not speak them right. At last, with much ado, she spoke them, and presently she came out of her Fit, and was very well. The same Words were used to another in a Fit, and likewise prevailed.

  The next Day at Dinner, Mrs. Elizabeth being into her Fit, was pointed to say Grace, and when she had half gone through it, presently her Mouth was shut up, that she could not finish it. Then Mr. Throckmorton called for Agnes Samuel, and desired her to charge the Spirit to open her Mouth again, that she might finish her Grace, which she did, and the Child went through to the end of it. Then Mr. Throckmorton endeavoured to teach Agnes Samuel a short Grace, and though the Children told her it, two or three times a Day, she could not learn it.

  On Thursday following, Mrs. Mary, who had been well ever since the Sessions Day at Huntington, was somewhat uneasie in the Morning, and about Nine-a-Clock fell into a great trembling and quaking, and could not hold a Joint of her without any known Cause. Soon after the fell into a very troublesome Fit, which held half an Hour, and at the last growing better, she said, is it true? Do you say, this is the Day that I must scratch the young Witch? I am glad of it, I will pay her home both for my self and Sisters. Mr. Edward, and Mr. Henry Pickering, and several others standing by, caused the Maid to be brought into the Chamber where the Child was, to see what would be the issue of it, knowing the Maid was able to keep her self from scratching, if three such as the Child should set upon her. As soon as the Maid came into the Chamber where the Child was, she cry'd; Art thou come, thou young Witch, who hath done all this Mischief. Agnes Samuel seemed to stand amazed at these Words, not being accustomed to hear such Expressions from the Child, so one in the Company desired her to take her in her Arms, and carry her down, for her Legs were taken from her.

Mrs. Mary let her take her up very quietly in her Arms, and clasped her Hands about her Neck; but as she began to lift her up, she fell a scratching her so eagerly and fiercely, to the Amazement of those that stood by, saying, I will scratch you, you young Witch, and pay you home for punishing me and my Sisters; the Thing tells me I should have had no more Fits, but been well, but for you. The Maid stood still holding down her Head (for the Child kneeled upon her Knees) and cried out pitifully; yet either would not, or could not once pluck away her Head. Nay, says the Child, I know you cry, but the Spirit said I should not hear you, because I shou'd not pity you; and it is he that holdeth you that you cannot get away from me.

The Child scratched till the Skin came off the Breadth of a Shilling, but no Blood, but Water. At last the Maid brought her down into the Parlour, where the Child sitting a while on her Stool, seemed to be very sorry, and said, I would not have scratched Nan Samuel so; but the Thing bid me do it, and forced me to it, stretching forth my Arms, and straining my Fingers, whether I would or not, and made me scratch her, which indeed appeared to be contrary to the Nature of the Child. The Child continued in her Fit till an Hour after Dinner, and when she was out would not believe what she had done till she saw her Face, and then cried and was sorry for it.

The next Day, being Friday, Mrs. Mary was in a very mild Fit all the Morning, and a-little before Dinner, said to her Sisters that were in their Fits, I am glad, and very glad, but would not tell why. Presently she said to the Thing that stood by her, but I know you will lye to meas you have often done. Nay, says the Thing, I use not to lye: Nor do, said she, Who are you, pray? The Thing answered, Smack. What, says she, are you that Smack that uses to come to my Sister Jane, and tells her so many things?

Yes, said he, adding that he never told her Sister Jane any Lye yet, neither was this a Lye that he told her now: Then Mrs. Mary told her Sisters, all of them being in their Fits, what Smack told her, which was that after Dinner she should come out of her Fit, and never have any more, because she had scratched Agnes Samuel, which happened accordingly.

  The same Day, being the Second of February, Mrs. Jane fell into her Fit, being in Bed, and it seemed Smack had been with her, and told her something, which he afterward declared to her Sisters being in their Fits; and going down into the Parlour to them, when she had sate a while by the Fire, she spoke to something by her; I will not look on you, for you never come but you bring ill News; for I was sick the last time you were here, and I wonder who sent for you? The thing answered, You were sick the last time I was here, but now you shall be much worse. Do your worst, said she, for God will preserve me. I fear you not. I wonder, said she, how your Leg doth? I think Smack spoke with you when he broke your Leg. Said he, I pray you don't tell Smack that was here. Do you pray me, said she, I do not know that Smack, but if I did, I would tell him that he might break your Neck too. The thing answered, Yes, you know him well enough, for you made him break my Leg; but I would not for any thing that he should know that I was here, said the Thing; but I will make you pay for all this Week that comes in. Will you, said she, I will lay with you what you will, that I shall not be sick this Week if I will, for one thing I know. Said he, I know very well that Smack was with you this Morning; but do both of you what you can, you shall have a sick Week of it, and that you shall find; for you shall be so sick next Week, that your Body shall be sore all the Week after, for I will course you as well as Smack hath coursed me. Why said she, do you revenge your self upon me and not upon Smack. He said he durst not deal with him, for he was too hard for him.

  After a little Silence, she asked her Sisters if they did not see Catch, who talked with her just now, they said No. Then perhaps he is gone said she, for I cannot see him. Then she began to talk softly with them, as if no Body should hear, saying, this Morning Smack was with her, and told her, she would have a very bad Week the next Week, which he could not help; but he had so beat Pluck, that he will never come at me again; and if he doth, he says, he will kill him; but he said, if you will go to some Friend's House, and stay all the Week, then you shall be well; but I told him I had no Friend's House to go to, nor to none I would go, do what he would: Then he desired me to go to Sommerson, a Town two Miles from Warboyse, where she had been very well with an Uncle of hers; but said she, I wonder how he knows Sommerson, I think he knows all the Country round; but I told him I would not once stir my Foot for him, do what he could. Then they asked when Smack would come again; she said, he told her he would come again after Supper. In the mean time some Strangers came in who were desirous to see her out of her Fit, which was upon the Account of Agnes Samuel, as she was charged with being a Witch, and consented to the Death of the Lady Cromwell.

At Night a little before Supper she fell into her Fit again, and so continued till Supper was ended. When the Company was risen from the Table, and set by the Fire, Smack came to her again, and told her that she could not avoid those Fits next Week, except she would go from home. She told him she would not, and bid him do his worst. Then said he, when was Catch, with you? Said she to Day, and threatned to punish her strangely next Week with sick Fits, he said, because I had caused you to break his Leg; but I hope you will break his Neck, and some Body will break yours, for you are all naught. Smack said he would course Catch for it, and would warrant he would never come again to her, when he had done with him. Then, said she, tell me when my Fits begin, and when they shall end? He said, that on Monday Morning they wou'd begin and end that Day seven Night in the Morning. You will have a Week I suppose then said she? Yes, says he, and you will be sore of your your Body next Week after. On Saturday, which was the next Day, she had several Fits, and was brought out of them by Agnes Samuel's Charge, and so on the Sunday.

On Monday, when her troublesome Fits were to begin, in the Morning the grew very sick and uneasie, and had her Senses all the Week; Mrs. Elizabeth too was troubled this Week with very sudden and extraordinary Fits, her Body being more severely twisted than of several Months before, which made us conclude something more than ordinary was a working it being impossible she should bear such violent Passions long.

On Saturday the Tenth of March, as she sat at Supper it seemed, by the Motion of her Hands and Head, and her Humming, as if she had a Mind to speak to something on the Table, but her Mouth was shut up; then she lamented sadly, but could not express her Grief. Soon after she fell into so troublesome a Fit, that she could not sit on her Stool; then Agnes Samuel was desired to hold her, which she did, and in a little time she began to grow more quiet. And her Sister Grace was more troubled than she was, so the set down the one, and took up the other; and as she was holding Mrs. Grace in her Arms, Mrs. Elizabeth, who sat hard by her, said on a sudden, with a great deal of Anger, now I can see the young Witch in my Fit, which I never could do before in a Fit. The Company wondered to hear the young Child call the Maid a Witch, who never before gave her or her Mother, or any Body else, an ill Word, either in or out of her Fit, and therefore concluded something extraordinary was a working; then she said, my Sister Jane's Devil told me as I sat at Supper, that I must scratch the young Witch. As soon as the had said so, she slipped from the Bench and fell upon her Knees, for she was not able to stand, and caught the Maid by the Hand that stood next to her, and which was holding her Sister, and scratched one of her Hands violently, and said it was she that had bewitch'd her and her Sisters, or they had been well long before; O thou young Witch! O thou young Witch! Fie upon thee, fie upon thee; who ever heard of a young Witch before.

When she had breathed a while, she fell upon her again, and said this was her Sister Jane's Devil that used not to lye that bid her scratch her; for said she, I would not have scratched you, and it is against my Will; but the Devil makes me scratch you, and holdeth forth my Arms, and bends my Fingers, otherwise I would not do it, as I am now my self. All this while the Maid held the other Child still in her Arm, never offering to pull her Hand away from her, but cryed out sadly, desiring the Lord to pitty her. Then one that sat by desired her to speak, whether she thought the Child scratched her of her own accord or not; she answered, she thought not; nay, says she, I know she did not, and that it is not her own Mind to scratch me thus. When the Child was weary of scratching the second Time, she put out her Hands, and said, Look you here, the Devil says I must scratch her no more now, for my Fingers are bent out so straight that I cannot bend them, which appeared when she held out her Hand. Then she rubbed her Hand upon the Maid's Hand that bled little, and wiped the Blood upon her own Hands, which she did often whilst the talked with her.

Presently, when the Scratching was ended, the Child began to weep, and crying, said to the Maid, I would not have scratched you, but the Devil made me whether I would or not: Oh that you never had deserved to be thus used, complaining as if she had done some great Offence.

When this weeping Fit was over, the began to exhort her, raising her voice with so much desire for her Amendment, that the like was never heard out of a Childs Mouth. Oh, said the Child, that thou hadst Grace to repent thee of thy Wickedness, that thy Soul might be saved, for thou haft forsaken thy god, and given thy self to the Devil. Oh. Oh! that thou hadst known what a precious thing thy Soul was, thou never wouldst have given it to the Devil. Thou hadst need to pray Night and Day for Gods Favour again, otherwise thy Soul shall be damned in Hell for ever. Thou dost often pray here at home when we pray, and likewise at Church, but thou prayest in vain, because thou prayest not with thy Heart; but I will pray for thee with all my Heart, and I will forgive thee, and desire all my Sisters, and all my Friends to forgive thee, if thou wilt confess thy Fault; but thou hast a hard

Heart, and the Devil holdeth thy Heart, and will not suffer thee to confess it; but thou must confess it, whether thou wilt or no, when thy Time is come: But Oh! that thou wouldst now confess it, that thy Soul might be saved.

When she used these Words, she would repeat them at least three times over, with so much Earnestness, and never leave expressing them as long as her Breath would serve. Then she would tell her, my Sister Joan's Devil standeth here before my Face, and points with her Finger to the Place, and telleth me that thou shalt one Day confess it, or else thou shalt be hanged; for before thou dost confess it, or be hang'd, we shall not be well; but if thou wilt now confess it, we shall be presently well; therefore defie the Devil and confess it, that God may forgive thee and thy Soul may be saved.

If thou wouldst think of the Torments of Hell, and that thou must burn in Hell Fire, except thou dost confess and repent, thou wouldst not stand so strictly in the Denial of it as thou dost; but thou art a wicked Child, and hath been a Witch this four or five Years and more; thou hast done more Mischief than to me and my Sisters; thou hast killed my Lady Cromwell and more, the Devil that standeth here telleth me so; and thou wouldst have killed my Sister Joan in this sick Week, but God will not let thee: What a wicked Heart hast thou, that nothing will content thee but our Death?

Thou and thy Father were the Cause, said the, why thy Mother did deny what she confessed; she was in a good way, and if your Mother's Soul be damn'd, you and your Father must answer for it. Your Mother had confessed and was sorry for her Naughtiness, and every Body would have forgiven her, and prayed for her. Oh! that she had never gone home, that her Soul might have been saved: Thy Mother is a Witch, they Father is a Witch, and thou art a Witch, and the worst of all, thy Mother would never have done so much Hurt as she hath, done but for thee, and so the Devil hath told me.

Oh! that thy Father were now here, for the Devil says that I should scratch him too, he is a Witch and a naughty Man. Oh!

that he were here that I might speak to him. Then Mr. John Pickering and Mr. Henry Pickering were desired to see if they could perswade the old Man to come to the House, which they doubted he being a churlish man; however they went, and were not twenty paces from the house before they saw him comeing as fast as he could to wards it, and watching him in, followed him.

When they were come into the Hall, near the Parlour door, where the Child was, the Child cried out, he is come, he is come, I will go and scratch him; and pressed forwards on her knees towards the Parlour door, though she was in such a part of the Parlour that she could not see into the Hall, and therefore could not see the Man. Then Mr. Dorrington, who was present, stopped her, and caused him to be called into the Parlour; when he came in she still pressed to wards him and said, I must scratch him, I must scratch him, but presently stopped, and said, I must not scratch him, shewing her fingers close shut up together. If he had come here just now, said she, the Devil said I must have scratched him, but now I must not.

Then Mr. Throckmorton, asked him why he came to the House, he answered, that he heard his Daughter was sick. Mr. Throckmorton and Mr. Dorrington then asked him who told him, but he said, he would not tell them; but at last he said, that his Brothers Daughter came to the House and told him, that she saw Mr. Dorrington and Mr. Throckmortons Man come to this House together, and then thinking there was something to do about his Daughter, he came to see what was the matter; but this they thought could not bring him, since before he would not come without a Precept from the Justices.

The Child still continued to cry out upon him, and said, that he was a naughty Man and a Witch, and but for him and his Daughter his Wifes Soul might have been saved; and repeated a great deal to him, of the Exhortations she gave his Daughter, advising him to prayer, and to ask forgiveness. But he was so rude and loud, that the Child could not be heard, and told her and the rest of the Company, that they lyed in calling him a Witch; and said the Child was above seven years old, though indeed not twice seven; but he would not be silent, nor hear her till obliged to it by her Father, though the Child could not hear him or answer to any of his Speeches, nor did she stop speaking for his talking, in any thing she designed to say to him; but though she could not hear him, yet she saw him and his Daughter, and none else in the Company.

When the Child had thus exhorted the Father and the Daughter for an hour and a half, Mr. Throckmorton told John Samuel that his Daughter Agnes, by a Charge which he had, commanded the Spirits to depart from his Children, and they had departed; he therefore desired him to use the same Words which his Daughter before had used, to see what would come of it; he said he would not, neither should any make him speak them, nor would he be brought to it for any thing. Then Mr. Throckmorton told him, that since he came to his House unsent for, he should not go away till he had said them, as long as the Child continued on her Fit, if it were a Week first. The Mr. Dorrington to encourage him spoke the Words before him, as did also two or three of his Neighbours, but he would not be perswaded, till he saw Mr. Throckmorton was resolute, not to let him depart till he had spoken them; the Words were, As I am a Witch, and consenting to the Death of the Lady Cromwell, so I charge the Spirit to depart from Mrs. Elizabeth Throckmorton at this present, and to suffer her to be well. The Man had no sooner spoken the Words but the Child arose, and was very well, wondring to see so much Company there. Then the Child was asked if she knew of any thing that was done or said, and several Particulars were named to her, but she knew of no such thing, saying she had been asleep, and was ready to weep, because they had charged her with such things. The Company then departing she went to Bed very well.

In the next place, we shall relate how Mrs. Joan Throckmorton was handled in the sick Week that was threatned by the Spirit. On Sunday Night she went to Bed very well and merry, but in the Morning when she waked, she complained of every part of her Body, saying, That she was very full of Pain, especially in her Head and Stomach, and that there was something under her Sides that twitched her, that she could not fetch her Breath. All that Day, as well as the Week following, she was strangely tormented, crying out of Pain in every part of her; her Stomach was taken from her, so that all the Week she eat scarce enough to sustain Nature; her Legs were very sore and full of Pain, having little or no use of them all the Week; her Hands were continually cold and benumbed; but her greatest and continual Pain lay in Head, which mightily disturbed her Rest, she doing nothing but cry and groan all Night, most part of the Week.

  Besides this continual Pain, she had several Fits every Day, as well as in the Night, so violent, that one would scarce have thought it possible for her to escape with her Life; for she would lie upon her Bed scrieking and starting for an Hour together, and sometimes four or five, without any Intermission; sometimes she would lie as in a Swoon or a Trance, holding her Breath a quarter of an Hour or longer; so that one could not perceive that she breathed at all, yet at last she would rise up with her Belly, and fetch a deep Sigh, and so loud and doleful a Groan, as if she had been dying, which sort of Fit was customary Night and Day, and held her the longest of any other, and always the longer when any of her Friends stood by and endeavoured to comfort her; sometimes it would rise up into her Head, and there resting a while, it would raise up her Body and her Head very strongly, till she almost stood upright; and with so much Strength, that no Body could hold her down. In which Fit she desired to have her Head holden, otherwise she said it would tear it in Pieces; and always a little before she felt the Fit coming, she would cry hold; and all the while she was rising with her Body, it would hold her Breath, until she came to the highest, and then she would fetch a great Groan, and falling down suddenly, would settle her self in the Chair again; and though she was all the Week in this continual Danger, and was at the Point of Death every Hour, yet on Saturday all Day, especially in the Night, she was in the greatest Hazard, no Body expecting her Life, the Fits were so extremely violent and dangerous; yet before Morning it pleased God to give her some Ease, though as the Devil had told them before, Nan Samuel would have had him to have killed her this Bout, as she did the Lady Cromwell. And one thing observable was, that all the Week long she had her perfect Senses, as the Spirits foretold; but though the could always hear, yet her Breath was so stopped, that very often she was not able to speak. And another thing was, that she could never abide the Company of Nan Samuel all that time, being always more grievously tormented while she stayed.

When the Week was ended, and Monday Morning came again, she said, she felt her self reasonably well, and all that Day had no Fit at all, but complained that she was sore in her Body and in her Legs, as if she had been beaten. All the next Week she continued pretty well, yet not without many Fits, and great Soreness in her Legs, especially towards Night, as it was common to them all to be worse against Night.

On Monday after that, which was the 19th of March, Smack came to her again, and she presently said, I trust one Day God will revenge me on you, and all your Company, for punishing me thus, and all my Sisters. Why, said he, had you a sick Week of it? It is no matter to you, said she. Why, I told you, said he, I could not help it, except you would have gone abroad to some Friend's House. Go you, said she, whither you will, and do what you can, I will not stir my Feet out of Doors for your Pleasure; I know you would kill me if you could, and you use all the Means you can to kill me and my Sisters, but I trust God will not give you leave; and if he does, I shall be content rather than live in this continual Pain. You have often told me, I should scratch the young Witch before the Assizes, now tell me when shall it be; for I would fain scratch her, I cannot abide her of late, whatever is the matter. God, I think, hath set my Heart against her, for I cannot eat my Meat if I see her, it goes so much against my Stomach. But tell me, said she, what Day I shall scratch her; He told her, it should be two or three Days before the Assizes. Tell me, said she, on which Day it shall be? On Monday, said he, which is this Day Fortnight. Well, look that it be, for I will keep my Nails unpared for her. I will scratch one Side for my self, said she, and the other for my Aunt Pickering, who was one of the Twelve that were bewitched, Wife to John Pickering, of Ellington in Huntington. Well, said Mrs. Joan to Smack, I will lay it on whenever I scratch, that all the World may see that she is a Witch. Saith Smack, They that think otherwise of her, are deceived, and I will prove it. How will you prove it, said she? By compelling you to scratch her. Will you compell me? Then I will not scratch her. But you shall scratch her, said he, so they had many Words about it. At last, she said she had a good mind to scratch her, but would not if she could otherwise choose. Smack said that she must scratch her as well as the rest had done, and that there were two more besides her to do it. When they had ended their Talk, she called for Agnes Samuel, and said she should not come out of her Fit till she had charged the Spirit to depart, which the Maid did, and she was presently well.

Within two Days after, Mrs. Grace, as she sat in the Maids Arms, in a very troublesome Fit, suddenly fell a scratching the Maid's Hand, very fiercely, but was not able to speak, her Mouth being shut up, yet she groaned and wept, as if she had been doing something against her Will; but her Nails were so short, and her Strength so small, being youngest of all, that she could not raise the Skin upon the back of her Hands. Several Things were remarkable in this Child, as her Mouth being generally shut up during the Fit, yet she had a great many, and was scarce ever clear of them, and hath set whole Days in her Chair, or on her Stool, groaning and lamenting.

The 25th of March at Night, when Supper was ended, Mrs. Joan fell into her Fit, having had many that Week; but Smack never came to talk to her till now. And it seemed that he talked to her a good while before she would listen to him, or give him an answer, yet by her Countenance and Gesture it might be perceived, that something talked to her; for she would turn away her Face, and shake her Head, as if she liked not of it. On a sudden she said, Go to, if what you say be true, let us see what you will do. So Mrs. Joan called for her Sister Elizabeth, who was in her Fit too, and told her that Smack was come, and will tell her a great deal before Nan Samuel's Face: Smack, saith she, calleth her nothing but young Witch to begin with, very likely he is angry with her. Therefore she called for Nan Samuel, and told her, that she must be present and hear what Smack would say to her, yet, saith she, I cannot hear you, but I can see you. By-and-by she said, That Smack saith you must say these Words, and I shall presently come out of my Fit, but I shall fall into it again and shall have many Fits to Night, and come forth of them again, at your Words; the Words which the Maid must first speak, are these; As I am a Witch, and would have bewitched Mrs. Joan Throckmorton to Death in her last Week of great Sickness, so I charge the Spirit to depart, and, to suffer her to be well at this present. And as soon as they were expressed, Mrs. Joan came out of her Fit, and was well, and being ready to arise, she suddenly fell down into her Fit again; so resting the while, she said to her, The thing says that you must say, As I am a Witch, and have bewitched Mrs. Pickering of Ellington, since my Mother hath confessed, so to charge the Spirit to depart from me, and I shall be well, for the Thing says, That my Aunt Pickering would have been well before this time, had not you bewitched her again since your Mother confessed. Alas! says she, poor Aunt Pickering, how have you deserved this Usage? And then she began to weep for her, which moved Tears in those that stood by; after she had done weeping she wished the Maid to use that Charge, upon the use of which she was well, but was soon in the Fit again. Then, saith Mrs. Joan to the Maid, The Spirit saith that you must say, As I would have bewitched Mrs. Joan Throckmorton lame, since I could not bewitch her to Death, as I would have done in her last Week of her great Sickness, so charge the Spirit to depart from me, and I shall be well, and presently fall into my Fit again, all which was presently done, and found true.

Then said Mrs. Joan, the Spirit says you have bewitched all my Sisters overagain, since your Mother confessed, or else they had been now well; and to prove this to be true, you must charge the Spirit to depart from me, as you have bewitched them all severally, and I must have so many several Fits, and run out of them at your several Charges. So the Maid began with them one after another, saying, As I have bewitched Mrs. Mary Throckmorton since my Mother confessed, so I charge the Spirit to depart from you, and after went to the rest of the Sisters; so Mrs. Joan had four several Fits, and came out of them at four several Charges, which the Maid used to her. Then said Mrs. Joan, the Spirits say, That now I also must start and struggle, and be pained in my Body as well as my Sister Jane is, whensover you shall name God, or Jesus Christ, or any good Work, though I cannot hear you, yet he doth hear you, and he will make me start. Then Mr. Throckmorton, with others that were in Company, perceiving the Spirit to be willing to declare so many things of the Maid, desired her in the Name of God to answer her to certain Questions, which she should ask, and not to lye. The Maid gave their Charge to the Spirit, and the Spirit told Mrs. Joan, the young Witch chargeth me to tell the Truth in certain Questions that she shall ask me; I said, Mrs. Joan, and see that you do tell the Truth, and not lye in any one thing: The Spirit answered, That he does not use to tell so many Lyes as the young Witch does; which Words Mrs. Joan repeated over after the Spirit. Then said Mr. Throckmorton to the Maid, Charge the Spirit to tell you, in what part of your Body Mrs. Joan shall scratch you; which the Maid did, and the Spirit said to Mrs. Joan, The young Witch would know in what part of her Body you shall scratch her. Yes, says Mrs. Joan, in what part of her Body shall I scratch her? The Spirit answered, You shall scratch her on the Face, the right Cheek for your self, and the left for your Aunt Pickering of Ellington. Then said Mrs. Jane, I'll surely scratch the left Cheek well for my Aunt, if that will do her any good, whatever I do for my self. Yes, said the Spirit, do so; and the young Witch had as good take it patiently at first, for you shall have your Pennyworth of her before you have done. Then the young Maid was desired to ask the Spirit whether her Mother would confess at the Assizes, all that she had already confessed. The Spirit answered, Yes, if she have no evil Counsel, and confess that this young Witch her Daughter is a worse Witch than her self; for, saith the Spirit, when the old Witch had bewitched the Lady Cromwell, and would have unbewitched her again, and could not, she put it to her Husband, and bid him help her; and when he could not, she put it to this young Witch her Daughter; and when she could not help her neither, then she counselled her Mother to kill her.

And to prove, saith the Spirit, that all this is true, Mrs. Joan, whenever any Strangers come to this House, before the Assizes, you shall fall into your Fits, and you shall have three several Fits, and shall come out of them at three several Charges by the young Witch. The first Charge that she must use is, As she is a Witch, and a worse Witch than her Mother, in consenting to the Death of the Lady Cromwell, so I charge the Spirit to depart, and you shall be well. The second is, That as she hath bewitched Mrs. Pickering of Ellington since her Mother confessed. And the Third is, As she would have bewitched Mrs. Joane Throckmorton to Death, in her last Week of great Sickness, after which you shall be well; so the Maid used these three several Charges to Mrs. Joane at that Time, and she came out of three several Fits, and presently fell into her Fits again.

Then the Maid was desired to ask the Spirit, whether Mrs. Jane should have these Fits before my Lord Judge, if she were carried to the Assizes; she asked the Question, and the Spirit said she should have all the Fits that ever she had. Then she was desired to ask whether Mrs. Jane should have any more Fits after the Assizes; to which the Spirit answered, That neither they nor none of the Kindred would be able to hurt them after that time. Then the Spirit was asked the like Question in relation to her Sisters, but he said their Spirits must answer those Questions. Then it was asked, how many Spirits her Mother had, to which it was answered Nine at the first, naming them all severally. He said further, that she had them of an old Man who was now dead, but his Name he would not tell. Three of these Spirits were named Smacks; the Fourth, Pluck; the Fifth, Blem; the Sixth, Catch; the Seventh, White; the Eighth, Callicot; and the Ninth, Hardmane.

Mrs. Jane Throckmorton had the first of the Smacks; Mrs. Mary had his Cousin Smack; Mrs. Elizabeth had the other Smack; Mrs. Jane had Blew; Mrs. Grace had White; and the old Woman had Hardmane, still with her in the Jayl and what was become of the rest he could not tell. Then the Maid asked, Whether the old Woman did reward them with any thing, or no: The Spirit answered, That she did, with Blood from her Chin. Then Mrs. Jane asked the Spirit, Whether John Samuel was a Witch, or no; the Spirit answered that he was, and would be a worse than either of them, when they two were hang'd; for then all the Spirits would come to him: For, saith the Spirit, he hath already bewitched a Man and Woman; and to prove this, if the young Witch shall charge the Devil to depart from you at this present, even as her Father hath bewitched two Parties, you shall be presently well; so Nan Samuel did, and Mrs. Jane was well, and fell into her Fit again. Then Mrs. Jane asked the Spirit, Who those two were whom the Man had bewitched; the Spirit answered, He would not tell, except the young. Witch went out of the Parlour, for she must not hear: So Mrs. Jane desired Nan Samuel to go out, and the Spirit said let her be watched, that she do not hear when she is gone. Then the Spirit told Mrs. Jane that it was Chappel and his Wife, which were the old Man's next Neighbours, and were at some Varience and Contention with him, and suspected the Matter very much. A little before that time, being not able to stir herself, the Woman and the Man, for a Fit or two, was just in the same Condition that these Children were in. Yet, said the Thing, if Chappel will beat the old Witch well, perhaps he may never be more troubled with him. The old Witch, said the Spirit, would once have broken his Neck, by giving him a Fall on the Causway in the Street, as he met him, causing both his Pattens to be broken suddenly; and if he had fallen on the Stones, as he fell in the Dirt, he had been maimed. This Fall was not known to any in the House at that time; and Mrs. Jane being asked about it, when she came out of her Fit, said, that she never heard of any such thing: But when it enquired after of Chappel himself, he confess'd that he had once such a

Fall, as he met with old Samuel in the Streets, both his Pattens being broke at an Instant; and because he would not fall upon the Stones, he cast himself on one Side into the Myre, where he was sadly dirtied; and if another had not been with him, he had been in more danger.

This was told by the Spirit to Mrs. Jane, and Mrs. Jane repeating the Spirits Words, declared it to them that stood by.

Then the Maid was called into the Parlour again, and desired to ask the Spirit, whether Mrs. Jane should be well in the Way she went to the Assizes, or not; and whether she should be better at the Assizes, or at Home: The Spirit answered, Better there; but it should be worse for the young Witch if Mrs. Jane went, and she should be well all the Way she went, till she took her Chamber, and then she should fall into her Fit, The Spirit told her further, that she should have three several Fits on the Assize Day, and the young Witch must bring her out of them, by three several Charges; the First must be as she is a worse Witch than her Mother in bewitching the Lady Cromwell to Death; the Second as she bewitched Mrs. Pickering of Ellington since her Mother confessed; and the Third, as she would have bewitched Mrs. Jane Throckmorton to Death in her last Week of great Sickness; and the Spirit said all this is true, and shall be proved true hereafter. And in Token thereof, Mrs. Jane, you shall be very well all Day to Morrow, and have never a Fit, let the young Witch do what she can, except some Stranger come, and then you must have three several Fits to prove her a Witch, and so you shall have them when ever any Strangers come. But this you must remember in any Case, to pair your Nails when you have scratched the young Witch. Why, must I do so, said she? Because the young Witches Blood will stick upon your Nails, and you must burn her Blood lest you be worse afterwards. Said Mrs. Jane, do you put me in Mind of it, if I forget it; so I will, said he, and then the Spirit departed: And Mrs. Jane said, she must not come out of her Fit, except Nat Samuel helped her out by one of her Charges, which she did, and then she went to Bed very contentedly and well, and the next Day continued without any Fits at all, no Stranger coming to the House.

On Tuesday following Dr. Dorrington with one of his Brothers, and Mr. John Dorrington coming into the House, Mrs. Joan fell into her Fit: Then the called for the Maid, Nan Samuel, and one of the Company desired her to say the Lord's Prayer and the Belief, which she did; and whenever she named God or Jesus Christ, or the Holy Ghost, Mrs. Jane started and struggled very much, so that she could scarce sit upon her Stool; and at last the Maid brought her out of her Fit three several times, by her three several Charges, as the Spirit said.

The next Strangers that came to the House were Mr. Henry Cromwell, one of Sir Henry Cromwell's Sons, and one of Sir Henry's Men with him, which was upon Thursday the Twenty-ninth of March. When they came into the House Mrs. Joan was well, but in a quarter of an Hour's time she fell into her Fit; and she, as well as her Sister Jane, were very severely handled whenever the Maid named God or Jesus Christ; but at last she was brought out of her Fit three several times, by the three several Charges above-mentioned. Many Strangers came to the House that Week, and she had these several Fits.

On Monday following, which was the Day appoint for Scratching, Mrs. Joan fell into her Fit a little before Supper, and continued so all Supper-time, being not able to stand on her Legs. As soon as they began to give Thanks after Supper, she started up upon her Feet and came to the Table side, and stood with her Sisters that were saying of Grace; and as soon as Grace was ended, she fell upon the Maid, Nan Samuel, and took her Head under her Arms, and first scratched the right Side of her Cheeks; and when she had done that, now, said she, I must scratch the left Side for my Aunt Pickering, and scratched that also till Blood came on both Sides very plentifully. The Maid stood still, and never moved to go from her, yet cried pitifully, desiring the Lord to have Mercy on her. When she had done Scratching, Mrs. Joan sat her self upon a Stool, and seemed to be out of Breath, taking her Breath very short, yet the Maid never struggled with her, and was able to hold never a Joynt of her, but trembled like a Leaf, and called for a pair of Scissars to pair her Nails; but when she had them, she was not able to hold them in her Hands, but desired some Body to do it for her, which Dr. Dorrington's Wife did.

Mrs. Joan saved her Nails as they were paired, and when they had done threw them in the Fire, and called for some Water to wash her Hands, and then threw the Water into the Fire: Then she fell upon her Knees, and desired the Maid to kneel by her, and prayed with her, saying the Lord's Prayer and the Creed; but Mrs. Joan seemed as if she did not hear the Maid, for the wou'd say amiss sometimes, and then the Company would help her out; but Mrs. Joan did not stay for her, so that she had ended before the Maid had half done hers.

After this Dr. Dorrington took a Prayer-Book, and read what Prayers he thought fit; and when he had done Mrs. Joan began to exhort the Maid, and as she was speaking she fell a Weeping extreamly, so that she could not well express her Words, saying, that the could not have scratched her, but the was forced to it by the Spirit.

As she was thus complaining, her Sister Elizabeth was suddenly seized with a Fit, and coming hastily upon the Maid, catched her by one of her Hands, and fain would have scratched her, saying, the Spirit said the must scratch her too; but the Company desired the Maid to keep her Hand from her, so they strove a great while till the Child was out of Breath: Then, said the Child, will no Body help me? twice or thrice over. Then said Mrs. Joan, being still in her Fit, shall I help you, Sister Elizabeth? Ay, for God's sake Sister, said the: So Mrs. Joan came and took one of the Maid's Hands and held it to her Sister Elizabeth, and she scratched it till Blood come, at which she was very joyful. Then she paired her Nails, and washed her Hands, and threw the Pairing and the Water both in the Fire. After all this, before the Company departed, the Maid helped Mrs. Joane out of her Fit three several Times one after the other, by three several Charges; and likewise brought Mrs. Elizabeth out of her Fit by saying, as she hath bewitched Mr. Elizabeth Throckmorton since her Mother confessed.

But to pass to Mrs. Jane, who was first afflicted, and who first discovered the Author of their Afflictions, crying out that it was Mother Samuel that bewitched them, for which reason she had been the most severely handled; and not only tormented, but tempted to dangerous and mortal Attempts, as to cast her self into the Fire, and into the Water, and to cut her Throat. Upon which Occasions she was aware of the Temptations, and desired the Lord to strengthen her; and what was a wonderful Effect of Providence; these Temptations never offered themselves when she was alone, but had Company to prevent the ill Consequences.

On Friday the 15th of March 1592, Mrs. Jane was very much troubled with her Fit, sitting at the Table at Dinner; and it seemed as if something sat upon the Table and talked to her about Nan Samuel, for she would listen a while to it, and then look back with a heavy Countenance towards the Maid, shaking her Head as if some Sorrow was at Hand. Now Mrs. Jane had been often told by her other Sisters in their Fits, that the Spirit had told them, that she should also scratch Nan Samuel before the next Assizes, let what would happen; but she would often tell the Spirit that she would not do it. At Night, as she sat at Supper with the rest of her Sisters, she fell into a very severe Fit, bowing and bending of her Body, as if she would have broken her Back, shaking of her Hands so that she could not hold her Knife; and many times it would thrust it against her Arm. When this Fit was ended the Spirit seemed to talk to her again, as at Dinner; for she used the same Jestures to Agnes Samuel as before, and rather gave greater Tokens of Sorrow. On a sudden she rose from the Table, and went to the upper End of it, casting a heavy discontented Look at the Maid, so that she must have something in her Mind she could not utter. The Maid then asked her how she did; and presently she opened her Mouth and answered, the worse for you, you young Witch, turning away her Face from her, as if she loathed to look at her. It was a little strange to the Maid to have such Language from her, and therefore she continued asking of her Questions, but she turned her Face from her, and stopped that Ear which was next to her saying, she could not abide to hear her nor see her. The Maid then asked, what was the Matter; she answered, That the Spirit said she must scratch her; When must you scratch me, said the Maid? But immediately the Child's Mouth was shut up that she could make no Answer. Then the Child began to weep, yet with so much Anger towards the Maid, that when she looked upon her, she would suddenly turn away her Face, and gnash her Teeth with a Voice that expressed the most inveterate Dislike: Continuing so a quarter of an Hour, the Maid asked again, When she should scratch her; she could not speak, but answered by Signs, holding her Finger up at I, and down at No, by which they understand that she would scratch her after Supper, as soon as Grace was said. Then the Maid asked in what Place she should scratch her; she answered, by Sign upon her right Hand, which the Opposite to which her Sister Elizabeth had scratched a Week before.

  Then Mr. Throckmorton caused Dr. Dorrington, and some other Neighbours in the Town to be sent for, and told them what the Child had said of the Maid; it was half an Hour before they came; all which time the Child continued pensive and heavy, weeping extreamly, and often starting from the Place where she sat towards the Maid; then one of the Children gave Thanks; and as soon as it was ended, Mrs. Jane sunk down upon her Knees, and fell upon the Maid with such Fierceness and Rage, as if she would have pulled the Flesh of her Bones, yet was scarce able to raise the Skin, saying to the Maid, that the Spirit that stood there by her, told her that Pluck held her Heart and her Hand, and would not suffer the Blood to come. When the Child was weary of Scratching, she breathed a little, and told her, that she must have the other Fit at her. Then Dr. Dorrington moved the People to pray with him, all which time she kneeled very quietly; but as soon as Prayers were ended, she began to scratch again, and with Tears running down her Cheeks, said, I would not scratch you, but the Spirit forces me saying, I must scratch you as well as my Sister Joane before the Assizes, it being then about three Weeks to them.

The Maid, when she began to scratch, seemed to go from her, but the Child still followed still upon her Knees, saying, she might as good take it now as at another time, for she must fetch Blood of her, and must have her Penny-worths, saying she knew she cried, though she did not hear her, lest she should take pitty on her. When the Child was weary, and left scratching, Dr. Dorrington began to instruct the Maid, and to tell her, that surely God would not suffer her to be cried out upon by these Spirits, and to be afflicted by these innocent Children against their Wills, if she were not concerned in, or consenting to those wicked Practices her Mother had confessed: The Maid denied all, and wished God might send some sudden Token upon her, that they all might know whether she was guilty of these Matters, and presently her Nose began to bleed very much: But she said she had bled that Day before, wishing that Bleeding so often might foretel no Evil to her.

At last the Child said of her self, The Thing that now stands by her, tells her, that she must not come out of her Fit till John Samuel came and pronounc'd some Words to her, which she must tell him. Then they asked her what these Words must be, but the Child could not hear any Body; but by and by she said of her self, What is her Father come to his reckoning now? And shall I never come out of my Fit till he speaks these Words? Even as he is a Witch, and consented to the Death of Lady Cromwell, so to charge the Spirit to depart from me, and then shall I be well, and not before. I did not think, said she, that he had been as bad as the rest. Then Mr. Throckmorton sent frequently to desire him to come, but he would not, and so the Child continued in its Fit even till the Assizes.

The Sunday after, being the Eighteenth of March, the Spirit came to her again; and then she said, the Spirit tells me now I should both hear and see the young Witch, if she were here; and also see the Thing I never did see, all of them together : Then was the Maid sent for, and asked her what the Thing said to her; says she, the Thing tells me now, that I must start as well as Sister Joane doth, when she named God; and that I must not come out of my Fit this Week nor next, and perhaps never except one of these three Things comes to pass, which are, either your Father must come and speak these Words to me. Even as he is a Witch and hath consented to the Death of the Lady Cromwell, or you must confess that you are a Witch, and have bewitched me and my Sisters, or must be hanged. Then the Maid was desired to ask her, whether she should come out of her Fit, if her Father spoke these Words to her; which she asked the Spirit, and he said she should; and then he went away, leaving her in her Fit, which was after this manner; sometimes she would fit in the House all the Day together, as if she was melancholly, neither speaking to any Body, nor desirous of Company; sometimes she was very lightsome and merry, and would play with her Sisters a great part of the Day, yet could neither hear nor see anyBody, nor speaking to them : When any Body passed by, she would say, yonder goes such a colour'd Gown, I wonder it goes alone. Yonder is a pair of Stocks, or a Hat, or a pair of Shoes, or a Cloak of such a Colour ; but I can see nothing else : And if one shewed her a Ring upon their Finger, she could see the Ring and nothing else; and would say, she wondered how it hung in the Air. And often fitting at Dinner or Supper, she would suddenly have he Mouth shut ; and if Agnes Samuel had then held a Knife to her Mouth, and put it betwixt her Lips, her Mouth would be presently opened, and not before, and thus the Spirit served her five or six times in Dinner-time; and in this Fit she continued three Weeks within a Day, till the Assizes.

    But to come to the Assizes, which were on Wednesday the 4th of April, Mrs. Joan went to Huntington, and continued well till within half an Hour after she had been in her Chamber in the Inn; and then she fell into her Fit, and several coming to see her, finding her sit so quietly, would scarce believe any thing was the matter with her. Then some of them turning to Agnes Samuel, and asking her Questions concerning her Faith and Service of God, she answered, That she served God as other

People did. When she named God, Mrs. Joan began to start and struggle with her Arms, which the Company percieving, brought her nearer, and desired her to say the Lord's Prayer, and her Belief; which the Maid begun to do, but before she had gone half through, the Company desired her to leave off, Mrs. Joan being so grievously tormented in her Body, so that they were all amazed, and saw plainly, that Mrs. Joan was far from being in a good Condition of Body. So the Company continued their Discourse to the Maid, but whenever God or Jesus Christ was named, Mrs. Joan startled and struggled with her self, shivering and shaking with her Arms and Shoulders after such a manner, that it was impossible any Body should do so of themselves; and when no Body took Notice of the Maid's naming God, Mrs. Joan's struggling would put them in Mind of it; and if the Maid doubled the Name of God; as saying the God of Heaven and Earth. or Jesus Christ the Son of God, it would not suffer her to sit on her Stool. If she desired the God of Heaven and Earth to help her ; or Jesus Christ the Son of God to be merciful to her, it would so torment her, that it moved every Bodies Wonder and Compassion.

Then a Gentleman in the Company desired the Maid to say to her, My God help you, or my God preserve and deliver you, or the God whom I serve defend you, and be merciful to you, which she did; but those Expressions did not move Mrs. Joan; but if she said Jesus Christ deliver you, or the God of Heaven and Earth help you, then she would struggle, and fill all the Chamber with her Groans. And this was tried several Times by Hundreds.

The same Evening, after Court was broken up, Justice Fenner, who was then Judge, had a Mind to see Mrs. Joan Throckmorton, who was at the Sign of the Crown in Huntington, where the Judge lodged, and to that end he went into the Garden to her, where she was with other Women, with a great Number of Justices and other Gentlemen. They met her in a fair Ally, being then out of her Fit, and perfectly well. After the Judge had had a little Discourse with her, she fell into one of her ordinary Fits, her Eyes closed up; shaking her Shoulders, and Arms stretched right out, ready to fall on the Ground, but for her Father, who assisted her. Being not able to stand, she was led into an Harbour, the Judge and the rest of the Company going along with her, where they saw her most grievously tormented, and made a great many good Prayers for her, but to no purpose. Then Mr. Throckmorton told the Judge, that there was one in the Company, Agnes Samuel, who if she said but some certain Words, by way of Charge, that Mrs. Joan would presently be well. Then the Judge ordered Agnes Samuel to come nearer and to repeat the Words, which were these, As I am a Witch, and a worse Witch than my Mother, and did consent to the Death of the Lady Cromwell, so I charge thee, Devil, to let Mrs. Joan Throckmorton come out of her Fit at this present. But before Agnes Samuel spake the Charge, the Judge, Dr. Dorrington, Mr. Throckmorton, and others, spoke it; but Mrs. Joan had small ease by what they said; then they all made Prayers and Petitions to God for her Amendment, but none appeared. Then the Judge commanded Agnes Samuel to make some good Prayers to God for her Ease, which she did, but whenever she used the Name of God or Jesus Christ, the Maid was worse than before; God Almighty being not pleased that his Name should be used in the Mouths of such wicked Creatures. Then Agnes Samuel was commanded to say, As I am a Witch, neither did consent to the Death of the Lady Cromwell, I charge thee, Devil, to let Mrs. Joan come out of her Fit at this present; but this was to no purpose. Then Agnes Samuel was commanded to say the right Charge, As I am a Witch, and worse Witch than my Mother, and did consent to the Death of the Lady Cromwell, so I charge thee, Devil, to let Mrs. Joan Throckmorton come out of her Fit at this present. Upon which she immediately wiped her Eye, and came out of her Fit, and pay'd her Respects to the Judge, and continued well about half a quarter of an Hour, and then she fell into another kind of Fit, first shaking one Leg, and then the other; then one Arm, and afterwards the other; and then her Head and Shoulders, with other extraordinary Passions. Upon which the

Judge and the rest, lamenting her Case, and makeing some good Prayers for her, commanded Agnes Samuel to repeat another Charm, viz. As I am a Witch, and would have bewitched Mrs. Joan Throckmorton to Death in the last Week of her great Sickness, so I charge thee, Devil, to let Mrs. Joan come out of her Fit at this present. And as soon as Agnes Samuel had said these Words, she was presently well. Then the Judge asked her where she had been. She answered, I have been asleep. I pray God, said the Judge, send you no more such Sleeps. Soon after she fell into one of her other ordinary Fits, with a most strange and terrible kind of Sneezing, and other Passions, which were so vehement and pitiful to be heard, that it moved all the Company to pray to God to save her, fearing her Head would burst asunder, or her Eyes start out of it: so the Judge made no Delay, but commanded Agnes Samuel to speak the other Charm, which was, As I am a Witch, and did bewitch Mrs. Pickering of Ellington since my Mother's Confession, so I charge thee, Devil, to let Mrs. Joan come out of her Fit at this present: Which Words being said, Mrs. Joan was presently well, and continued well to this Day.

The next Day, being Thursday, there were three several Indictments made, and delivered to the great Inquest, whereof the one was against Samuel, old Mother Samuel, and Agnes their Daughter; for bewitching unto Death the Lady Cromwell, Wife of Sir Henry Cromwell, of Finchbrook in the County of Huntington, Knight, contrary to God's Laws, and a Statute made in the xvth Year of the Queen's Reign, &c.

The other two Indictments were framed upon the said Statute, for bewitching Mrs. Joan Throckmorton, and others, contrary to the said Statute. The Indictments being delivered to the Grand-Jury, the Evidence was given them privately by Dr. Dorington, Parson of Warboyse, Gilbert Pickering, of Tichmersh in the County of Northampton, Esq; Robert Throckmorton, Esq; Father of the said Children, Robert Throckmorton, of Brampton in the County of Huntington, Esq; John Pickering, and Henry Pickering, and Tho. Nut, Vicar of Ellington. The Grand Jury made no great delay; but found them all guilty, and about eight of the Clock, the Evidence was openly delivered in Court, to the Jury of Life and Death; and with great Patience of the Judge it was continued till one of the Clock in the Afternoon.

So many of these Proofs, Presumptions, Circumstances, and Reasons, contained in this Relation, were delivered at large, as that time would admit, which was five Hours, till the Judge, Justices and Jury said the Case was apparent, and their Consciences were well satisfied, that the said Witches were guilty, and had deserved Death; and then the Gentlemen ceas'd to give any further Evidence.

And what was remarkable was, That Mrs. Jane Throckmorton, on Friday the xvi of March last, being in one of her usual Fits, said, That the Spirit told her, she should never come out of her Fit, till old Father Samuel had said these Words, As I am a Witch and consented to the Death of the Lady Cromwell, so I charge thee, Devil, to suffer Mrs. Jane to come out of her Fit. This she published in the hearing of many, and her Father endeavoured to get John Samuel to come to the House, but could not prevail; therefore she continued in her Fits till the 4th- of April, which Day Mrs. Jane was brought to Huntington, and set in her Fit before the Judge, where several Questions were asked her; but she answered to none, for the Devil would not suffer her to speak; her Eyes were open, yet such Mists were before them, that she neither knew nor saw her Father that was next her, nor any of her Friends. Then the Judge ordered old Samuel to be brought nearer to the upper Bar, near where the Clarks sat, where Mrs. Jane stood, And the Judge being told, That if old Samuel spoke the Words above-recited, she would be well, he asked Samuel whether he could by any means cause the said Jane to come out of her Fit. He denied he could. Then the Judge told him, he was informed, that he had a Charm that would make her well, therefore the Judge recited the Charm, and desired him to speak the Words; but he refused it, and said he would not speak them. Then to encourage him, the Judge, Dr. Dorrington, and others, repeated them, yet he refused. Then the Judge desired him to pray to God for the Comfort of the Child, which he did;

but when he named God or Jesus Christ, the Child's Head, Shoulders and Arms were sadly shaken, and worse than before.

Then the Judge told him, That if he would not speak the Words of the Charm, the Court would bring him in guilty of the Crimes he was accused of; so that at last he was prevailed on to say, in the hearing of them all, As I am a Witch, and did consent to the Death of the Lady Cromwell, so I charge thee, Devil, to suffer Mrs. Jane to come out of her Fit at this present; upon which she wiped her Eyes, and came out of her Fit; and then seeing her Father, asked him Blessing, and pay'd her Respects to her Friends, and said, O Lord! Father, where am I?

Then the Judge said, You see all she is now well, but not with the Musick of David's Harp. Then old Mother Samuel's Confession was read, which she made before the Bishop of Lincoln; as also her Confession made before the said Bishop, Francis Cromwell, and Richard Toyce, Esq; Justices of the Peace in the County of Huntington.

When these were read, it pleased God to raise up more Witnesses against these wicked Persons, as Robert Poulton, Vicar of Brampton, who openly said, That one of his Parishioners, John Langley, at that time being sick in his Bed, told him, That one Day being at Huntington he did in Mother Samuel's hearing, forbid Mr. Knowles of Brampton to give her any Meat, for she was an old Witch; and upon that, as he went from Huntington to Brampton in the Afternoon, having a good Horse under him, he presently died in the Field, and within two Days after, he escaped Death twice very dangerously, by God's Providence; and though the Devil had not Power over his Body at that time, yet soon after he lost many good and sound Cattle, to Mens Judgment, worth Twenty Marks, and that he himself not long after, was very severely handled in his Body; and the same Night of the Day of Assize, the said John Langley died.

Mr. Robert Throckmorton, of Brampton also said, That at Huntington, and other Places, he having given very rough Language to the said Mother Samuel, on Friday the 10th Day following, one of his Beasts, of two Years old, died; and another the Sunday following. The next Friday after a Hog died, and the Sunday following a Sow which had sucking Pigs died also; upon which he was advised, the next Thing that died, to make a Hole in the Ground, and burn it. On Friday the fourth Week following, he had a fair Cow, worth sour Marks, died likewise, and his Servants made a Hole accordingly, and threw Faggots and Sticks on her, and burnt her; and after, all his Cattle did well. As to the last Matter, Mother Samuel being examined the Night before her Execution, she confessed the bewitching of the said Cattle.

Then the Jaylor of Huntington gave his Evidence, That a Man of his, finding Mother Samuel unruly whilst she was a Prisoner, chain'd her to a Bed-Post, and not long after he fell sick, and was handled much as the Children were, heaving up and down his Body, shaking his Arms, Legs and Head, having more Strength in his Fits than any two Men had, and crying out of Mother Samuel, saying she bewitched him, and continuing thus five or six Days, died.

And the Jaylor said, that not long after one of his Sons fell sick, and was much as his Servant was, whereupon the Jaylor brought Mother Samuel to his Bed-side, and held her till his Son had scratched her, and upon that he soon mended.

In the Afternoon the Jury of Life and Death found all the Indictments Billa vera, which when old Father Samuel heard, he said to his Wife, in the hearing of several, A Plague of God light upon thee, for thou art she that hath brought us all to this, and we may thank thee for it.

Then the Judge came to Sentence, and asked old Father Samuel what he had to say, why Sentence of Death should not be pronounced on him. He said he had nothing to say, but the Lord have Mercy on him. Then the Judge asked old Mother Samuel what she had to say to stay Judgment: She answered, that she was with Child. At which every Body laughed, and she her self most, hoping it would save her. The Judge perswaded her to wave that, but she would not. Then a Jury of Women was sworn to search her, who gave their Verdict, That if she was with Child, it was with the Devil. She was near Fourscore Years of Age. After she was found guilty, Mr. Henry Pickering went to her, and perswaded her to confess the Truth, and amongst other Things she confessed, that William Langley, who gave her the Spirits, had carnal Knowledge of her Body when she received them.

After this, the Judge asked Agnes Samuel what she had to say why Judgment should not be given. One that stood by her urged her to say she was with Child. No, says she, it shall never be said that I was both Witch and Whore. So the Judge, after good Divine Counsel given to them, proceeded to Judgment, which was to Death.

The next Day a great many Godly Men went to the Prison, to perswade them to Repentance, and to confess their Sins, and ask God Pardon. And Mother Samuel being asked by John Dorrington. Esq; one of the Justices of the Peace for that County, whether she did bewitch the Lady Cromwell, she said, No, forsooth, I did not; but her Husband, old Father Samuel, standing behind, and hearing her deny it, said, Deny it not, but confess the Truth, for thou did'st it one way or another.

The Confession of the Old Woman Alice Samuel, unto certain Questions that were demanded of her by Dr. Chamberlin, at the Time and Place of Execution, being upon the Ladder.

Being asked what were the Names of those Spirits she bewitched with. She said, Pluck, Catch and White. Being asked whether she had bewitched the Lady Cromwell to Death or not; she answered, She did. And being asked with which of the Spirits, she said with Catch. Being asked why she did it, she said, Because the Lady had caused some of her Hair and Hair-Lace to be burnt; and she said Catch asked her to be revenged of the Lady, and upon that she bad him go and do what he would; and being asked what he had done when he came back, he said, he had been revenged of her. And she further owned, That she was guilty of the Death of the said Lady.

Being asked whether she bewitched Mr. Throckmorton's Children, she confessed that she had done it; and being asked with which of her Spirits, she said with Pluck. Being asked what she said to him when she sent him on that Errand; she said, she bid him go and torment them, but not to hurt them. Being asked how long they should be in that Condition, she said she could not tell, and that she had not seen Pluck since Christmas last. Being asked what she did with White, she said she never did hurt with him, and that she had sent him to Sea, and that he had sucked on her Chin, but the other Two had no Reward. She confessed further, That she had these Spirits of one Langeley, but where he dwelt she knew not. Being asked whether her Husband was privy to the Death of the Lady Cromwell, she said he was.

Being asked whether her Husband was a Witch, and what Skill he had in Witchcraft, she said he was one, and could bewitch and unbewitch She would confess nothing of her Daughter, but endeavoured to clear her. As for the Daughter, she would confess nothing, but being desired to say the Lord's Prayer, when she stood upon the Ladder, and the Creed, she said the Lord's Prayer till she came to Deliver us from Evil; but could not pronounce those Words. And in the Creed she missed very much, and could not say that she believed the Catholick Church.

When the Execution was over, and these Three Persons were dead, the Jaylor, whose Business it is to see them buried, stripped off their Cloaths, and found upon the Body of Alice Samuel, a little Lump of Flesh, like a Teat, about half an Inch long, which being near her Private Parts, they covered them, and let several People see it. The Jaylor's Wife squeezing it with her Hand, a Mixture of yellowish Milk and Water issued out of it, then clear Milk, and at last Blood it self.

To conclude this Relation, since the Death of these Persons, the Children have continued well, without any Fits at all, enjoying their perfect Health.

Though this Relation is so well attested, and by all Circumstances carries along with it the undeniable Evidence of Truth, yet being willing to be fully satisfied about the same, we have made what Enquiry we could about it, and are informed by a very worthy Person, the Reverend Mr. Baker, now Fellow of St. John's College in Cambridge, 'That upon the Occasion of this Discovery at Warboyse, there is a Sermon preached annually at Huntington, on Lady-day, (being their Fair Day) by one of Queen's-College in that University; for which Sermon the Preacher receives annually forty Shillings of that Corporation; so much being answered for, and charged upon the Town, by the Family of the Cromwells soon after this Occasion happened.'

CHAP. IV.

Containing an Account of the Possession, Dispossession, and Repossession of William Sommers, &c. with some Depositions taken at Nottingham about the same Matter.

William Sommers of Nottingham, about Nineteen or twenty Years of Age, about the beginning of October 1597, began to be strangely tormented in his Body, and so continued for several Weeks, to the great Astonishment of those that saw him; so that there were evident Signs of his being possessed with an evil Spirit.

  The Mayor and Aldermen of Nottingham being acquainted with this Matter, and hearing of Mr. Dorrel, Minister at Asbby, who had by Prayer and Fasting restored eight or nine Persons, who had been tormented after the same Manner, sent for Mr. Dorrel to come to Nottingham, to use his Endeavours with this Man. But at the first he refused it, taking upon him no more in such Cases, than what belonged to any other godly Minister, which was to entreat the Lord, in the Name of Christ Jesus, to dispossess the Person of that wicked Spirit; yet being frequently importuned by Letters and Messengers he condescended to their Desires, and came to Nottingham the Fifth of November.

  The seventh Day of November, being Monday, was appointed for the Exercise of Prayer and Fasting, that the said Sommers might be dispossessed, which Almighty God, at the Prayers of Mr. Dorrel and others, being about 150 Persons, brought to pass: Whereupon Mr. Dorrel was retained as Preacher in Nottingham, that populous Town having had no settled Preacher, before this time, since the beginning of her Majesties Reign.

  When Sommers was dispossessed, he discovered several Witches, one of which was Doll Freeman, related to one Freeman an Alderman of Nottingham. This Freeman offended that his Kinswoman should be called in Question, threatned Sommers, and said he was a Witch, who upon that was committed to Prison, where the Devil appeared to him in the Form of a Mouse;

and threatned Sommers, that if he would not suffer him to re-enter, and say that all he had done whilst he was tormented, was counterfeit, he should be hanged; but if he complied with him, he should be saved. Thus a new Bargain being made betwixt them, the Devil entered; and afterwards Sommers pretended that all he had done before was counterfeit; yet upon his Repossession he was as much tormented as before, which appeared from the Depositions of several.

To know the Truth of this Matter, a Commission was awarded from the high Commissioners for the Province of York, to certifie the Matter to Twelve of the principal Persons threreabouts. Mr. Dorrel had taken the Names of threescore Persons, who were ready to make Oath concerning the Manner the said Sommers was handled in; Seventeen of which being sworn, examined, and their Depositions taken, Sommers himself was called before them to be examined, who told them all that he did was but counterfeit. The High Sheriff exhorted him in the Name of God to tell the Truth, upon which he was suddenly cast into one of his Fits before them all, and tumbled up and down the Chamber where they were, very strangely. They thrust Pins into his Hands and Legs to try if he counterfeited, or not; but he was sensless, and no Blood followed. At last coming to himself as one out of a Sleep, they asked him what he had done, but he could not tell. They asked him whether he had been pricked with Pins, and he said Yes; but being asked where, he shewed them the wrong Hand. When he was asked how the Hole came into his other Hand which was pricked, he said it was there before; and being asked why he fell down, he said a Qualm came over his Stomach; being then taken away, he was worse tormented than before.

They brought him back again to know if he would confess who perswaded him to say he had counterfeited; and as he was going up a Pair of Stairs through a Gallery, if he had not been prevented he had broken his Neck. When he was brought before the Commissioners, he was more terribly handled than before, which convinced them that he was really possessed, and proceeded to examine Witnesses, Mr. Walton Archdeacon of Derby being present, and an Enemy to Mr. Dorrel, who confessed that this Case was occasioned by a supernatural Cause.

This occasioned a great deal of Joy in Nottingham, that the Truth appeared so evident when it came to a Tryal. When the Commission was returned to York, and Sommers was committed to the Care of some honest Persons, where he was tormented as before; in his Fits he acknowledged how the Devil appeared to him in Prison in the Form of a Mouse; and that the Devil, as well as other Persons, had advised him to say, that he did but counterfeit, and what Promises were made him. He also gave them an Account of Things that happened elsewhere, without being informed by any Body; which was taken in Writing by those that heard him, which they offered to take their Oaths of. And when he came to himself he acknowledged his Possession, and said he would forfeit both Body and Soul to the Devil if he dissembled.

The Archbishop of York, when the Depositions came to his Hand, was satisfied that Sommers was possessed; yet he took occasion to silence Dr. Dorrel, because he proposed to dispossess the Devil by Prayer and Fasting; though he told the Bishop it was his Opinion, and would alter it, if better informed.

Having thus given a brief Account of the Possession of William Sommers, we shall next subjoyn the Depositions taken at Nottingham about the same Matter, by Virtue of a Commission from the Right Reverend Father in God Matthew Archbishop of York, the 20th of March 1597, before John Therold, Esq; High-Sheriff of the County of Nottingham. Sir John Byron, Knt. John Stanhop, Robert Markham, Richard Parkins, Esqs; and Peter Clerk Mayor of the Town of Nottingham; Miles Leigh, Official of the Archdeaconry of Nottingham; John Ireton, Parson of Legworth; John Brown, Parson of Loughborough; Robert Evington, Parson of Normanton upon Some, and Thomas Bolton, Ministers, Commissioners appointed for taking of the same.

And First, Thomas Hais of Kirby in Ashfield, in the County of Nottingham, Clerk, and Preacher of God's Word, being sworn and examined, faith, That being at Nottingham upon All-Saints Day, and intreated to come to William Sommers his House by his Mother, he there found the said Sommers strangely tormented, and frequently at the Name of Jesus cast upon the Ground, the one Leg being bended crooked towards him, and not being able to straighten the same: In which Leg he saw something run, and out of that into the other, and from thence into his Belly, very much swelling it; from thence it appeared in his Throat, his Tongue, and thence into his Cheek near his Ear, which seemed to be in Quantity as big as the Yelk of an Egg, and laying his Hand upon it he found it soft. Upon which he went to Mr. Atkinson of Nottingham, who had been acquainted with Melancholy People, or such as had been afflicted with Temptations, to find out whether it proceeded from a natural Cause. But after he had discoursed of Convulsions, Falling-Sickness, &c. he could not find that it proceeded from any such Cause; upon which he got Mr. Evings and Mr. Aldridge to come to him, in whose Presence he had several Fits as before, saying it was no Disease, but the Devil.

Secondly, Robert Aldridge, Vicar of St. Mary's in Nottingham, sworn and examin'd, said, That when he first came to William Sommers, on Thursday the Third of November, he found him lying upon a Bed, without any thing upon him, but his Stockings, and saw a Thing run up his right Leg about the Bigness of a Mouse; and he praying to God, it presently moved out of his right Leg into his left; and when he laid his Hand upon it, it presently moved into his Belly, which was presently swelled very much, being twice as big as before; from thence it moved into his Breast, being there as big as his Fist; from thence into his Neck, and then under his Ear, where it continued as big as a Walnut, without changing its former Colour, and remained there a Quarter of an Hour; and that Sommers lying upon his Back, was held by Two all the Time he was there.

The same Witness said further, that he heard a strange hollowish Voice say, that he was his; upon which the Witness examined said, he lyed, he was God's, and that he had made a Promise in Baptism that he would be his; to which the Voice answered, that he was God, Christ and a King; and that he made Baptism, and that he made him his by a new Covenant; for he had given three Pence, and that it was in the Boy's Sleeve; but that being searched, it could not be found; then it said again it was in his Glove.

He further said, That the 17th of November, from Seven in the Morning till Three in the Afternoon, he was strangely tormented, and after a different manner; and was so strong, that five Men had much adoe to keep him down, all which time he was extreamly swelled, scrietching and roaring, and gnashing his Teeth, and foaming at his Mouth. And on the 18th of November, betwixt Seven and Eight in the Morning, he went into the House of Robert Cooper, where William Sommers lay, to enquire how he had done the Night before; and standing in the Hall, he heard a great Knocking in the Parlour where the Boy lay, and going suddenly in, he found the Boy lying upon his Bed alone in his Fit, with his Face upwards, and his Mouth drawn awry, and his Eyes staring as if they would have started out of his Head: And kneeling down to Prayer, he heard the Knocking again as if it were under his Knees. And in the Bed, under the Coverlet, he saw, in Appearance, Shape and Bulk, five Things; and after he saw the Bed-cloaths at the Feet move and shake like the Leaves of a Tree moved with the Wind.

Next William Hind of Nottingham, Taylor, swore, that coming to the said Sommers, he found Mr. Aldridge there, and saw a Swelling in his Neck as big as a large Walnut, from whence it moved to the Bone of his Cheek, appearing there as big as a Hazel Nut; from thence it moved to his Eye, and the Skin of his Eye grew black. He further said, that when he laid his Hand upon his Cheek, the Swelling there trembled, and was very soft, but in that place did not change the natural Colour of the Skin.

Next, Thomas Westfield in the County of Nottingham, Minister, swore, That on Sunday Night, being the Sixth of November, desirous to see what he had heard of the said Sommers, he came to him with Master Dorrel, and found a great Swelling under the left Ear, as big as a Walnut, which removed from thence to the Eye, which was not so large there, but caused a Blackness in his Eye, and laying his Hand upon it, he felt a Motion, and his Eye came to its natural Colour immediately, and so changed eight times betwixt Three and Six a Clock in the Morning.

William Aldred of Collwick swore, That he, along with the Major of the Town and others, coming to Sommers about seven a-Clock in the Evening, on the sixth Day of November; after Prayers made to God, exhorted such as were there disposed, to meet the next Morning about seven a-Clock, and to consecrate that whole Day with Prayers and Fasting, and departed at that time. The next Day about 150 met, and the said Aldred began first, and after Prayers preached against the Sins of those Times. The Boy at the same time was strangely tormented with Fits, heaving up his Body, and hawling his Lips awry, one towards one Ear, and the other towards the other, opening his Mouth wide, as if it were four Square, thrusting out his Tongue, and putting it double again into his Mouth, with dreadful Scrietches and Cries, and sometimes lay silent.

When the said Aldred had ended his Sermon, Mr. Dorrel began with Prayer, at which time the Boy's Fits seemed as violent again; and Mr. Dorrel perceived the same Signs of Possession mentioned in the Ninth of Mark very violent, for he scrietched with a loud Voice, and foamed very much, gnashing with his Teeth, and his Body distracted several ways: And when Mr. Dorrel came to these Words, All things are possible to him that believeth; the Boy answered, thou liest; and with a terrible Countenance, staring with his Eyes, and gaping with his Mouth, stretched out his Hands with bended Fingers like Eagles Claws towards the Preacher, leaping up with his Body, and other threatening Postures, only he was restrained by those that held him.

Thus Mr. Dorrel continued his Discourse of Faith; but when he came to discourse of the Signs of Dispossession, Sommers his Torments again began to be violent; and Mr. Dorrel going on with his Discourse, He came out of him; William Sommers at the same time seeming to vomit, and then the whole Congregation joyning in fervent Prayer to God, in a Quarter of an Hour's Time, the Devil came out of him, and being thrown upon the Bed he lay quietly at rest; and when they returned Thanks to God for this Deliverance, the Boy going upon his Knees returned Thanks likewise, and when the Service was ended returned home with his Master well.

Joan Pye, Wife of Robert Pye, swore, That about a Week ago Mr. Dorrel was sent for to William Sommers, being Saturday before All-Saints Day, and at Night she coming to the House where the Boy lay, after a while he fell into a Fit of Laughing, and was suddenly thrown to the Bed's Feet, his Body doubled, and his Head betwixt his Legs; then suddenly he was drawn round in a Heap, and rowling on the Bed, was cast up like a Ball three or four times together about half a Yard high; the Coverlet being so fast wrapped about him, that all the Company could not pull it from him.

And the same Witness says, that she hath often seen Sommers handled with so much Violence, that four or five Persons could not hold him down; and notwithstanding they held him, he would move his Legs, Arms and Head with so much Violence, as if he would have beat his Brains out, And further, the same Witness says, That on Allhallow-even about Noon, she and several others being present, the same Boy sitting in a Chair about two Yards from the Fire-side, he was suddenly cast towards the Fire; and three or four taking him up to save him from burning, they could not set him in his Chair again; his Legs being so bent that they could not straighten them; and he was so heavy that they could scarce lift him; and that neither his Head, Hair, nor any Part of his Body was hurt, or burnt by the Fire. And she said further, That there was a small Line which tied up a painted Cloth, which was hung over the Bed, to which Sommers stretched his Hand, but could not reach it; and then he appeared to them taller than the tallest Man in the Town, and suddenly got his Chin over the Line, and with his Hands got it so fast about his Neck, that they who stood by had much adoe to save him from hanging. And she further said, That the Boy in one of his Fits said, the Night before Mr. Dorrel came, that Dorrel was coming, when he nor any Body she knew had certain Intelligence that he was coming; the Messengers sent to him, bringing Word that he designed not to come till next Week. And she further said, That the same Day Mr. Dorrel came to Town, he was worse handled than before; and many times with his Mouth wide open said, I will use W. S. his Tongue, and Members for three Days, without moving or stirring his Tongue or Lips in speaking any of those Words, and that the Speech was in the ordinary Voice of W. Sommers.

And the same Witness further said, That an Hour and a half before Mr. Dorrel came to Town, the Boy fell into an extreme Fit, so that they thought he had been dead; for he lay senseless, and speechless, his Eyes being out of his Head like Walnuts, his Face black after a strange manner, and all his Body cold on a sudden for an Hour; and being asked when the Fits were past, whether he remembred the Extremity, or any part of it, he denied it; and whatever they gave him to recover him out of these Fits was of no Effect. And when Mr. Dorrel came to Town, the Boy said, I have but a short time to stay now, but I will shortly return. And when Mr. Dorrel came in at the Back-side of the House he foretold his coming, and had several times foretold Mr. Aldridge his coming.

She further said, That several times when he was in his Fits, she smelled a Smell like Brimstone; and that several times in his Fits, she had seen a Swelling in his Foot, which removed from Toe to Toe, and from thence into his Leg, and from thence to his Body, and so to his Throat, as big as a Rat, and thence to his Ear as big as a Walnut, and in his Eye-brows like a black Clock, and so removed from Place to Place, which she and others have both seen and felt.

And she further said, That after he was dispossessed he discovered several to be Witches, particularly Milicent Horselie, who lived at Bridgford, whom Mr. Dorrel and Mr. Aldred carried to Mr. Parkins to be examined; and about One a-Clock the same Day the Boy said, Now they have her, and are examining her, and she says she does all by Prayer, and now she is saying her Prayer.

And she further said, That several Times she had heard a Clapping in his Bed, as if Hands had been clapped; and that she had often seen a Motion in the Bed, as if it had been three Kitlings creeping, which she and others have endeavoured to take hold of, but never could, it vanishing when they offered to take hold of it. At other times they heard a Knocking, as if it were at the Bed's Feet under the Bed, and in some of those Fits he would cry, Now she comes, now she comes, now she will break my Neck; and presently his Neck was thrown about as if it had been broken, his Mouth being drawn sometimes on one side, and sometimes on the other.

Richard Newton, of Nottingham, swore, That coming to the said Sommers in his Fit, he heard him say plainly, with his Mouth wide open, his Tongue drawn into his Throat, so that nothing but the Root of it could be seen in his Mouth, and neither his Lips nor Chaps moving, Ego Sum Rex, Ego Sum Deus, with other Words which this Witness did not understand.

Henry Nussie, Blacksmith, swore, That sitting up with the said Sommers about Ten or Eleven-a-Clock at Night, he saw him with his Mouth wide open, and he spoke several Words to John Wigan in Latin, which he understood not, neither his Chaps nor Tongue moving, and at the same time he came very near him, that he might see it the better.

William Langford, of Nottingham, Surgeon, swore, That the same Day he was dispossess'd, he gnashed with his Teeth, wallow'd, and foam'd at such a rate, that the Foam hung down from his Mouth to his Breast, though it was wiped away continually with Cloaths, which continued for the Space of an

Hour; which was the stranger, he having taken nothing from Six-a-Clock in the Morning till Five in the Afternoon; and that he scrietched with three several Voices, so hideously, that it was not like a human Creature, but like a Bull, the second Voice like a Bear, and the third was a small Voice, such as could hardly be counterfeited.

This Witness further said, That he was so strong, especially on the 17th of February, that three of them could not hold him, and that feeling his Temples and Arm, he could feel no Pulse, but that he was senseless, like a dead Man, and that all the outward Parts of his Body were cold; nor did he pant or breathe much, as he could perceive. He further said, That he head him sing with a small Tuneful Voice, and that he could not sing so out of his Fit. And that the 7th of November, the Day appointed for his Dispossession, finding him on his Knees at Prayer, and some others along with him, he being then designed to be carried to the Place appointed, he was suddenly thrown a-thwart the Bed, and that Five or Six of them had much adoe to carry him to the Place; and that he alone holding of his Head, it was sometimes forcibly taken from him. And being extreamly tormented that Day, and his Buttons opening, he saw a Rising or Swelling in the bottom of his Belly, which moved the Cloaths; and his Breast and Stomach being bare, he saw the same Swelling the Bigness of a Goose Egg, which ascended from his Breast up to his Throat, with Motions to Vomit, which continued till he was dispossess'd, and then suddenly he was thrown over, by what Means no Body could imagin.

Thomas Graie, of Graies Langlie in the County of Leicester, Esq; swore, That the third of November, he saw the said Sommers lie upon a Bed, several Persons holding him at his Feet and Head, so that he seemed to be in a Fit, though his Countenance did not shew it, and immediately praying to God that some Token of the Reality of his being possess'd might appear to him, he saw something move under the uppermost Covering of the Bed, not far from the Small of his Leg, which lay in a round Lump, panting; which he pointing at said, what is that?

Some said it was his Feet, but others said they had his Feet there, and held them; then he laid his Hand upon it, and felt it move, and clasping his Hand together, he perceived it to yield like Wind or Air; and when he opened his Hand, it filled it up again; and when he took away his Hand, the Cloaths settled very softly down, like a Bladder blown with Wind, which falls down when prick'd, and presently the same Sort of moving was on the other Side; and laying his Hand upon it, he found something move very sensibly under his Hand like the Foot of a Kitling.

John Wood of Lenton swore, That on Friday the 17 of February, being told, That William Sommers was very much tormented with strange Fits; going there with other Company, he found, that three or four Men could scarce hold him; and to try whether the Boy's Strength was so great or not, he had a mind to try how he could deal with him himself, and stepping behind him, got fast hold of his Arms, as if he would have pinnion'd him; but finding that he could not hold him, but that he would slip out of his Hands, he let go his Hold there, and clapped his Fingers one betwixt the other, round his Body; but he was soon so tired that two of the Standers by laid hold of him, one, holding one Leg, and the other the other Leg, he still holding his Body; but he tired them all in an Hour's Time, so that others that stood by were forced to relieve them.

Upon this, this Witness stepped before him, to see if he was out of Breath himself or panted, and found his Eyes and Lips close shut up, and so far from panting, that he could not perceive him draw his Breath, nor did he sweat the least, nor was there the least Redness in his Cheeks.

The same Witness said further, That hearing it reported that the said Sommers dissembled, and was delivered to Nicholas Shepherd and John Cooper, as his Keepers at Lenton; therefore taking a Friend along with him they openly asked him before Witnesses, whether he remembred what was done to him in some of his preceding Fits? To which he answered, He did. And then John Wood asking him, Whether he could remember what he did to him, he told him he could, and that he nipped him by the

Finger with his Thumb-Nail, and made a Sign with his own Thumb-Nail, upon his own Finger, saying, He nipped him thus; but being desired in the Name of God to tell the Truth and shame the Devil, he confessed, that he did not nip his Finger, and at last confessed, that he could not tell any thing he did.

Next John Setwellie swore, That coming to the said Sommers in the Presence of Mr. Dorrel, and others, he found him in a Fit, and so strong, that several Persons were soon tired with holding him. And another Time finding him well, and exhorting him out of the Word of God, he was suddenly thrown from the Place he sat, and his Head knocked to the furthest Post of the Chimney, that they thought it had been broken, he being so heavy, that it seemed impossible for any Natural Body to be of so great a Weight; and being laid upon the Bed, and lying there half an Hour, several strange Accidents happen'd, as his Neck being doubled under him, and being likewise tormented in his inward Parts; one of his Legs being very heavy, and a little Thing seemed to move in every Part of him, swelling his Body, and rising in several Parts of his Face as big as a Walnut; and afterwards coming to himself again, and continuing well a small Time, he was suddenly seized with a Fit again, and cast into the Fire, and being taken out again without any Hurt, he began to foam, wallow, and gnash with his Teeth, scrietching and roaring, and tormented in his Body, with several Swellings both in his Body and Face, as before, saying several strange Things, his Mouth being wide open, and his Tongue drawn into his Throat.

Richard Mee likewise swore, That coming to the said Sommers to watch with him, between Three and Six a-Clock in the Morning, he heard a Voice, saying, That he would have his Right Eye, and then he would have his Left; and presently a great Blackness was in his Left Eye. And the same Witness says, That a Day or two before, and several other Times, he saw a Swelling in his Arms and Legs, as big as a Walnut, removing from one Place to another in his Body, and that he felt in his Body the Bigness of a Six-penny-Loaf, and so hard, that he could not press it down with his Hand.

The same Deponent says, That he hath seen him often turn his Face quite backwards, and moving his Body; and that his Eyes were as big as Beasts Eyes, seemingly ready to start out of his Head. The same Deponent further says, That he hath seen him fall down before them, and that one of his Legs would be crooked with the Fall, which could not be pulled straight by any means. He hath likewise seen his Mouth strangely distorted, and that his Tongue would be thrust out of his Mouth, as big as a Calve's Tongue. He hath also seen him laugh very strangely, and suddenly scrietch like a Swine when it is sticking, also wallow and gnash with his Teeth, and foaming at the Mouth, being senseless; and sometimes he would be cast into the Fire, standing a Yard and half off, and neither his Cloaths burned nor his Hair singed.

He further says, That in many of his Fits he sometimes would be so strong, that Six Men could scarce hold him without being out of Breath with struggling; and sometimes a loud Voice would come from him, saying, that there was no God; that he was God; that he was King and Prince of Darkness. And in saying the Lord's Prayer he could not be perswaded to say, Lead us not into Temptation, but lead us into Temptation. And further he says, That he hath smelled such sweet Smells in the Room where he was, that he could not bear the Sweetness of them.

Elizabeth Milward swore, That the Day Mr. Dorrel came to Town, William Sommers was extreamly tormented, so that for an Hour and a half he lay as dead, being senseless and speechless, and to Appearance without Breath; being presently as cold as Ice, and his Hands black: nor would any Cordials revive him, but he was so heavy that they could not lift him up; and the first Words he said, were Dorrell comes, Dorrel comes, he will have me out, but I will come again, for Nottingham and Lenton are Jolly Towns for me. And the first time he called any of his Neighbours to help him, she heard a thumping and knocking in his Bed, and putting her Hand into the Bed, she felt the knocking at a hollow Place above the Chest of his Body, which she heard as she went down the Stairs, being so much afraid that she durst not stay with him.

John Pane of Plumtree, Minister, swore, That about Nine of the Clock before Noon, the Day-set apart for Fasting and Prayer, he staid till three in the Afternoon before he could see the Boy, whom he found groveling on the Bed on his Face, and a Swelling under his Cloaths, as big as a Mouse, which removed from Place to Place in his Body. He also heard a Thumping and Beating in three several Places in the Boys Bed at the same time, and putting his Hand into the Bed, felt it knock sensibly under his Hand.

John Clark of Nottingham swore, That going to see the Boy the sixth of November, he found him in a Fit, in which he said the following Words to Edward Garland, Edward Garland, Art thou there? how do thy Children? I will have one of them, even the youngest. To which Garland answered, I defie the Devil, for he can have no Power of me nor my Children. And a little Time after the Boy came to his Senses, and being asked whether he would rise, when the Cloaths were taken off, he saw a Swelling upon his Breast as big as a Mouse, which he took hold of, and found it very soft, and endeavouring to take hold of it presently went away, and the Boy said it was gone down into his Leg, and he said he saw him several times when his Legs and Arms were inflexible, and very heavy.

W. Hunt likewise swore, That he saw William Sommers in his Fit, lying for dead, when he heard a Voice come from him when his Lips were quite closed, he neither moving his Lips or Jaws, as he perceived, yet he continued speaking a Quarter of an Hour. And he said further, That in the same Fit he saw a Thing about the Bigness of a Walnut, running in the Flesh of the said Sommers, about his Face, Forehead, and Eyes, and to his Ear.

CHAP. V.

Containing a further Account of the Works of the Devil, without the Assistance of Man; also by Witchcraft, Sorcery, &c.

That the Works of the Devil are often put in Practice without the Assistance of Magicians, Witchcraft and Sorcery, as well as by those Wicked Instruments, is evident from Scripture; the Devil in the Body of a Serpent, being able to speak to, and dispute with Eve; his Voice being manifestly perceived and heard by her, there being at that time no Body born to act the Part of a Witch. Another Example of the Devil's acting without the Assistance of Witches was, when our Saviour was carried and set upon the Pinacle of the Temple; nor was it less visible, how the Devil, by a supernatural Power, brought down Fire from Heaven, and burnt so many Thousands of Job's Sheep, and caused whole Herds of Swine to run headlong down into the Sea.

  The Scripture likewise gives us Examples, how the Devil himself tormented the Bodies of Men; Mark the 1st, Luke 4, Matthew 17, and Mark the 9th; the Devil being heard to cry out of the Bodies of the possessed Persons after a strange and wonderful manner, in which Cases the Devil was sole Agent without the Help and Assistance of Witches or Sorcerers.

  This is confirmed not only by sacred, but other faithful Historians, and the Reports of Ethnick Writers, who lived in different Ages, several Authors of approved Credit having told us, how the Devil not only spoke out of the Bodies of Men possessed, but also out of Trees, Caves of the Earth, Images and Statues. The Truth of the first appears from what hath been delivered concerning the Python's speaking out of the Bellies of several Persons: The second is also confirmed by the several Relations, which were continued for some hundreds of Years, before the Birth of our Saviour, concerning the Oracle of Delphos, the Oak of Dodona, and the Statue of Memnon. And Petrus Gregorius Tholosanus, writing of some Statues at Alexandria tells us, That they fell on the Ground suddenly, and with a loud Voice declared the Death of the Emperor Mauricius, at the same Time that he was slain at Rome.

And as the Devil shews himself by Voices and Sounds, in Trees, Caves, Statues, so he does in several other outward Shapes, and in the Forms of other Creatures. Thus the Devil spoke to Eve in the Form of a Serpent; and Orpheus mentions six Kinds of visible Spirits, viz. Spirits inhabiting the heavenly Regions, such as rule in the Air, in the Water, in the Fire, in the Earth, and under the Earth. The Spirits in the Air, Plato says, are Presidents of Divination, of Miracles, and of Chaldaick Magick; the Spirits in the Earth, and under the Earth, are such as appear in the Shapes of Dogs and Goats, moving Men to foul and unlawful Lusts. And the same Author tells us, that Spirits make use of airy Bodies or Substances that they may appear to Men.

Upon this Occasion we might recite the Apparition that appeared to Athenodorus the Philosopher reported by Pliny; and Brutus his Genius, after the Death of Julius Cæsar, appearing and speaking to him; as also those Representations, which in the Shape of Men appeared to Lucius Domitius, returning towards Rome, Suetonius reporting that it touched his Beard, which immediately was turned from a perfect Black to a lively Yellow, and therefore afterwards he was called Ænobarbus; but not to mention such, later Times have furnished us with Examples of this kind.

It is reported by John de Serres the French Chronicler, that the late K. of France, Henry the 4th, being out a Hunting, a Devil presented him and the whole Company with the loud Cry of Hounds, and Winding of Horns. The King commanded Count Soissons to go and see who it was, wondering who durst interrupt his Game: The Earl still advancing to wards the Noise, heard it, but came no nearer. At last a big black Man appeared in the thickest of the Bushes, and speaking some few Words to the Earl suddenly vanished. And Mr. Fox in the Life of Martin Luther, tells us of the Apparition and Conference of the Devil with a young Man, who, upon Contracts agreed between the Devil and himself, delivered his Bond to the Devil for the

Performance of the same. And Speed in his Chronicle, within the Time of Henry the Fourth, makes Mention of the Apparition of the Devil in the Habit of a Minorite Fryar at Dunbury Church in Essex, with such Thundering, Lightning, Tempests, and Fireballs, that the Vault of the Church broke, and half of the Chancel was carry'd away.

And as the Devil, without the Assistance of human Instruments, hath frequently exercised his Power, so he hath done it frequently by making Covenants with Man.

Livy reports, that the Roman Claudia, a vestal Virgin, actually appeared, to be able alone with Ease and Facility to draw a mighty Ship along by a small Line or Girdle, which was so large and heavy, that a great many Men could not move it, though assisted by the Strength of a great many Cattle accustomed to draw very heavy Burthens. Tuccia also a vestal Virgin, is reported by repeating a certain Prayer to keep Water within a Sieve or a Riddle. And Camerarius mentions a Man who armed only with certain Charms, would receive upon his Body, without Harm, Bullets or Shot fired out of a Cannon; and he mentions another, who would undertake to lay his Hand upon the Mouth of a Cannon when it was fired, and stop both the Fire and the Shot from going out of it; and it is recorded, that Decius Actius the Augur told Tarquinius the Roman King the Time intended for his most secret Designs. And it is written of the Enthusiastes or Prophetesses of Diana in Castabola, a Town of Cilicia, that they would frequently and voluntarily walk with their bare Feet upon burning Coals, without any Hurt or Alteration by the Fire. And it is said of Pythagoras, that by certain Words he could compel an Ox or Bullock to leave off eating. Others report, that he could command the wild Beasts and Birds to come to him and grow tame and follow him. It is also said of him, that he was once seen at the same Time in the City of Thurium, and the Town of Metapontum. Apollonius is said to have been translated in the Twinkling of an Eye from Smyrna to Ephesus.

It is said of Apollonius, That he foretold the Day, the Hour of the Day, and the Moment of the Hour, wherein

Cocceius Nerva the Emperor should die, a long time before, and being in Places far distant from him. And it is further said of him, That being asked of one how he should grow rich, Apollonius appointed him to buy a certain Field, and to be careful in Tilling and Plowing of it; which when he had done, he found a great Treasure, and so became rich. The same Apollonius likewise told Titus Vespasian the Time and Manner of his Death.

To these we may add, what was said of that famous and renowned British Wizard Merlin, and his high Esteem amongst Princes for his Prophecies, being able to foretel for many succeeding Ages, the Successes and Events of several Princes Affairs in their several Reigns.

And it is reported of that infamous Woman amongst the French, Joan of Arc, who foretold a great many wonderful things to King Charles the Seventh, that upon her Encouragement and Assurance of Success, the French after encountered the victorious English, and contrary to all Reason and Expectation to their great Terror and Amazement suddenly confounded them, though at last she was taken Prisoner by the English, and executed and burnt for her Witchcraft. And the same Historian reports, That a Wizard foretold Duke Biron of his Death, and that he should die by the Back-blow of a Burguignan, who afterwards proved his Executioner, being that Country-man.

Philip de Commines tells us of one Fryar Hierome, and of his admirable Predictions, concerning the Affairs of the King of France; nor could any Body deny him to be a Witch or Wizard, who, as Mr. Speed testifies, in the Reign of Richard the Usurper foretold, that upon the same Stone where he dashed his Spur going towards Bosworth Field, he should dash his Head upon his Return, which proved accordingly true; for being slain in the Battle, and carry'd naked out of the Field, his Head hanging low by the Horse's Side, behind him that carried him off, it struck against the same Stone he had struck his Spur against as he went; to which we might add several Relations of the like Kind.

In the Malleus Maleficorum there is an Account of a German Sorceress, who commonly cured not only those that were bewitched, but all kind of diseased People, so far beyond the Power of Nature or Art, that the Use of Physicians was wholly left off, and People of all Countries, both far and near, resorted so much to her, that the Governour of that Country only imposing a Penny upon every one that came to her, raised by that Means a vast Treasure.

To these Historical Relations we shall add, that it was once objected against a Witch in Northampton-shire at the publick Assizes, that a Rat was often observed to resort to her privy Parts, and with her Consent to suck, which was not only proved by sufficient Testimony, but acknowledged by her own Confession. What strange Effects have been produced by the Power of Witchcraft, in a great Measure appears from the foregoing Relations to which we shall add, That it hath been observed, that several Persons in the Time of their Fits have been seen to vomit crooked Iron, Coals, Brimstone, Nails, Needles, Pins, Lumps of Lead, Wax, Hair, Straw, &c. and several sick Men have in the Time of their Sickness declared Words, Gestures and Actions done in distant Places, even in the Time of their being done, acted or spoken.

And besides the different Actions of Witches already mentioned, it is not unknown that several have undertaken to reveal hid Treasures, Goods lost or conveighed away, and the Works and Guilt of other Witches, good Fortunes and ill Fortunes in several Affairs, Designs or Attempts; as also by Enchantment to lead Captive the Minds and Wills of Men, either towards extraordinary and unreasonable Desires and Lusts, Hatred or Love, to or against particular Persons, or particular Things.

Franciscus Picus Mirandula reports, that a famous Magician in Italy, in his Time, kept the Skull of a dead Man, out of which the Devil would give Answers to any Questions proposed, the Wizard first repeating some Words, and turning the Skull towards the Sun.

Some in the Execution of their Diabolical Works, never undertake any thing without Mumblings, Whisperings, and secret

Sounds and Words heard grumbling in their Mouths; as Theophrastus tells us of certain Magicians, who used that Practice in gathering of Helleborus and Mandragora. And Galen tells us of a certain Sorcerer, who by uttering and muttering but one Word, would immediately kill or cause to die, a Serpent or Scorpion. And Benivenius affirms, that some kind of People have been observed to do hurt, and to surprize others by using only certain sacred and holy Words. Others have accomplished their devilish Ends by Apparitions, raised or conjured into Glasses. Others put their devilish Designs in Execution by inchanted Herbs, which they mix and gather with brass Hooks, or by Moonshine; and sometimes with their Feet bare and naked. Hollingshead takes Notice in his Chronicle of several Traitors, who were executed for conspiring the King of England's Death by sorcerous and magical Pictures of Wax: And the same Author takes Notice, That in the twentieth Year of Queen Elizabeth, a Figure-Caster being suspected as a Conjurer or Witch, suddenly dying, there was found about him the Picture of a Man wrought in Tin; and several late Writers have observed, that Witches, by such Pictures, have caused the Persons they represented to consume away secretly, which hath been proved by several Witches executed in Yorkshire and Lancashire: Others put their infernal Designs in Execution by Medicines taken out of the Bodies of dead Men, and murdered Infants.

Some practise Witchcraft by tying Knots, as St. Jerome witnesseth of a Priest of Æsculapius at Memphis. Some make use of touching with the Hand or Finger: Some make use of Parchment made of the Skins of Infants, or Children born before their Time, as Serres reports of Witches detected in the Reign of King Henry the Fourth. And some make use of living Creatures to minister to them, or of Devils and Spirits in their Likeness. And Theocritus in his Pharmaceutria induces a Sorceress, who by the Power of her Bird, forced her Lover to come to her.

And it seems not impossible for a Witch to act by a Multitude of living Shapes, which the Devil in former Ages hath assumed; as Fauns, Satyrs, Nymphs, familiarly conversing with

Men: Some bring their wicked Sorcery to an end, by sacrificing to the Devil some living Creatures, as Serres witnesseth, from the Confession of Witches in King Henry the Fourth's Time, one of which confessed that she offered a Beetle to the Devil or evil Spirit.

And in former Times living Creatures were not only sacrificed to Devils, but even Men, with which the Heathens pleased their Gods, which were no other than Devils. And rather than the Devil will want Worship, he is sometimes willing to accept of paring of Nails, as Serres reports from the Confessions of several French Witches.

Some Authors testify, that some Kind of Sorcerers fix their Magical Effects and Works on Men, by conveighing or delivering to the Persons whom they mean to assault, certain Sorts of Meat or Drink, as appears from the Magick Cups of Filtra or Love-draughts. St. Augustin mentions a Woman who bewitched others by delivering only a Piece of Cheese. And some Witches have been observed to work their Mischief on them they sought to destroy, by obtaining some Part of their Garments, or of their Excrements; as their Hair, or the like.

Thus much being said of Witchcraft and Sorcery, we shall briefly take Notice of some of the Ceremonies and Rites of Diviners. Some in former Times used to divine by the Flying of Birds, by Viewing of Lightning, by Monsters, by Lots, by the Inspection of the Stars, and by Dreams. Some declared their Divinations out of Tubs, or Vessels of Water, into which were cast thin Plates of Silver and Gold, and other precious Jewels, by which the Devils were allured to answer to their Demands, Doubts and Questions. Some derived their Divinations from Looking-Glasses, where the Devil answered their Demands, by Figures and Shapes appearing in them. Some take their Divinations from Lots taken from Points, Figures, Characters, Words, Syllables, Sentences, Fire, Water, Earth and Air; also by Sieves, Riddles, and the Guts and Bowels of the Dead: Devils also are sometimes conjured by several Sorts of Stones, Heaths,

Woods, Creatures, Times and Rites, Spirits delighting in Signs and Creatures, as they betoken Honour and Respect.

CHAP. VI.

Containing the wonderful Discovery of the Witchcrafts of Margaret and Philip Flower, Daughters of Joan Flower, by Beaver Castle, and executed at Lincoln the 11th of March 1618.

WHEN the Right Honourable Sir Francis Manners succeeded his Brother in the Earldom of Rutland, and took Possession of Beaver-Castle, and the rest of the Revenues belonging to the same Earldom; he took such honourable Measures in the Course of his Life, that he neither displaced Tenants, discharged Servants, nor denied the Access of the Poor, but making Strangers welcome, did all the good Offices of a Noble Lord, by which he got the Love and Goodwill of the Country; which he did the more heartily, his Noble Countess being of the same Disposition; so that Beaver-Castle was a continual Place of Entertainment, especially to Neighbours, where Joan Flower, together with her Daughters was not only relieved at the first, but quickly after entertained as Chair-woman, and her Daughter Margaret admitted as a continual Dweller in the Castle, looking to the Poultrey abroad, and the Wash-house at home; and thus they continued till found guilty of some Misdemeanour, which was discovered to the Lady.

And though such honourable Persons want not all Sorts of People to bring them News, Tales or Reports, and to serve them in all Offices; yet in this Family there were neither Busie-bodies, Flatterers nor Underminers, or Supplanters of one another's good Fortune; each doing their Duty, and regarding the Interest of the Earl and his Lady, which encouraged them to give more Heed to their Complaints.

The first Complaint against Joan Flower, the Mother, was, that she was a monstrous malicious Woman, full of Oaths, Curses, and irreligious Imprecations; and as far as appeared, a plain Atheist: Besides of late her Countenance was strangely altered, and her Eyes very fiery and hollow, and her Speech fallen and altered, and envious, her Behaviour very strange likewise; so that there were great Suspicions of her being a Witch; and some of her Neighbours affirmed, that she dealt with familiar Spirits, and terrified them all with Curses and threatning Revenge, upon the least Cause of Displeasure or Unkindness.

As for Margaret, she was accused of frequently going from the Castle, and carrying Provisions away in unreasonable Quantities, and returning at such unreasonable Hours, that they could not but conjecture at some Mischief amongst them, and that their extraordinary Expences tended both to rob the Lady, and served to maintain some debauched and idle Company which frequented Joan Flower's House, and especially her youngest Daughter.

As for Philip, she was accused of being lewdly transported with the Love of one Thomas Sympson, who presumed to say, that she had bewitched him, having no Power to leave her, and as he thought strangely altered both in Mind and Body since he knew her.

These Complaints began to be made many Years before their Conviction, or publick Apprehension; nevertheless the Earl and his Lady were so honourable, and this monstrous Woman carry'd it so slily and cunningly towards them, and the Devil was so subtle in bringing what he designed to pass, and her Malice was attended with so much Wit and malicious Envy, that every Thing passed on smoothly for a long Time, 'till the Earl, by Degrees, entertained some Dislike of her, and used not that Freedom, nor familiar Conferences with her as usual: At last one Peale offered her some Wrong, and upon that she made her Complaint, but found they took no Notice of her clamorous and malicious Information. And after one Mr. Vavasor forsook her Company, either suspecting her lewd Life, or misliking such base and mean Creatures as no body but the Earl's Family loved.

In some Time the Countess misliking her Daughter Margaret, and discovering some Indecencies in her life, and the Neglect of her Business, discharged her from lying any more in the Castle, yet gave her forty Shillings, a Bolster, and a Matress of Wool, commanding her to go home; so that at last her frequenting the Castle not so much as usual, turned her Love towards this honourable Family into Hate and Malice; and being offended, that she should be so much slighted and reproached by her Neighbours upon her Daughter's being put out of Doors, she grew past all Shame, and several times cursed all those that were the Occasion of her Discontent, and made her unacceptable to her former familiar Friends, and beneficial Acquaintance.

The Devil perceiving the ill Disposition of this Wretch, and that she and her Daughters might easily be made Instruments to enlarge his Kingdom, he grew more familiar with them, and began to offer them his Service, and told them that they should command what they pleased, and that he would attend them in the Form of a Dog, or a Cat, or a Rat, that he might be less frightful to them, and less suspected by others: At last they agreed, and gave away their Souls for the Service of such Spirits as he had promised them; which Promises were ratified and confirmed by abominable Kisses, and an odious Sacrifice of Blood, making use of certain Charms and Conjurations, with which the Devil deceived them, that nothing might seem to be done without some Ceremony and Form.

When thus they were deceived and caught in the Snares of the Devil, they grew proud of their cunning and artificial Power to do what Mischief they pleased, having learned the Art of Enchanting, Spells and Charms; so that they could kill what Cattle they pleased, and dissemble their Malice with Flattery, and a Shew of kind Entertainment. Then they began to threaten the Earl and his Family with a terrible Tempest, which through the devilish Devices of these Women fell upon him, when he neither suspected nor understood any Thing of it; for both the Earl and his Countess began to be subject to Sickness, and extraordinary Convulsions, which they took with Patience, as submitting to the Hand of God, glorifying their Creator in Heaven, and willingly bearing his Crosses on Earth.

But at last these wicked Women growing still more malicious and revengeful, his Family were more sensible of their, wicked Dispositions: For first his eldest Son, Henry Lord Rosse, was taken sick after a strange Manner, and in a little time died; and after Francis Lord Ross was severely tormented by them, and inhumanly tortured by a strange Sickness: And presently after the Lady Catharine was set upon by their devilish Practices, and very frequently in Danger of her Life, in strange and unusual Fits. And as they confessed, both the Earl and his Countess were so bewitched, that they should have no more Children. Yet the Earl attended his Majesty both at Newmarket and Whitehall, bearing his Loss with a great deal of Patience, and little suspecting it proceeded from Witchcraft, 'till God Almighty would suffer them no longer to go on in their Wickedness, but bring them to Shame for their wicked and villanous Practices.

About Christmas they were apprehended and carried to Lincoln Jayl, after due Examination before sufficient Justices and discreet Magistrates. Joan Flower, before her Conviction, called for Bread and Butter, and wished it might never go through her if she were guilty of the Matter she was accused of; and upon mumbling of it in her Mouth she never spoke more, but fell down and died as she was carried to Lincoln Jayl, being extremely tormented both in Soul and Body, and was buried at Ancaster.

When the Earl heard of their Apprehension he made haste down with his Brother Sir George, and sometimes examining them by themselves, and sometimes employing others, he referred them to their Tryal, before the Judges at Lincoln, where they were convicted of Murder, and executed the 11th of March.

To demonstrate the Justice of their Suffering, and the horrible Practices they were guilty of; we shall subjoin their own Examinations and Evidences against them selves, which apparently discover their ill Practice of that abominable Art of Witchchraft.

The Examination of Anne Baker of Bottesford in the County of Leicester Spinster, taken March the First 1618, by the Right Honourable Francis Earl of Rutland, Sir George Manners, Knight, two of his Majesty's Justices of the Peace for the County of Lincoln, and Samuel Flemming Doctor of Divinity, one of his Majesty's Justices of the Peace for the County of Leicester.

SHE says that there are four Colours of Planets, Black, Yellow, Green and Blue, and that Black is always Death; and that she saw the Blue Planet strike Thomas Fairborn, the eldest Son to William Fairborn of Bottesford aforesaid, by the Pinfold there, in which Time the said William Fairborn beat her and broke her Head, whereupon the said Thomas Fairborn did mend; and being asked who sent that Planet, she answered it was not I.

    She said further, That she saw a Hand appear unto her, and that she heard a Voice in the Air say to her, Anne Baker save thy self, for to Morrow thou and thy Master must be slain; and the next Day she and her Master were in a Cart together, and suddenly she saw a Flash of Fire, and said her Prayers, and the Fire went away, and presently after a Crow came and picked upon her Cloaths, and she said her Prayers again, and bade the Crow go to whom he was sent, and the Crow went unto her Master, and did beat him to Death, and she with her Prayers recovered him to live, but he was sick a Fortnight after, and saith, That if she had not had more Knowledge than her Master, both he and she and all the Cattle had been killed.

    Being examined about a Child of Anne Stannidge, which she was suspected to have bewitched to Death, she said, the said Anne Stannidge delivered her Child into her Hands, and that she laid it upon her Skirt, but did not Harm to it: And being charged by the Mother of the Child, that upon the Burning of the Hair, and the Pairing of the Nails of the said Child, the said Anne Baker came in and sat her down, and for the Space of an Hour could say nothing; she confesses that she came into the House of the said Anne Stannidge in great Pain, but did not know of the

Burning of the Child's Hair and Nails, but said she was so sick that she did not know whether she went.

Being charged that she bewitched Elizabeth Hough, the Wife of William Hough to death, because she made her angry for giving her Alms of her second Bread; she confesses that she was angry, and said that she might have given her of her better Bread, for she had gone too often of her Errands, but she confessed no more.

She confess'd that she came to Joan Gill's House, her Child being sick, and that she was entreated to look on the Child, and he tell her whether it was fore-spoken or no; and the said it was fore-spoken, but when the Child died she could not tell.

And being asked concerning Nortley carrying his Child home to his own House, where the said Anne Baker was; she asked him who gave the Child that Loaf, and he told her Anthony Gill, to whom she said, he might have had a Child of his own, if he would have sought in Time for it, which Words she confessed she did speak.

Being blamed by Henry Mills after this Manner, a Fire set on you, I have had two or three ill Nights; she answered, You should have let me alone then; and this she confess'd.

The said Anne Baker, March the 2d, confess'd before Doctor Flemming, that about three Years ago she went into Northamptonshire, and that at her coming back again, one Peak's Wife, and Dennis's Wife of Beloyre told her that my Lord Henry was dead, and that there was a Glove of the said Lord's buried in the Ground; and as the Glove did rot and waste, so did the Liver of the said Lord rot and waste.

Further she said, March the Third, before Sir George Manners, Knight, and Samuel Flemming Doctor of Divinity, that she had a Spirit which had the Shape of a white Dog, which she called her good Spirit.

Samuel Flemming, Test.

The Examination of Joan Willimot, taken the 28th of February, in the 16th Year of the Reign of our Lord James over England, King, &c. and over Scotland the 52d, before Alexander Amcots, Esq; one of his Majesty's Justices of the Peace of the said Parts and County.

SHE confesses that Joan Flower told her that my Lord of Rutland had dealt badly with her, and that they had put away her Daughter; and that though she could not have her Will of my Lord himself, yet she had spied my Lord's Son, and had stricken him to the Heart; and she says that my Lord's Son was stricken with a white Spirit, and that she can cure some that send unto her; and that some reward her for her Pains, and of some she taketh nothing.

She further says, that on Friday Night, her Spirit came to her and told her, that there was a bad Woman at Deeping who had given her Soul to the Devil; and that her said Spirit did then appear unto her in a more ugly Form than it had done formerly; and that it urged her much to give her something, though it was but a Piece of her Girdle, and told her that it had taken a great deal of Pains for her; but she says that she would give it nothing, and told it that she had sent it to no place, but only to see how my Lord Ross did, and that her Spirit told her that he would do well.

The Examination of the said Joan Willimot, taken the second Day of March, before the said Alexander Amcots.

BEING examined, she said That she had a Spirit which she called to duty, which was given to her by William Beary of Lingholm in Rutlandshire, whom she served three Years; and that her Master, when he gave it to her, desired her to open her Mouth, and he would blow into her a Fairy which would do her good; and that she opened her Mouth; and that he did blow into it; and that presently after there came out of her Mouth a Spirit, which stood on the Ground in the Form of a Woman, and enquired about her Soul, which she promised to list at her Master's Desire. She further confessed, that she never hurt any Body, but helped several that sent for her, which were strucken or fore-spoken; and that her Spirit came weekly to her, and would tell her of several that were stricken and fore-spoken. And she says, That the Use she had of the Spirit, was to know how those did whom she had undertaken to mend, and that she helped them by certain Prayers which she used, and not by her own Spirit; neither did she employ her Spirit in any thing, but to bring her Word how those did whom she had undertaken to cure.

And she further says, That her Spirit came to her last Night in the Form of a Woman, mumbling, but she could not tell what it said; and being asked whether she was not in a Dream, or Slumber when she thought she saw it; she said, No, and that she was as much awake as at that present.

Alexander Amcots,
Thomas Robison, Test.

The Examination of Joan Willimot of Goodby in the County of Leicester, Widow, taken the 17th of March by Sir Henry Hastings, Knight, and Samuel Flemming Doctor of Divinity, Two of his Majesty's Justices of the Peace of the said County.

SHE confessed that she told one Cook's Wife of Stathorne in the said County, Labourer, that John Patchett might have had his Child alive, if he would have sought out for it in Time, and if it were not Death stricken in her Ways; and that Patchett's Wife had an evil Thing within her, which should make an end of her, and that she knew by her Girdle.

    She said further, That Gamaliel Greete of Waltham in the said County Shepherd, had a Spirit like a white Mouse put into him, in his Swearing; and that if he did look upon any Thing with an Intent to hurt, he could hurt; and that he had a Mark on his left Arm, which was cut away; and that her own Spirit told her all this before it went from her.

    She said further, That Joan Flower, Margaret Flower and she, met about a Week before Joan Flower's Apprehension in Blackborrow Hill, and went from thence home to the said Joan Flower's House; and there she saw two Spirits, one like a Rat, and the other like an Owl; and that one of them sucked under her right Ear, as she thought; and the said Joan told her, that her Spirits did say, that she would neither be hang'd nor burnt.

    Further she saith, That the said Joan Flower took up some Earth and spat upon it, and worked it with her Finger, and put it up into her Purse, and said, Though she could not hurt the Lord himself, yet she had sped his Son which is dead.

H. Hastings,
Sam. Flemming.

The Examination of Ellen Green of Stathorne in the County of Leicester, taken the 17th of March, by Sir Henry Hastings, Knight, and Samuel Flemming Doctor of Divinity, Justices of the Peace for the said County.

SHE says, that Joan Willimot of Goodby came about six Years since to her in the Woods, and perswaded her to forsake God, and to betake her self to the Devil, and she would give her two Spirits, to which she gave her Consent; upon which Joan Willimot called two Spirits, one in the Likeness of a Kitlin, and the other of a Moldwarp; the first, the said Willimot called Puss, the other Hiffehiffe, and they presently came to her; and then she departing left them with the said Green, and they leaped upon her Shoulder, and the Kitlin sucked under her right Ear on her Neck, and the Moldwarp on her left Side in the like Place.

After they and sucked her she sent the Kitlin to a Baker of that Town, whose Name she remembered not, who had called her Witch and stricken her, and bid her Spirit go and bewitch him to death; the Mold warp she bid go to Anne Dawes of the same Town and bewitch her to death, because she had called her Witch, Whore and Jade, &c. and in a Fortnight's Time they both died.

And the said Ellen Green further said, That she sent both her Spirits to Stonesby, to one Willison a Husbandman, and Robert Williman a Husbandman's Son, and bid the Kitlin go to Willison and bewitch him to death, and the Moldwarp to the other and bewitch him to death, which they did, and within ten Days they died. These Four were bewitched whilst the said Green lived at Waltham.

About three Years since, the said Green removed thence to Stathorne where she now dwelt. Upon a Difference between the said Willimot, and the Wife of John Pacchet of Stathorne, Yeoman; the said Willimot called her the said Green to go and touch the said John Pacchet's Wife and her Child, which she did accordingly, touching the said John Pacchet's Wife in her Bed, and the Child in the Nurse's Arms, and then sent her Spirits to bewitch them to death, which they did, and the Woman lay languishing for a Month and more, but the Child died the next Day after she was touched.

And she further confessed, That the said Joan Willimot had a Spirit sucking on her, under the left Flank, like a white Dog: And she said further, That she saw the same sucking on her, last Barley Harvest, being then at John Willimot's House.

And as to her self the said Ellen Green further says, That she gave her Soul to the Devil to have the said Spirits at command; for a Confirmation of which, she suffered them to suck her always, as above-mentioned, about the Change and Full of the Moon.

H. Hastings,
Sam. Flemming.

The Examination of Philip Flower, Sister of Margaret Flower, and Daughter of Joan Flower, before Sir William Pelham, and Mr. Butler Justices of the Peace, Feb. 4. which was brought in at the Assizes, as Evidence against her Sister Margaret.

SHE said, that her Mother and Sister bore Malice to the Earl of Rutland, his Countess and their Children, because her Sister Margaret was put out of the Lady's Service as Laundress, and exempted from other Services about the House; whereupon her Sister, by her Mother's Command, brought from the Castle the Right-Hand Glove of the Lord Henry Rosse, which she delivered to her Mother, who presently rubbed it on the Back of her Spirit Rutterkin, and then put it into hot boiling Water; afterwards she pricked it often, and buried it in the Yard, wishing the Lord Rosse might never thrive; and so her Sister Margaret continued with her Mother, where she often saw the Cat Rutterkin leap on her Shoulder, and suck her Neck.

  She further confessed, That she heard her Mother often curse the East and his Lady, and upon that would boil Feathers and Blood together, using many devilish Speeches and strange Gestures.

The Examination of Margaret Flower, Sister of Philip Flower, about the 22d of January, 1618.

SHE confessed, That about four or five Years since, her Mother sent her for the Right-hand Glove of Henry Lord Rosse; and afterwards her Mother bid her go again to the Castle of Beaver, and bring down the Glove or some other Thing of Henry Lord Rosse; and then she asked, for what? Her Mother answered, to hurt my Lord Rosse; upon which she brought down a Glove, and delivered the same to her Mother, who stroked Butterkin her Cat with it, after it was dipped in hot Water, and so pricked it often; after which Henry Lord Rosse fell sick in a Week, and was much tormented with the same.

She further said, That finding a Glove above two or three Years since, of Francis Lord Rosse, on a Dung-hill, she delivered it to her Mother, who put it into hot Water, and afterwards took it out and rubed it on Butterkin the Cat, and bid him go upwards; and after her Mother buried it in the Yard, and said a Mischief light on him, but he will mend again.

She further confessed, That her Mother and she and her Sister agreed together to bewitch the Earl and his Lady, that they might have no more Children; and being asked the Cause of their Malice and Ill-will, she said, that about four Years since, the Countess taking a Dislike to her, gave her forty Shillings, a Bolster and a Matress,

Page 214

and bad her lie at home, and come no more to dwell at the Castle, which she not only took ill, but grudged it in her Heart very much, swearing to be reveng'd. After this her Mother complained to the Earl against one Peake, who had offered her some Wrong, wherein she perceived that the Earl took not her Part, as she expected; which Dislike, with the rest, exasperated her the more against him, so that she waited for an Opportunity of Revenge; upon which she took Wool out of the Matress, and a Pair of Gloves which were given her by Mr. Vavasor, and put them into warm Water, mingling them with some Blood, and stirring it together, then she took the Wool and Gloves out of the Water, and rubbed them on the Belly of Butterkin the Cat, saying the Lord and the Lady would have more Children, but it would be long first.

She further confessed, That by her Mother's Command, she brought to her a Piece of a Hankerchief of the Lady Catherine's, the Earl's Daughter, and her Mother put it into hot Water, and then taking it out, rubbed it upon Rutterkin, bidding him fly and go; whereupon Rutterkin whined and cried Mew; upon which she said Rutterkin had no Power of the Lady Catherine to hurt her.

The Examination of Philip Flower the 25th of February 1618, before Francis Earl of Rutland, Francis Lord Willoughby of Ersby, Sir George Manners, and Sir William Pelham.

SHE confessed, that she had a Spirit sucking on her in the Form of a white Rat, which keeps to her left Breast, and hath done so this three or four Years; and as to her Agreement betwixt her Spirit and her self, she confessed that when it came first to her, she gave her Soul to it, and it promised her to do her good, and cause Thomas Sympson to love her, if she would suffer it to suck her, which she agreed to; and so the last Time it sucked was on Tuesday at Night, the 23d of February.

The Examination of Margaret Flower at the same Time, &c.

SHE confessed, That she had two familiar Spirits sucking on her; the one White, the other Black spotted: The White sucked under her lest Breast, and the Black spotted within the inward Parts of her Secrets. When she first entertained them, she promised them her Soul, and they covenanted to do all things which she commanded them, &c.

She further saith, That about the 30th of January last past, being Saturday, four Devils appeared to her in Lincoln Jayl, at eleven or twelve a-Clock at Midnight: The one stood at her Bed's Feet, with a black Head like an Ape, and spoke to her, but what, she could not well remember; at which she was very angry, because he would speak no plainer, or let her understand his Meaning; the other three were Rutterkin, Little Robin and Spirit, but she never mistrusted them, nor suspected her self till then.

There is another Examination of the said Margaret Flower, taken the Fourth of February, to this Effect.

Being asked what she knew concerning the Bewitching of the Earl of Rutland, his Wife and Children, she said, that it was true, that her self, her Mother and Sister were all displeased at him, especially with the Countess, for turning her out of Service; upon which, four Years agoe, her Mother commanded her to go to the Castle, and bring her the Right-hand Glove of the Lord Henry Rosse, the Earl's eldest Son; which Glove she found on the Rushes in the Nursery, and delivered the same to her Mother, and put it into hot Water, prick'd it often with her Knife, and then took it out of the Water and rubbed it upon Rutterkin, bidding him height and go, and do some Hurt to Henry Lord Rosse; whereupon he fell sick and soon after died, which her Mother hearing of said it was well; but after she had rubbed the Glove on Rutterkin, the Spirit, she threw it into the Fire and burnt it.

These Examinations were taken and carefully preserved, as Evidence against them: And when the Judges came to Lincoln, about the First of March, being Sir Henry Hobbert, Lord Chief Justice of the Common-Pleas, and Sir Edward Brombley one of the Barons of the Exchequer, they were presented to them, who both wondered at the Wickedness of those Persons, and were amazed at their horrible Contracts with the Devil to damn their own Souls.

And though the Right Honourable the Earl of Rutland had sufficient Cause of Grief for the Loss of his Children, yet he could not but be amazed at their Wickedness and horrible Contracts, hearing them exclaim against the Devil for deluding them, and now breaking his Promise, when they stood most in need of his Help. And notwithstanding all these Aggravations, yet this generous Nobleman urged nothing against them but their own Confessions, and left them wholly to the Censure of the Law, their own Actions and Confessions bringing them to deserved Death.

CHAP. VII.

Containing Histories of Visions, Apparitions, Spirits, Divinations, &c.

IT is reported of Melampus, Tiresias, Thales, and Apollonius Tyanæus, that they understood the Language of Birds: The latter of them sitting amongst his Friends, seeing a great many Sparrows upon a Tree, and another coming in chirping amongst the rest, told them that it told its Fellows that there was a Sack of Wheat spilt in such a Place near the City, and they going to see found it true. And it is said of Democritus, that he could name the Birds, whose Blood being mixed together would produce a Serpent; of which whosoever should eat would understand the Voices of Birds. Hermes says, That whoever goes to catch Birds on a certain Day of the Calends of November, and boils the first Bird they catch with the Heart of a Fox, that all that eat of that Bird should understand the Voices of Birds and all other Creatures.

It is also reported of Rabbi Johena, the Son of Jochabod, that after a certain Manner he enlightened a rude Country-man, called Eleazer; being altogether illiterate; so that being encompassed about with a sudden Brightness, he unexpectedly preached such high Mysteries of the Law to an Assembly of wise Men, that he did even astonish all that were near him.

The Sibyl in Delphos was wont to receive the Devil two Ways, viz. either by a subtil Spirit and Fire, which did break out of the Mouth of the Cave, where she sitting in the Entrance, upon a brazen three-footed Stool, dedicated to a certain Deity, was presently inspired and uttered Prophecies; or a great Fire flying out of the Cave, surrounded the Prophetess, and enabled her to prophesie, which Inspiration she also received as she sat upon a consecrated Seat, breaking forth presently into Predictions.

There was a Prophetess in Branchi which sat upon an Ex-tree, and either held a Wand in her Hand, given her by some infernal Deity, or washed her Feet, and sometimes the Hem of her

Garments in the Waters, upon which she was presently filled with the Spirit of Prophecy, and unfolded many Oracles.

In the Country of Thracia there was a certain Passage consecrated to Bacchus, from whence Predictions and Oracles were wont to be given, the Priors of whose Temples having drank Wine abundantly, did strange Things.

There was once at Pharis, a City of Achaia, in the Middle of the Market, a Statue of Mercury, where he that went to be informed, having fumed Frankincense, and light Candles which was set before it; and that Country Coin being offer on the right Hand of the Statue, whispered into the right Ear of the Statue, whatever he desired to know, and presently his Ears being stopped with both his Hands, made what Haste he could from the Market-place; which when he was past, his Ears being open, the first Voice he heard from any Man was observed for an Oracle.

Zoroastres, the Father and Prince of the Magicians, was said to attain to the Knowledge of natural Things as well as divine, by twenty Years Solitude, when he wrote and did very strange Things concerning the Art of Divining and Sooth-saying.

Simon Magus, who was the Prince of Hereticks, and the Father of the first Heresies after Jesus Christ, giving himself out to be a great one, taught that himself was he, who should appear to the Jews as the Son, and in Samaria he should descend as the Father, and to other Nations should appear as the holy Ghost. He set himself forth for a God, at least for the Son of a Virgin: He bewitched the People, with his Sorceries or Magick, to say, This Man is the great Power of God: And in Administration of his Magical Operations, they set up a Statue with this Inscription; To Simon the holy God. His Image was made after the Figure of Jupiter, and the Image of Salena, or Helena, his Harlot (whom he affirmed to be the first Conception of his Mind, the Mother of all, by whom, in the Beginning he conceived in his Mind, to make the Angels and Archangels) was made after the Figure of Minerva, and these they worshipped with Incense, Victims, Offerings and Sacrifices. Notwithstanding, this Magical Sorcerer imitated the

Christian Faith, and was baptized, supposing that the Apostles healed by Magick, and not by the Power of God; and suspecting the holy Ghost to be given by Magical Science, he offered Money for the Gift, which being denied him, he studied all Manner of Magick, so much the more, and to make himself seem so much the more glorious in the Emulation; and to make himself famous in his Contest against the Apostles, vented his Heresies, and boasted of his Sorcery. And instead of the holy Ghost he got him a Devil for a Familiar, which he said was the Soul of a slain Child, and that he had adjured it for his Assistance, in doing whatever he commanded. His Priests and Proselytes were also taught to use Exorcisms and Incantations, and Charms and Allurements; and had also their Familiars, and studiously exercised all manner of curious Superstitions and unlawful Arts.

Elymas, the Sorcerer or Magician, sought to turn away the Deputy from the Faith; Menander the Successor and Disciple of Simon Magus was possessed with a Devil, and being instructed with Demoniacal Power, was not inferior to the other in Diabolical Operations; and having attained to the Height of Magical Science, which he said he had from his Euvoja, and by her was taught, and gave it to others, deceiving and deluding Abundance by his prodigious Art. And this he said it was he founded his prodigious Heresies upon; affirming himself to be the Saviour sent from Olympus or Heaven, or from the invisible World, for the Salvation of Men: Teaching also, that the Angels, the invisible Operators of this World, cannot be otherwise bound, compell'd, or conquered by any, unless by learning the deceitful, or proving the experimental Part of the Magical Art, which he taught, and by receiving the Baptism which he himself delivered, which whosoever had been Partakers of, they should by it obtain everlasting Immortality, and die no more, but remain everlastingly happy by themselves or with him, and be ever free from old Age and be immortal.

Saturninus and Basilides were notorious Impostors in all Magical Arts, using Images, Incantations, Invocations, &c. They invented 365 Heavens, making one another by Succession and

Similitude, and the Lowest begetting the Creatures here below; and the Chief or Highest of them, which they call Abrafax or Abraxas, they pretend to have not only the Number of 365, but the Vertues of them all.

  Carpocrates, and his ear-marked Disciples, practised all manner of Magical Arts; used Incantations, Philtres, Paredrials, &c. They set up Schools of Magick, and taught prestigious Operations in publick, saying, That by Vertue of these they had got Dominion over Princes, and Fabricators of this World; and not only over them, but all that are made therein; teaching that those that will attain to their Mystagogie, may dare to do any Thing; Yes, and must do any filthy Thing, otherwise they cannot escape the Prince of this World, except by such secret Operations they pay their Debt to all; the Absolving of which Debt was, a wicked Coition of Men and Women, and an abominable Operation of Incantations, and other ill Practices.

  Marcus was very skilful in all Magical Arts, by which he seduced a great many Men and Women, making them believe he had got great Vertue from invisible and unknown Powers and Places: For feigning himself to say Grace over a Cup of White-wine, by his long Invocations and Incantations, he turned it to Red, or made it so appear, that it might be thought by that Grace he distilled his own Blood into the Cup, through that Invention; making those that stood by desirous to taste of that Cup, that the Grace the Magician invoked might distill upon them, or what the Magician called Grace. He had likewise a Devil his Paredrial or Assessor, by which he himself seemed to prophesie, and so many Women, as he thought to be worthy to partake of his Grace, he made to prophesie; especially he was very industrious about Women that were noble, rich, and well dressed; and thus he would flatter them and delude them. I wish that thou wouldst partake of my Grace, because the Father sees every Angel of thine before his Face always: Now the Place of thy Greatness is in us, and it's fit we should unite in one, receive from me, and by me Grace first, and be thou prepared as a Spouse, to entertain her Well-beloved, that thou may be as I, and I as thou: Place thou in thy Chamber the Seed of Light, and take from me thy Well-beloved, and receive thou him, and be received of him; behold Grace descendeth upon thee, open thy Mouth and prophesie. Thus she being enticed, seduced and puffed up, and her Heart beating and burning within her, out of a Hope or Presumption to prophesie; and after that, speaking any Thing vainly and boldy, she takes her self for a Prophetess, and returns Thanks to Mareus, who hath communicated his own Grace to her, and rewards him not only with her Wealth, but the Enjoyment of her self.

    To manifest further the wicked Designs and Practices of Magicians, and such Sort of Diabolical Actions, we shall add the following Relation of Simon Magus and St. Peter out of Ecclesiastical History. Simon Magus, by his Fascinations, having gained the Heart of Nero, by promising him Victory, Dominion, long Life and Safety, by his Art, was afterwards detected by Peter, and the Art he practised so much exposed, that he was scorned and derided, which moved him both to Malice and Envy. And though he knew Peter's Power in other Parts (for under Claudius Cæsar he was struck with Madness, having dealt maliciously against the Apostle in Judea, and wandered up and down) and coming to Rome he boasted, that he could raise the Dead: Upon which it happening that a noble young Man, a Kinsman of Cæsar's, died at that Time, to the Grief of all; most of them advised that an Experiment should be made, whether he could be raised again from the Dead. And though Peter was very famous for such Works, yet as yet the Gentiles had no such Faith; yet some of them, moved with the Excess of their Grief, sent for Peter and desired that Simon Magus might be sent for likewise; both of them being come, Peter bid Simon Magus raise him if he could, and if he could not, he would endeavour to do it by the Name of Christ. Simon proposed, That if he should raise the Dead, Peter should be put to death for opposing, so great a Power as his: And on the contrary, that if Peter did it, he should have the same Revenge upon Simon. Both being agreed to this, Simon drew near to the Deadman's Bed; and when he began to mumble his Charms, the dead Body began to move his Head;

upon which the Gentiles cried out, that he was already alive and spoke to Simon, and shewed a great deal of Indignation towards Peter, that he should affront so great a Power; upon which, says Peter, if the Dead is restored, let him rise, walk and speak: To which he adds, that this was only a Delusion; and that if Simon was called from the Bed-side no such Thing would appear, which was accordingly done, and then there appeared not the least Motion in the dead Man. Then Peter standing at a Distance, and praying earnestly, cried out with a loud Voice, Young Man arise, the Lord Jesus healeth thee, and presently he arose and walked, and spoke, and eat Meat. Then the People rose up to stone Simon; but Peter said, let him yet live, and see the Kingdom of Christ encrease. The Magician being inflamed with this Glory of the Apostles and his own Disgrace, summons up all the Force of his Charms, and told the People, that since he was so much affronted with a People that he had so much defended, he would leave the City. He then appointed a Day when he would fly away, saying, That the Heavens were open to him when he pleased; and upon the Day appointed he went to the Capitoline Mount, and casting himself from the Top of a Rock, he began to fly; upon which the People began to worship and wonder, saying, It was the Power of God and not of Men to fly with a Body, and that Christ himself did no such Thing: Whereupon Peter praying Christ to magnifie his own Power, by detecting the Vanity of such tempting Arts, Simon's Wings were forthwith clipt and he fell down head-long, and died in the Place, or soon after. Nero being concerned for the Loss of so good a Friend and a Familiar, persecuted Peter to Martyrdom.

  Cynops, a great Magician, opposed St. John, and inveighed against his Doctrine, detracting from the Miracles wrought in the Name of Christ, and defamed his Person, assisted by the false Accusations of Apollo's Priests: And provoking him to admire his Power, in raising the Dead out of the Sea (which were only Devils in the Form of Men) whilst he was diving himself to fetch up more dead Men, the Sea making a great Noise, with loud Acclamations of the superstitious bewitched

People; St. John praying, the Sea made a terrible Noise, and swallowed up Cynops amongst his Dead, so that he never appeared above Water again. He then commanded those Devils to depart thence to their own Place, having first confessed the mutual Compact or Agreement betwixt them and Cynops; and expelled Devils out of several Places, for which Domitian commanded him to be banished into the Island Pathmos.

Wardacheus King of Babylon being foretold by his Diviners of the great Danger and Loss which he should suffer in his War against the Indians, and being dejected, the Apostles Simon and Jude smiling told him, they had brought Peace into his Kingdom, and bid him not be afraid, for the Indians would be glad to make Peace with him. But the Magicians derided both what they said and themselves, and bad him not believe those vain Men, for it should be as they had said; but the Event proved contrary. Those Apostles were also derided by Zaroes and Arphaxat, two Magicians; but at the Hour of their Martyrdom, the Magicians were struck dead with Thunder and Lightning.

Maruthas Bishop of Mesopotamia being sent Embassador to Isdigerdes King of Persia, he was much honoured for his singular Piety, and be began to attend to his Doctrine. But the Persian Magicians fearing he should perswade the King to receive the Christian Faith, and envying him because he had cured the King of a Pain in his Head by his Prayers, which had proved too hard for all their Spells and Charms, they contrived to hide one under Ground who should presage and proclaim, as the King was at his Devotion, that he should be turned out of his Kingdom for giving Ear to a Christian Priest. Hearing this, though he had a great Esteem for Maruthas, he was inclined to remove him, rather than run so great a Hazard; but Maruthas discovering their Fallacy, he caused every Tenth Magician's Head to be cut off. Maruthas departed from Persia, but afterwards returned again, and then the Magicians began to play their Tricks, causing a noisome and poysonous Stink in the Place when ever the King and Maruthas met together.

All the Sophisters, Magicians, Necromancers, &c. gathered themselves together against St. Athanasius, alledging that nothing could be done in their Art 'till he was taken out of the Way, and excited Julian against him; and another Time accused him of the same devilish Art they made use of themselves.

Thus the Devil always makes use of these Instruments to bring about his Designs, and to oppose God Almighty. The Magicians pursued Daniel with Envy, Calumny and Treachery, before Cambyses, or Cyaxares, 'till they brought him to the Lyon's Den; yet when they had done the Devil's Work, God Almighty delivered Daniel and they were cast into it. Theoteclinus a Magician of Antioch, under Maximinus, by Magical Power, caused an Image of Jupiter to pour forth Oracles, such as served to exasperate the Emperor, and to continue the Persecution against the Christians.

Vitellius having commanded by his Edicts, that the Chaldeans, Magicians and Diviners, should depart the City of Rome, and be banished all Italy within the Kalends of October; upon that they set up an Imprecatory Libel, threatning that Vitellius Germanicus, the same Day of the Kalends should be no where in Being. And Domitian having decreed the Banishment of the Astrologers, they told him what Time he should die; and Ascletarion told him of his Death to his Face, at which Domitian demanded of him, what Death he should die himself, to which he answered, That he should be eaten up with Dogs, which happened accordingly, those Dogs being Devils. And Apollonius Tyanaus disputing at the Schools in Ephesus, stopped suddenly, with his Eyes fixed down, and a distracted Countenance, crying out (at the same Time that Domitian was slain at Rome) well done Stephanus kill the Tyrant; that Tyrant Domitian is even now wounded, slain and dead.

Pope Sylvester the Second of a Monk became a Magician, and insinuating himself into Familiarity with a Necromantical Saracene, stole from him a conjuring Book, and studying that Art, by the Devil's Assistance obtained the Popedom. As soon as he had arrived to that Dignity, he dissembled his black Art, under his holy Garments, but kept a brazen Head in a secret Place, from which he sought and received divining Answers: And enquiring of the Devil how long he should live in the Papal Dignity; he answered, That he should live long if he came not at Jerusalem. Now in the fourth Year of his Pontificate, as he was sacrificing in the Church of the holy Cross in Jerusalem at Rome, he was suddenly seized with a violent Fever, and then was convinced how the Devil had deceived him, and that he must die.

Cornelius Agrippa, in his Youth, wrote a Magical Book of occult Philosophy, but afterwards another of the Vanity of Sciences; yet towards his Death he said to his black Dog, away wicked Beast, thou hast utterly undone me. Roderick of Toledo hoping to find a Treasure, caused a Palace to be opened, which had been kept shut for many Years, where he found nothing but a Coffer, and in it a Sheet, with a written Prophecy; that after the Opening of it, Men like those painted in the Sheet, should invade Spain and subdue it; upon which the King being concerned, caused the Coffer and Palace to be shut up again.

Gyges living in all Manner of Felicity, would needs consult Pythian Apollo, if any mortal Man enjoyed more Happiness than himself. It was averred by a poor Arcadian, who lived contented in his own poor Cottage, that he was far more unhappy than he; upon which he would needs throw away his enchanted Ring, and after that fell into extream Misery.

A young Man living in Garioch, not far from Aberdeen, was haunted mightily with a spectrous Apparition of a beautiful Woman, inticeing him to Lewdness, which he discovered to the Bishop, who advising him to Fasting and Prayer, he was delivered from this Temptation.

A young Gentlewoman of the Country of Mar, suspected by her Parents, and examined severely, confessed, that a young Man kept her Company by Night, and sometimes in the Day; but how he came in or went out she could not tell: But one Day, having watched, they spied a horrible monstrous Thing in their Daughter's Arms; which a Priest, knowing the Scriptures and of honest Life, caused to vanish.

Immediately before the Destruction of Jerusalem, there was seen a Comet hanging over the Temple in the Similitude of a fiery Sword; and many Nights together there shone a Light about the Temple and Altar, as if it had been Day. A Heifer also ready to be sacrificed, brought forth a Lamb in the Middle of the Temple; and the brazen Gate divers Nights together, unlocked or opened of it self, and could not be shut again without a great deal of Difficulty. In the Clouds were suddenly seen, a little before Sunset, whole Troops of armed Men. In the Feast of Pentecost, the Priest entring into the Temple at Night to celebrate their accustomed Sacrifices, they first felt a Motion, then heard a Sound, and after that heard a Voice distinctly crying, Depart we hence. Four Years before, Jesus the Son of Ananias a Country Man, cried out in a Prophetical Spirit, the City being then in Peace and Plenty; a Voice from the East; a Voice from the West; a Voice from the four Winds; a Voice upon Jerusalem, and upon the Temple; a Voice upon the Bridegrooms, and the Brides; a Voice upon all the People. This enraged the Elders, who caused him to be punished; but neither Fear, not Stripes, nor Threats, nor Perswasions could influence him to alter his Voice; every Stripe, crying out, Woe to Jerusalem. At last, weary with punishing him, they gave him over as a Madman that knew not what he said; but he still continued the same Tune 'till the Beginning of the Siege, and then left off. But when the Fire was begun in the City and the Temple, going about the Wall, he began to cry again; Woe to the City, the People and the Temple; and Woe also to me; and so being struck with something that was slung at him, he died.

Spurina admonished Cæsar to take Heed of some Danger that was before him, which would not be deferred beyond the Ides of March. When the Day came Cæsar derided Spurina, saying the Ides of March are come, and yet he saw no Hurt; says the Augur, they are come indeed, but they are not past; before which Time the Conspiracy of Cæsar's Death took Effect.

Alaricus having besieged Rome, some heathenish People had sent for certain Tuscan Magicians, who confidently promised to make him raise the Siege; but Innocentius, then Bishop there, drove them out, thinking it better and safer for the City to be taken, than to be delivered by such devilish Means.

Gotschaltus and Wierus tell us, That a certain Woman, extremely troubled with sore Eyes, met with a Scholar, to whom she complained of her Infirmity, and desired his Assistance, promising to reward him; upon which he took a Piece of Paper, and wrote such Kind of Characters in it, as never were seen before, and underneath wrote the following Words in great Letters; The Devil pull out thy Eyes, and stop up the Holes with Dung. This he folded up and wrapped it in a Piece of Cloth, and tying it about her Neck, bid her have a great deal of Care it was not taken away, nor opened or read by any; all which she observed exactly, and her Eyes were cured. About a Year or two after, she let it fall, either by Chance, or was desirous to see what was contained in it; and the Charm being opened and read, and the cursed Contents understood and abhorred, it was thrown into the Fire; which being done, her sore Eyes returned as bad as before.

Nectanebus an Ægyptian King and great Magician, coming into Macedonia in King Philip Time, was so skilful in the Art of Magick, that he caused Olympias Philip's Wife, to dream that the should be carried to Jupiter Hammon, and should conceive a famous Child by him. Upon this Olympias sent to Nectanebus to learn what would become of her, since it was reported, that King Philip was inclined to leave her and take another; he told her that he received a Command from the Oracle as he came out of Æypt, to go and help a neglected Queen, whom Jupiter Hammon greatly loved and intended to embrace. The following Night he caused her to dream of the same, and caused the like Imagination in Philip, who was now absent in War: This made Olympias mightily long for Jupiter, and the next Day sent for Nectanebus again, and asked when the expected Time must be. He bid her adorn her Bed fit to receive so divine a Lover, and told her he would come in the Shape of a Dragon, with a Goat's Head and Horns. Hearing this she was much afraid; but he told her, that if she would make her a Bed hard by, he would secure her from all that Danger. At Night the Queen went to Bed, and as soon as all was silent, the Magician, by his Art, raised a great Noise, and caused an Apparition, and went to Bed to the Queen himself, and begot Alexander the Great.

A certain Ægyptian burning in Lust towards another Man's Wife, consults with a Magician or Sorcerer, how he might gain his Desire, who told him nothing could hinder but the mutual Love betwixt the Man and his Wife; upon which he hired the Magician to stir up Dislike betwixt them, which he did, by making the Woman appear to the Man, as if he had a shagged Mare in Bed with him.

A Paganish young Man in Gaza, loved a Virgin extremely that was a Christian, and all his Endeavours proving in vain, he went to Memphis, thinking to bring it about by Magical Art; where, after a Year's Attendance, he was instructed to put a Plate of Brass, with a portentous Figure under the Threshold where the Maid lived, and to recite certain Torments or Charms over it. Upon this the Virgin grew mad in Love with him, and did nothing but call for the young Man, Night and Day; but her Parents got her dispossessed of that Magical Fury.

Uter Pendragon coming into Cornwall, seeing Igrene, Wife of the Duke of that Country, he did all he could to prevail upon her, but could not: upon which he consulted Merlin, who using no small Charms, he altered the Face of the King so much in Appearance, that he had exactly the Features of Gonlois her own Lord; by which Means he soon violated the Lady's Chastity.

A Magical Monk in Spain was familiar with a Nobleman that had a fair Wife, who attempted her Chastity, but was repulsed; and upon his great and frequent Importunities, she acquainted her Husband, who consented he should be admitted again, and watched to trap him. At the Time appointed he came in a secular Habit and Equipage, yet she resolutely refused him; but the Night encouraging the Attempt, he endeavoured to force her: She resisted him and cried out, to alarm her Husband, and those that lay in Wait, but all in vain; for he had by Virtue of his Magick, charmed them all in a sound Sleep. As they struggled together, she spied a Dagger at his Back, and stabbing him with it, killed him. Then running into the Room where her Husband and the rest were, she found them so fast asleep, that all she could do could not awake them; and having none in the Family to help her or hear her, she went her self and cast the dead Carcass into the Street, which being found by those that passed by, the Matter was brought before the Corrigidor. The next Day the Prior of the Convent was desired to summons all his People together, who all came except the Gentleman who was dead; they knocked at his Chamber-door, but no Body answering, they broke open the Door, and there found a Torch burning very dimly in the Chimney; and neither the Husband, nor any of the Family could be awaked till that Torch was put out.

CHAP. VIII.

Of the Danger, Misery and Ruine of such at have favoured and consulted Magicians, &c. and the Punishments and Judgments that have fallen upon Magicians.

ANdronicus having made too severe an Edict, against Conjurers, and Necromancers; to retrieve the Ill-will he had got by it, he began to consult them himself; and enquiring about his Successor, the Magician making use of Water to play his Tricks in, he there saw, in Letters written backwards, (Si. for Is.) the two first Letters of his Successor's Name; signifying Isachius who slew him, and reigned in his Stead. Didius Julianus making the like Enquiry by a Glass, a Child looking in it, observed Julian's Slaughter, and the Succession of Severus. And Otho Sylvius was led on by his Diviners to Usurpation and Riot, and to kill himself desperately at the last. Maxentius likewise encouraged with Hopes of Victory, went on confidently, and so was vanquished and destroyed. Licinius also called together his Magicians and Necromancers, to enquire what should be his Success against Constantine, who foretold certain Victory. The Inchanters made Odes and Rhimes: The Augurs foretold Success and Victory by the Flight of Birds, and thus encouraged him to his Ruin and Confusion.

Italicus, a Christian Governour, having a customary Horse-race with a Pagan, came to Hilarion desiring his Prayers, because his Rival used sorcerous Imprecations to disable his Horses and animate his own. Hilarion thinking such an Occasion not worthy of Prayers, counselled him to sell his Horses, and give the Money to the Poor; but he answered it was a publick Custom, and that the other would not suffer it to be laid down; and that when they overcame the Christians they used to insult and domineer over them. Upon this, being importun'd both by him and others, he condescended to give him a Cup in which he used to drink, and bid him fill it with Water, and sprinkle his Horses with it, and so dismissed him: This was done, and he win the

Race, contrary to all Expectation; upon this Hilarion was looked upon as a Witch or Wizard by the Pagan Party, and punished.

Elianor Dutchess of Gloucester consulted so long with Wizards and Witches, 'till she came to be reckoned one her self, and died miserably.

In a Town within the Territories of Brunswick, they had hired a pied Piper to conjure away all the Rats and Mice, that troubled them very much; this he did by his Piping and Charming; but not being satisfied according to his Expectation, he piped and charmed again, and a 130 Children belonging to that Place followed him, whom he led to the Side of a Hill, and conjured them all into a gaping Cliff, so that both he and they were swallowed up, and never seen afterwards.

A Captain consulting with a Wizard about the next Day's Battle; was answered, the Day should be his, upon Condition he would not spare to kill the first Man he met in the Morning; which be performed accordingly, and got the Victory. Then returning home joyfully, he found to his Grief, that he had killed his own Wife, who out of her great Love, had come to him in Mens Cloaths, to take Part with him in that Day's Adventure.

Valerian, addicted to Predictions by Inspecting the Entrails of Men, Women and Children, was unfortunate in his Government, taken Prisoner by Sapor King of Persia, who used him as a Stirrup to get on Horseback, and afterwards caused him to be flayed alive.

One that had lost a Silver Spoon would needs go to a Magician to know the Thief; and it was agreed, betwixt the Parties, that he who had conveighed it away should lose one of his Eyes; and when he came home, he found that sad Mark inflicted on one of his little Children, that had carelesly laid it aside.

In the City of Como in Italy, the Official and Inquisitor having a great Number of Witches and Wizards in Prison, taking others with them, would needs urge them to shew them their Homages to the Devil, but were so beaten by him, that some of them died within fifteen Days; others renounced God, and vowed themselves Votaries to the Devil.

Lucrates seeing Pancrates an Ægyptian Magician do a great many Wonders, insinuated himself into his Friendship, and communicated all his Secrets to him. The Magician at length perswaded him to leave all his Family at Memphis, and to follow him alone; and after they came into their Inn, he took a Bar or a Broom, and wrapped it with Clouts, and by his Charms made it walk and appear like a Man, and made it serve them in several Respects, as in drawing of Water, &c. Then with another Charm he would turn it into a Bat, a Bar, or a Broom again. And one Day when Pancrates was gone abroad into the Market, Lucrates must needs imitate his Familiar, and dressed the Bar or Pestle, and muttered the Words, and commanded it to draw Water; and when it had drawn enough, commanded it to turn into a Bar or Pestle again; but it would not obey, but still drew Water, 'till he was afraid of drowning; then he took a Saw, and sawed the Bar in two, and then both Parts began to draw Water, and pour it in plentifully, 'till in comes Pancrates, and turned it into what it was at first, and so left his Fellow, and was never seen after of him.

John Faustus being among some of his Companions when they were half drunk, was desired to play some of his Tricks, which was to represent a Vine full of Grapes, as a great Novelty in the Winter Season. He consented to satisfy their Curiosity, upon these Terms, that they should keep Silence, and not stir out of their Places, nor offer to pluck a Grape 'till he bade them, otherwise it would be to their own Damage. The desired Sight appeared, and every one had his Knife drawn and hold of a Branch, but were not to cut 'till he spoke the Word. When he had kept them a while in Suspence, all suddenly vanished, and every Man appeared to have hold only of his own Nose, and ready to have cut it off, if the Word had been spoke.

Thraseus the Augur, telling Busyris the Ægyptian Tyrant, in a Time of Drought, that there was no other Way to procure Rain, but by Sacrificeing some Stranger to Jupiter, the King enquiring what Country-man he was, and finding him to be a Stranger, sacrificed him first.

A German being in Italy in the Wars, chose a Souldier that was a Conjurer to be his Mate, to shew him his Skill; the Circle being made, and the Imprecations express'd, the Spirit appeared in a most hideous Form, and being asked about the Success at Gowletta, confesses his Ignorance, and took Time to resolve it; and disappearing, left such a Terror and Stink behind, that they had like to have been poisoned with the Noisomness, and died for Fear.

But to recite the miserable and unfortunate Ends of Magicians, Necromancers, Sorcerers, &c. at large, would take up too much Time. Zoroastres the First of them was vanquished by Ninus, who burnt his Books: Some say that he himself was burned by the Devil, as he was Provoking him with his Magical Experiments. Simon Magus, as he would needs fly in the Air, had his magical Wings so clipped, that he fell down and broke his Neck. Cynops, as he went about to raise the Dead out of the Sea, was himself swallowed up, and died. Zaroes and Arphaxat were both burned by Fire. Chahebas died for Envy. Tullus Hostilius moving it to thunder, was strucken to Death himself. Nectanebus killed by his own Son. Ascletarian eaten up of Dogs as he went to Execution. Sempronius Rufus banished by Severus. Apuleius accused and condemned before Claudius Maximus Proconful of Africa, Amphiaraus swallowed up of the Earth. Aristæus was snatched away by an evil Spirit. Zito was fetch'd away quick by the Devil. Simon the blind Exorcist was slain by his own Wife possessed with a Devil. A Priest of Noremberg, who would needs conjure for a Treasure, and digging found a hollow Cave, in which was a Chest and a black Dog lying in it, where he no sooner entered, but the Cave closed up, and he perished in it. At Saltsberg a Charmer undertook to enchant all the Serpents within a Mile, which as he was a doing, a great old Serpent, bigger than the Rest, leaped upon him, wrapt his Tail about him, and drew him into the Ditch, where he was drowned. We might mention Hundreds of the like Examples; but these may be sufficient to shew what an ill End so ill a Master as the Devil brings his Servants to at the last.

CHAP. IX.

Containing a true and impartial Relation of the Confessions of three Witches.

The Information of Dorcas Coleman, the Wife of John Coleman of Biddiford aforesaid, Mariner, taken upon her Oath before Thomas Gist, Mayor of the Burrough, Town and Mannor of Biddiford aforesaid, and John Davie Alderman, two of his Majesty's Justices of the Peace within the same Burrough, &c. the 26th Day of July, Anno Dom. 1682.

THE said Informant upon her Oath says, That about the End of the Month of August, in the Year of our Lord God 1680, she was taken with tormenting Pains, Pricking in her Arms, Stomach and Heart, after a very violent Manner; upon which she desired one Thomas Bremincom to go to Dr. Bear for some Remedy for these Pains; and soon after the Doctor came to her.

When he came and saw her, he said it was past his Skill to ease her of her Pains, for she was bewitched.

She further said, That she continued after the same Manner ever since, more or less violently handled every Week. And when the said Susanna was apprehended upon the Account of Grace Barnes of Biddiford aforesaid, she went to see the said Susanna: And when the said Susanna was in Prison, she confessed to her, that she had bewitched her, and done her some bodily Harm by Bewitching her; and upon that she the said Susanna Edwards fell down on her Knees, and desired her to pray for her.

Thomas Gist, Mayor.
John Davie, Alderman.

The Information of Thomas Bremincom of Biddiford in the County aforesaid, Gent. taken upon his Oath before us, Thomas Gist, Mayor of the Burrough, Town and Mannor of Biddiford aforesaid, and John Davie, Alderman, Two of his Majesty's Justices of the Peace within the same Burrough, &c. the 26th Day of July, Anno Dom. 1682.

THIS Informant upon his Oath says, That about two Years agoe Dorcas Coleman, the Wife of John Coleman of Biddiford aforesaid, Mariner, was taken very sick; and in her Sickness, she apply'd her self to Doctor Bear for a Remedy for these Pains; and when the said Doctor Bear came to her, and saw how her Body was afflicted, he said it was past his Skill to relieve her, she being bewitched.

And he further saith, That after Dr. Bear left her, he the said Informant saw one Susanna Edwards of Biddiford aforesaid, Widow, come into her Chamber to visit the said Dorcas. And he further says, That as soon as Dorcas saw the said Susanna Edwards, she strove to fly in the Face of the said Susanna Edwards, but was not able to get out of the Chair she sat in. Then this Informant and John Coleman her Husband endeavoured to help her out of the Chair; upon which Susanna Edwards began to go backwards, in order to go out of the Room.

And he further says, That when she was almost gone out of the Room, the said Dorcas slided out of the Chair upon her Back, and strove to go after her. Upon that this Informant and her Husband endeavoured to lift her off the Ground, seeing her in such a sad Condition, but could not 'till Susanna Edwards was gone down Stairs.

And this Informant further says, That when her tormenting Pains were upon her, and when she could neither see nor speak, her Pains being so violent, he the said Informant hath seen her point with her Hand which Way Susanna Edwards was gone.

And he further said, That as soon as he was gone out of the Fore-door of the House where Dorcas lived, he saw the said

Susanna Edwards go the same Way, that Dorcas Coleman pointed with her Hand.

Thomas Gist, Mayor.
John Davie, Alderman.

The Information of John Coleman of Biddiford in the County aforesaid, Mariner, taken upon his Oath before Thomas Gift Mayor of the Burrough, Town and Mannor of Biddiford aforesaid, and John Davie Alderman, Two of his Majesty's Justices of the Peace within the same Burrough, &c. the 26th Day of July, Anno Dom. 1682.

THE said Informant upon his Oath says, That Dorcas Coleman his Wife hath been a long Time sick in a very strange and unusual Manner, and that he hath sought for Remedies far and near. He further says, That Dr. George Bear being advised with concerning her Sickness in his Absence whilst he was at Sea, the said Dr. Bear hath (as this Informant was told by his Wife, and his Uncle Thomas Bremincom, at his Return) said, That it was past his Skill to prescribe Directions for her Cure, because the said Dorcas was bewitched.

And he further says, That about three Months last past, his said Wife was sitting in a Chair, and being speechless, he the said Informant did see one Susanna Edwards of Biddiford aforesaid, Widow, come into her Chamber under a Pretence to visit her; at which Time the Informant's Wife strove to come at the said Susanna, but could not get out of the Chair; upon which the said Informant and Tho. Bremincom endeavoured to help her out of the Chair, and then Susanna Edwards went towards the Chamber-door; and when she was got to the Chamber-door, the said Dorcas Coleman slided out of her Chair upon her Back, and strove to come at Susanna, but was not able to rise from the Ground, 'till the said Susanna was gone down Stairs.

And he further says, That the said Dorcas hath continued in a strange and unusual Manner of Sickness ever since, with some Intermissions.

Thomas Gist, Mayor.
John Davie, Alderman.
Examined with the Original,
whereof this is a true Copy.
John Hill, Town-clerk.

The Information of Grace Thomas of Biddiford in the County aforesaid Spinster, taken upon her Oath the third Day of July, in the 34th Year of the Reign of our Sovereign Lord King Charles, by the Grace of God of England, Scotland, France and Ireland, Defender of the Faith, &c. before us Thomas Gist, Mayor of the Burrough, Town and Mannor of Biddiford aforesaid, and John Davie, Alderman, Two of his Majesty's Justices of the Peace within the same Burrough, &c.

THE said Informant upon her Oath saith, That upon or about the second Day of February, which was in the Year of our Lord 1680, this Informant was taken with great Pains in her Head, and all her Limbs; which Pains continued upon her 'till near the Beginning of August following, and then this Informant's Pains began to abate, and this Informant was able to walk abroad to take the Air; but in the Night-time she was in much Pain, and not able to take her Rest.

And she the said Informant further says, That about the 30th Day of September, now last past, she was going up the High-street of Biddiford, where this Informant met with Temperance Lloyd of Biddiford aforesaid, Widow; and she the said Temperance, did then and there fall down on her Knees to this Informant, and wept, saying, Mrs. Grace, I am glad to see you so strong again: upon which the said Informant asked her, Why dost thou weep for me? To which the said Temperance answered, I weep for Joy to see you so well again, as the said Temperance then pretended.

This Informant further says, That in that very Night she was taken very ill with sticking and pricking Pains, as if Pins and Awls had been thrust into her Body, from the Crown of her Head to the Soles of her Feet, and that she lay as if she had been upon a Rack: And she says further, That these Pains have continued upon her ever since, and that they are much worse in Night than in the Day.

And this Informant further says, That on Thursday the first Day of June last past in the Night, she, the said Informant, was bound and seemingly chained up, with all her sticking Pains gathered together in her Belly; so that on a sudden her Belly was swelled up as big as two Bellies, which caused her to cry out, I shall die, I shall die; and in this sad Condition she lay as though she had been dead for a long Space, which those Persons that were in the Chamber with her computed to be about two Hours.

And this Informant further says, That on Friday Night last, being the 30th Day of June, she was again pinched and pricked to the Heart, with such cruel thrusting Pains in her Head, Shoulders, Arms, Hands, Thighs and Legs, as if the Flesh would have been immediately torn from the Bones with a Man's Fingers and Thumbs.

And she says further, That she was almost plucked out over the Bed, and lay in this Condition for the Space of three Hours, as these that were in the Chamber told her. And this Informant further says, That upon the first Day of July, as soon as the aforesaid Temperance Lloyd was apprehended and put into the Prison of Biddiford, she, the said Informant, immediately felt her pricking and sticking Pains to cease and abate; and that she hath continued so ever since to this Time, but is still in great Weakness of Body.

And she further says, That she believes that the said Temperance Lloyd hath been an Instrument of doing much Hurt and Harm unto her Body, by pricking and tormenting of her, as this Information hath set forth.

Thomas Gist, Mayor.
John Davie, Alderman.

The Information of Elizabeth Eastchurch, the Wife of Thomas Eastchurch of Biddiford, in the County aforesaid, Gent. taken upon her Oath before us, Thomas Gist, Mayor of the Burrough, Town and Mannor of Biddiford, aforesaid, and John Davie, Alderman, two of his Majesty's Justices of the Peace within the same Burrough, &c. the Third of July, in the 34th Year of the Reign of our Sovereign Lord Charles the Second, Anno Dom. 1682.

THE said Informant upon her Oath saith, That upon the second Day of this instant July, the said Grace Thomas then lodging in the Informant's Husband's House, and hearing her complain of great pricking Pains in one of her Knees, this Informant see her Knee, and observed nine Places that had been pricked, and that every Place that had been pricked, seemed as if it had been pricked with a Thorn; upon which the said Informant, the second Day of July, did demand of the said Temperance Lloyd, whether she had any Wax or Clay in the Form of Picture, by Means of which she had pricked and tormented the said Grace Thomas; to which she answered, That she had no Wax nor Clay, but confessed that she had only a Piece of Leather which she had pricked nine Times.

Thomas Gist, Mayor.
John Davie, Alderman.

The Information of Anne Wakely, the Wife of William Wakely of Biddiford in the County aforesaid, Husbandman; taken the third Day of July, Anno Dom, 1682.

THE said Informant upon Oath says, That upon the second Day of July, she, by Order of the said Mayor, did search the Body of the said Temperance Lloyd, in the Presence of Honor Hooper, and several other Women; and upon Searching of her Body, she found in her secret Parts two Teats hanging near together, like a Piece of Flesh that a Child had sucked; and that each of these Teats was about an Inch long; upon which the Informant demanded of her, whether she had been sucked at that Place by the black Man? meaning the Devil.

She acknowledged that she had been often sucked there by the black Man; and that the last Time that she was sucked by the said black Man was the Friday before she was searched, which was the 30th Day of June last.

And this Informant further says, That she hath attended the said Grace Thomas about six Weeks now past; and that on Thursday last past, which was the 29th of June, in the Morning, she saw something in the Shape of a Magpye come at the Chamber Window, where the said Grace Thomas lodged; upon which this Informant demanded of Temperance Lloyd, whether she knew of any Bird that came and fluttered at the Window; to which she answered, That it was the black Man in the Shape of the Bird; and that she the said Temperance was at that Time down by Thomas Eastchurch's Door, being the House where Grace Thomas did lodge. Thomas Gist, Mayor. John Davie, Alderman. The like was deposed by Honor Hooper, Servant to Thomas Eastchurch, as appears by her Information, taken upon Oath the Day and Year abovesaid, before the said Thomas Gist, Mayor, and John Davie, Alderman, two of his Majesty's Justices of the Peace within the Burrough, Town and Mannor of Biddiford.

Thomas Gist, Mayor.
John Davie, Alderman.

Temperance Lloyd her Examination taken the third Day of July, in the 34th Year of the Reign of our Sovereign Lord Charles the Second, by the Grace of God of England, Scotland, France and Ireland, King, Defender of the Faith, &c. before us Thomas Gist, Mayor of the Burrough, Town and Mannor of Biddiford aforesaid, and John Davie, Alderman, two of his Majesty's Justices of the Peace within the same Burrough, &c.

THE said Imformant being brought before us by some Constables of the said Burrough, upon the Complaint of Thomas Eastchurch of Biddiford aforesaid, Gent. and charged upon Suspicion of having used some magical Art, Sorcery, or Witchcraft, upon the Body of Grace Thomas of Biddiford aforesaid, Spinster, and to have had Discourse or Familiarity with the Devil in the Shape of a black Man; and being demanded how long since she had Discourse or Familiarity with the Devil in the Likeness or Shape of a black Man; she says, that About the 30th Day of September last past, she met with the Devil in the Shape or Likeness of a black Man, about the Middle of the Afternoon of that Day, in a certain Street or Lane in the Town of Biddiford aforesaid, called Higher Gunstone-Lane; and then and there did tempt and sollicit her to go with him to the House of the said Thomas Eastchurch to torment the Body of the said Grace Thomas, which she at the First refused to do: but afterwards, by the Temptation and Perswasion of the Devil, in the Likeness of a black Man, she went to Thomas Eastchurch's House, and went up Stairs after the black Man, and confessed that both of them went in to the Chamber where the said Grace Thomas was; and that there they found one Anne Wakely, the Wife of William Wakely of Biddiford, rubbing and stroaking one of the Arms of the said Grace Thomas.

And the said Examinant does farther confess, That she did then and there pinch with the Nails of her Fingers the said Grace Thomas in her Shoulders, Arms, Thighs and Legs; and that after-wards they came down from the said Grace Thomas's Chamber into the Street together, and that there this Examinant did see something in the Form of a gray or braget Cat; and said that the said went into the said Thomas Eastchurch's Shop.

And the same Examinant further says and confesseth, being asked whether she went any more to the said Thomas Eastchurch's House; that the Day following she went again to the same House invisible, and was not seen by any Person, where she met with the braget Cat before-mention'd; and that the said Cat retired and leaped back into the said Thomas Eastchurch's Shop.

And being further asked when she was at the same Thomas Eastchurch's House the last Time, she said that she was there on Friday the 30th of June last, and that the Devil in the Shape of a black Man was there with her; and that they went up together into the said Chamber, where she found the said Grace Thomas lying in her Bed in a very sad Condition; notwithstanding which, she and the black Man tormented her again.

And she further confessed, That she had almost drawn her out of Bed; and that on purpose, that she might put an End to the said Grace Thomas's Life.

And she further says, That the black Man promised her, that no Body should discover her. And she further confesses, That the black Man did suck her Teats that she now hath in her secret Parts; and that she did kneel down to him in the Streets, as she was returning to her own House, and after they had tormented the said Grace Thomas, as above-mentioned. And being asked of what Stature the black Man was, she said he was above the Length of her Arm; and that his Eyes were very big; and that he hopped or leaped in the Way before her; and that he afterwards did suck her as she was lying down; and that when he sucked it was very painful to her; and afterwards he vanished quite out of Sight.

And she further confesses, That on the first Day of June last, whilst Mr. Eastchurch and his Wife were absent, she did prick and pinch the said Grace Thomas, the black Man assisting her, in her Belly, Stomach and Breast; and that they continued tormenting her so two or three Hours, with an Intent to have killed her.

And at the same Time she confesses, That she did see the said Anne Wakely rubbing and chafing of several Parts of Grace Thomas's Body; though the said Anne Wakely being present at the Time of her Examination says, That she did not see the said Examinant.

Thomas Gist, Mayor.
John Davie, Alderman.

WHEREAS the said Temperance Lloyd hath made such an ample Confession and Declaration concerning the said Grace Thomas, we the said Mayor and Justices were induced to demand of her some other Questions concerning other Witcheries which she had practised on the Bodies of several other Persons within this Town, viz. The said Examinant did confess, That about the 14th Day of March, which was in the Year of our Lord 1670, she was accused, indicted, and arraigned, for practising Witchcraft upon the Body of one William Herbert, late of Biddiford, Husbandman: And although at her Tryal for her Life, at the Castle of Exeter, she was there acquitted by the Judge and Jury; yet she now confesses, that she is guilty thereof, by the Perswasion of the black Man, and that she did prick the said William Herbert to Death.

Thomas Gist, Mayor.
John Davie, Alderman.

AND whereas upon or about the 15th of May, in the Year of our Lord 1679, she was accused before the present Mayor and Justices of the Town of Biddiford aforesaid, for practising of Witchcraft upon the Body of one Anne Fellow, the Daughter of Edward Fellow of Biddiford, Gentleman. And although her Body was then searched by four Women of the Town of Biddiford aforesaid, and the Proofs then against her not so clear and conspicuous, the said Mr. Fellow did not further prosecute against her; yet this Examinant does now confess, that the said black Man or Devil, or some other black Man or Devil, with her the said Examinant, did do some Bodily Hurt to the said Anne Fellow; and that thereupon the said Anne Fellow did shortly die, and depart this Life.

Thomas Gist, Mayor.
John Davie, Alderman.

WHEREAS we Thomas Eastchurch and Elizabeth Eastchurch his Wife, Honor Hooper and Anne Wakely, Yesterday, which was the Third of July 1682, did give in and deliver our several Informations upon our Oaths before Thomas Gist, Mayor of the Burrough, Town and Mannor of Biddiford aforesaid, and John Davie, Alderman, two of his Majesty's Justices of the Peace for the same Burrough, &c. of Biddiford, against Temperance Lloyd of Biddiford aforesaid, Widow, for using and practising of Witchcraft upon the Body of Grace Thomas of the same Town Spinster, as by our several Examinations it doth and may appear. But because we were dissatisfied in some Particulars, about a Piece of Leather which the said Temperance had confessed of unto the said Elizabeth Eastchurch, in such Manner as is mentioned in the said Elizabeth Eastchurch's Examination; and we conceiving there might be some Enchantment used in or about the Leather, therefore upon this fourth Day of June, we, with the Leave and Approbation of the said Mr Gist, Mayor, did bring the said Temperance in the Parish-church of Biddiford aforesaid, in the Presence of Mr. Michael Ogilby, Rector of the same Parish-church, and divers other Persons, where the said Temperance was asked, by the said Mr. Ogilby, how long since the Devil did tempt her to do Evil.

  Whereupon she the said Temperance did say and confess, that about twelve years ago she was tempted by the Devil to be instrumental to the Death of William Herbert named in her said Examination; and that the Devil did promise her that she should live well and do well: And she did then also confess, that she was thereupon an Instrument of the Death of the said William Herbert. And as to the said Grace Thomas, she further said and confessed, That on Friday was Sevenight, which was the 29th of June last, she the said Temperance came into the said Thomas Eastchurch's Shop in the Form and Shape of a Cat, and fetched out of the same Shop a Puppit or Picture, commonly called a Child's Baby, and that she carried the same up into the Chamber where the said Grace Thomas lodged, and left it about the Bed where she the said Grace lay, but would not confess that she had pricked any Pins in the said Puppit or Baby Picture, though she was asked that Question particularly by Mr. Ogilby. Also the said Temperance did then and there confess, that she was the Cause of the Death of the said Anne Fellow, the Daughter of Edward Fellow mentioned in her Examination. She also then confessed, That she was the Cause of the Death of one Jane Dalbyn, the late Wife of Simon Dalbyn of Biddiford Mariner, by pricking her in one of her Eyes, which she performed so secretly, that she was never discovered nor punished for the same. Also the said Temperance Lloyd did confess and declare, that she did bewitch unto Death one Lydia Burman of Biddiford aforesaid Spinster, because she had been a Witness against her the said Temperance, at her Tryal for Life and Death at the Assizes, when she was arraigned for the Death of the said William Herbert, and had deposed, that the said Temperance had appeared unto her in the Shape of a red Pig, at such Time as the said Lydia was Brewing in the House of one Humphery Ackland of Biddiford aforesaid. Being further asked in what Part of the House of the said Mr. Eastchurch, or in what Part of the Bed, whereon the said Grace Thomas lay, she left the Puppit or Baby Picture; she says, that she would not, nor must not discover; for if she did discover the same, that the Devil would tear her in Pieces. Afterwards Mr. Ogilby desired the said Temperance to say the Lord's Prayer and her Creed, which she imperfectly performing, Mr. Ogilby gave her many good Exhortations, and so left her. In witness whereof we have hereunto set our Hands this 4th Day of July, in the four and thirtieth Year of the Reign of our Sovereign Lord Charles the Second, &c. July the 4th 1682, Sworn before us,

Thomas Gist, Mayor.
John Davie, Alderman.

The Information of Thomas Eastchurch of Biddiford in the County aforesaid, Gent. taken upon his Oath before us, Thomas Gist Mayor of the Burrough, Town and Mannor of Biddiford aforesaid, and John Davie, Alderman, Two of his Majesty's Justices of the Peace within the same Burrough, &c. the third Day of July, Anno Dom. 1682.

THE said Informant says upon Oath, That Yesterday, being the Second of July, he heard the said Temperance Lloyd say and confess, that about the 30th Day of September last, as she was returning from the Bakehouse with a Loaf of Bread under her Arm, towards her own House, she, the said Temperance Lloyd, did meet with something in the Likeness of a black Man, in a Street called Higher Gunstone Lane within this Town; and then and there the said black Man did tempt her to go to the said Informant's House, to torment one Grace Thomas who is this Informant's Sister-in-law; but she refused it saying, That Grace Thomas had done her no Harm: But afterwards, by the further Perswasion and Temptation of the black Man, she did go to this Informant's House, and that she went up the Stairs after the black Man, and confessed that both of them went into the Chamber where this Informant's Sister-in-law was, and that there they found one Anne Wakely, the Wife of William Wakely of Biddiford, rubbing of one of the Arms and one of the Legs of the said Grace Thomas. And this Informant further says, That the said Temperance also confessed, that the black Man did perswade her to pinch the said Grace Thomas in the Knees, Arms and Shoulders, shewing with her Fingers how she did it; and that when she came down the Stairs into the Street, she saw a braget Cat go into the said Informant's Shop, and that she believed it to be the Devil. And the same Informant heard Temperance Lloyd confess further, That on Friday Night last, which was the 30th of June, the black Man met her near her own Door, about Ten a-Clock the same Night, and there did tempt her again to go to this Informant's House, and to make an End of the said Grace Thomas; upon which she went along with the black Man into the

Chamber where the said Grace Thomas Jay. And she confessed further, That she did prick and pinch the said Grace Thomas again in several Parts of her Body, shewing with both her Hands how she did it; and that when she did it, the said Grace cried out terribly; and she confessed, that the said black Man told her, that she should make an End of her, the said Grace Thomas. And the said Temperance further confessed, That the black Man promised her, that no one should discover her or see her. She also confessed, That about Twelve of the Clock the same Night, the black Man sucked her in the Street in her secret Parts, she kneeling down to him; that he had blackish Cloaths, and was about the Length of her Arm; that he had broad Eyes, and a Mouth like a Toad, and afterwards vanished clear out of sight.

And the said Informant says, That he heard the said Temperance confess further, that about the first Day of June last, the said black Man was with her again, and told her, that the same Night she should make an End of Grace Thomas: And she further confessed, That that Night she had griped Grace Thomas in her Belly, Stomach and Breast, and clipt her to the Heart; and that the said Grace cried out extremely; and that she tormented her for the Space of two Hours; and that Anne Wakely, with several other Women, were then present in the Chamber, but could not see her the said Temperance, and that the black Man stood by her in the same Room also. And this Informant further says, That he supposed, that the said Grace Thomas, in her Sickness, had been afflicted through a Distemper depending on a natural Cause, and went to several Physicians, but that the said Grace could never receive any Benefit by the Medicines prescribed by them.

Thomas Gist, Mayor.
John Davie, Alderman.

The Information of William Herbert of Biddiford in the County aforesaid, Blacksmith, taken upon his Oath the 12th Day of August, in the 34th Year of the Reign of our Sovereign Lord Charles the Second, &c. before Thomas Gist, Mayor of the Burrough, Town and Mannor aforesaid, and John Davie, Alderman, Two of his Majesty's Justices of the Peace within the same Burrough, &c.

THIS Informant upon Oath says, That near or upon the second Day of February, in the Year of our Lord 1670, he heard his Father, William Herbert, declare on his Death-bed, that Temperance Lloyd of Biddiford aforesaid, Widow, had bewitched his said Father to Death. And his Father further declared to him, That he and the Rest of his Relations should view his Body after his Decease; and that by his Body they should see what Prints and Marks the said Temperance Lloyd had made upon him. And he further says, That his said Father did lay his Blood to the Charge of the said Temperance, and desired the said Informant to see her apprehended for the same, which was accordingly done; for which she was accused and acquitted at the Assizes.

And the Informant further says, That the fourth Day of July he went to the Prison of Biddiford, where the said Temperance was; she being then in the Prison upon the Account of the said Grace Thomas, and demanded of her whether she had done any bodily Harm or Hurt unto the said William Herbert deceased; to which she answered, surely William, I did kill thy Father. This Informant demanded of her further, whether she had done any Hurt or Harm to one Lydia Burman late of Biddiford, Spinster; to which she confessed, that she was the Cause of her Death: And being asked why she did not confess as much last Time she was in Prison; she answered, That her Time was not expired, for the Devil had given her greater Power, and a longer Time. The said Informant likewise heard Temperance Lloyd confess, that she was the Cause of the Death of Anne Follow, the Daughter of Edward Fellow of Biddiford, Gent. And also that she the said Temperance was the Cause of the Bewitching out of one of the Eyes of Jane, the Wife of Simon Dalbin of Biddiford aforesaid, Mariner.

Thomas Gist, Mayor.
John Davie, Alderman.
Examined with the Original,
whereof this is a true Copy.
John Hill, Town-clark.

The Information of John Barnes of Biddiford in the County aforesaid, Yeoman, taken upon his Oath before us Thomas Gist, Mayor of the Burrough, Town and Mannor of Biddiford aforesaid, and John Davie, Alderman, Two of his Majesty's Justices of the Peace within the same Burrough, &c. the 18th Day of July, Anno. 1682.

THE Informant upon his Oath says, That upon Easter Tuesday, the 18th Day of May, his Wife was taken with very great Pains, Sticking and Pricking in her Arms, Stomach and Breast, as if she had been stabbed with Awls, being so described to him by the said Grace, so that she thought she should have died immediately, and in such a Condition, she hath continued 'till this Day with tormenting and grievous Pains. And on Sunday last, which was the 16th Day of this Instant July, about ten a-Clock in the Forenoon, the Informant's Wife was again taken worse than before, so that four Men and Women could hardly hold her. And at the same Time Agnes Whitefield, Wife of John Whitefield of Biddiford Cordwinder, being in this Informant's House, and hearing some Body out at the Door, she opened it, where she found Mary Trembles of Biddiford, single Woman, standing with a white Pot in her Hands, as if she had been going to the common Bake-house: Upon which this Informant's Wife asked of the said Agnes Whitefield who it was that was at the Door; to which Agnes Whitefield answered and said, that it was Mary Trembles. Then the Informant's Wife replied, and said, that she the said Mary Trembles was one of them that did torment her, and that she was now come to put an End to her Life. Thomas Gist, Mayor. John Davie, Alderman. Devon. ss.} Biddif. ss.} The Information of Grace Barnes, Wife of John Barnes of Biddiford in the County aforesaid Yeoman, taken upon her Oath before Thomas Gist, Mayor of the Burrough, Town and Mannor of Biddiford aforesaid, and John Davie, Alderman, Two of his Majesty's Justices of the Peace within the same Burrough, &c. the 2d Day of August, Anno Dom. 1682. THE said Informant upon her Oath says, That she hath been very much pained and tormented in her Body these many Years last past, and hath sought out for Remedies far and near, and never had any Suspicion that she had any magical Art or Witchcraft practised upon her Body, 'till about a Year and a half ago, being informed by some Physicians that it was so; upon which she suspected Susanna Edwards of Biddiford aforesaid, Widow, because the said Susanna would often come to the said Informant's Husband's House, upon frivolous or no Occasions at all. And she further says, That about the Middle of the Month of May last, she was taken with very great sticking and pricking Pains in her Arms, Breast and Heart, as if several Awls had been pricked or stuck in to her Body; and was in great tormenting Pain for many Days and Nights together, with a very little Intermission. And that on Sunday the 16th Day of July last she was taken in a very grievous and tormenting Manner; at which Time one Agnes Whitefield, the Wife of John Whitefield of Biddiford, was in this Informant's Husband's House, who opening the Door and looking out, found one Mary Trembles of Biddiford, single Woman, standing before the Door: and thereupon this Informant asked of the said Agnes Whitefield, who it was that stood at the Door; who answered, that it was the said Mary Trembles: Upon which this Informant was very well assured, that the said Mary Trembles, together with Susanna Edwards, were the very Persons that had tormented her, by using some magical Art or Witchcraft upon her Body, as aforesaid.

Thomas Gist, Mayor.
John Davie, Alderman.

The Information of William Edwards of Biddiford in the County aforesaid, Blacksmith, taken upon his Oath, before us Thomas Gist Mayor of the Borough, Town and Mannor of Biddiford aforesaid, and John Davie Alderman, Two of His Majestie's Justices of the Peace within the same Borough, &c. the 18th Day of July, Anno Dom, 1682.

THE said Informant upon his Oath says, That on the Seventeenth Day of July instant, he heard Susanna Edwards confess, that the Devil had carnal Knowledge of her Body, and that he had suck'd her in her Breasts, and in her Secret Parts. And further, that he heard her, Susanna Edwards say, That she, and one Mary Trembles of Biddiford aforesaid, Single-woman, did appear hand in hand invisible in John Barnes's House in Biddiford; where Grace, the Wife of the said John Barnes did lye in a very sad Condition. And the said Informant further says, that he then also heard the said Susanna say, That she and the said Mary Trembles were at that Time come to make an End of her the said Grace Barnes.

Thomas Gist, Mayor.
John Davie, Alderman.

The Information of Joane Jones, the Wife of Anthony Jones of Biddiford, in the County aforesaid, Husbandman, taken up-upon her Oath before us Thomas Gist Mayor, and John Davie Alderman, the 18th Day of July, Anno Dom. 1682.

THE said Informant upon her Oath says, That on the 18th Day of July instant, she being present with Susanna Edwards of Biddiford aforesaid, Widow; John Dunning of Great Torrington, came in to see the said Susanna, which said John Dunning asked Susanna Edwards, How, and by what Means she became a Witch? To which she answered, That she never did confess before, but now she would. And she further says, That she heard the said Susanna Edwards confess to John Dunning, that she was once out gathering of Wood, when she saw a Gentleman coming near to her; upon which she was in hopes to have a Piece of Money of him. And this Informant further says, That the said John Dunning asked Susanna, Where she met with the said Gentleman? To which she answered, In Parsonage Close. And after John Dunning was gone, this Informant heard Susanna Edwards confess, That on Sunday the 16th of July, she, with Mary Trembles, and by the Help of the Devil, did prick and torment Grace, the Wife of John Barnes of Biddiford.

And this Informant further says, That she heard the said Susanna Edwards and Mary Trembles say and confess, That they did this present Day, being the 18th of July, torment and prick her the said Grace Barnes again. And further, that she heard the said Mary Trembles say to Susanna Edwards, 0 thou Rogue, I will now confess all; for it is thou that hast made me to be a Witch; and thou art one thy self, and my Conscience must Swear it. Upon which, Susanna replied to the said Mary Trembles; I did not think thou wouldst have been such a Rogue as to discover it. And she further says, That the said Susanna did confess, That the Devil did carry about her Spirit oftentimes: And that she heard the said Susanna further confess, That she did prick and torment one Dorcas Coleman, the Wife of John Coleman of Biddiford aforesaid, Mariner. And she further says, That she heard the said

Susanna Edwards confess, That she was sucked in her Breast several times by the Devil in the Shape of a Boy lying by her in her Bed, and that it was very Cold to her; and that after she was suck'd by him, the said Boy, or Devil, had the Carnal Knowledge of her Body four several Times. And she further says, That Anthony Jones, observing her the said Susanna to gripe and twinkle her Hands upon her own Body, said to her, Thou Devil, thou art now tormenting some Person or other. Upon which the said Susanna was displeased with him, and said, Well enough, I will fit thee. And at that present Time, the said Grace Barnes was in great Pain with Prickings and Stabbings unto her Heart, as she afterwards affirmed. This Informant further says, That one of the Constables and her Husband, with some others, was sent by Mr. Mayor, to bring the said Grace Barnes to the Town-Hall of Biddiford aforesaid, which they did accordingly; and as soon as they had led, and with much ado brought the said Grace Barnes into the Town-Hall, the said Susanna Edwards turned about and looked upon her said Husband, and presently this Informant's said Husband was taken in a very sad Condition as he was leading and supporting Grace Barnes up the Town-Hall Stairs before the Mayor and Justices, so that he cried out, I am now bewitched with this Devil, Wife; meaning Susanna Edwards, and presently leaped and capered like a Madman, and fell a shaking, quivering and foaming, and for the space of half an Hour like a dying or dead Man; and at last coming to his Senses again, he declared to this Informant, that the said Susanna Edwards had bewitched him. And this Informant further says, That she never knew her said Husband Anthony Jones to be taken in any Fits or Convulsions, but a Person of a sound and healthy Body, ever since he had been her Husband.

Thomas Gist, Mayor.
John Davie, Alderman.

The Information of Anthony Jones of Biddiford, in the County aforesaid, Husbandman, taken upon his Oath, before us Thomas Gist Mayor of the Burrough, Town and Mannor of Biddiford aforesaid, and John Davie Alderman, Two of His Majesties Justices of the Peace within the said Burrough, &c. the 19th Day of July, Anno Dom. 1682.

THE said Informant upon Oath saith, That Yesterday, whilst Susanna Edwards was in the Town-Hall of Biddiford, concerning the said Grace Barnes, he observed the said Susanna to gripe and twinkle her hands, upon her own Body, in an unusual manner; whereupon he said to her, Thou Devil thou art now tormenting some Person or other: Upon which the said Susanna was displeased with him, and said, Well enough, I will fit thee: And at that present time Grace Barnes was in great Pains, with pricking and stabbing to her Heart; as the said Grace did afterwards affirm. And this Informant further says, That one of the Constables and he, with some others, being sent by Mr. Mayor's Order, to bring the said Grace to the Town-Hall of Biddiford; The said Susanna turned about, and looked upon this Informant and forthwith he was taken in a very sad Condition, as he was coming up the Stairs of the Town-Hall, before the Mayor and Justices, insomuch that he cryed out, Wife, I am now bewitched with this Devil Susanna Edwards.

Thomas Gist, Mayor.
John Davie, Alderman.

The Examination of Mary Trembles of Biddiford in the County aforesaid, Single Woman, taken before Thomas Gist Mayor of the Burrough, Town and Mannor of Biddiford, and John Davie Alderman, Two of His Majesties Justices of the Peace within the same Burrough, &c. the 18th Day of July, An. Dom. 1682.

THE said Examinant being brought before us, and accused for Practising of Witchcraft upon the Body of Grace Barnes, the Wife of John Barnes of Biddiford aforesaid, Yeoman; was question'd by us, how long she had practised Witchcraft? Who said and confessed, That about Three Years last past, Susanna Edwards of Biddiford, Widow, informed her, that if she would do as the said Susanna did, that this Examinant should do very well: Whereupon she yielded to the said Susanna Edwards, and said she would do as the said Susanna did. And the said-Mary Trembles farther confesses, That the said Susanna Edwards did promise that she should neither want for Money, Meat, Drink, nor Clothes. And that, after she had made this Bargain with Susanna Edwards, the Devil in the Shape of a Lyon, came to her and lay with her, and had Carnal Knowledge of her Body. And that after the Devil had had Knowledge of her Body, he sucked her in her Secret Parts, and that his Sucking was so hard, which caused her to cry out with Pain. And she further confesses, That on Tuesday in the Easter Week, which was the 18th Day of May last, she went about the Town of Biddiford to beg some Bread, and met with the said Susanna Edwards in her Walk; who asked her, Where she had been? To whom she answered, That she had been about the Town, and had begged some Meat, but could get none. Upon which, she with the said Susanna Edwards, went to the said John Barnes's House, in hopes that there they should have some Meat. But the said John Barnes not being at home, they could get no Meat or Bread, being denied by the said Grace Barnes, and her Servant, who would not give them any Meat: Whereupon the said Susanna, and this Informant, went away from the said Barnes's House. Afterwards on the same Day, Susanna Edwards bid the said Informant go to Mr. Barnes's

House again, for a Farthing-worth of Tobacco. Upon this she went, but could not have any, which she told Susanna Edwards of; who then said, It should be better for her, the said Grace, she had let her have had some Tobacco. And she further confesses, That on the 16th Day of this instant July, she with the said Susanna, did go to the said John Barnes's House in Biddiford, and went in at the fore Door invisibly, into the Room, where they did prick and pinch the said Grace Barnes almost to Death; and that she saw John Barnes in Bed with his Wife on the innerside of the Bed.

And being further asked, how many Times the Devil had Carnal Knowledge of her Body, besides the Time above-mentioned, she confesseth, That the Devil had Carnal Knowledge of her Body Three other Times, and that the last of the Three Times was upon the said 16th Day of July, as she was going towards the common Bakehouse. And that at that Time she, with the help of the Devil, would have killed the said Grace Barnes, if she had not spilled some of the Meat she was then carrying to the Bakehouse.

Thomas Gist, Mayor.
John Davie, Alderman.

The Examination of Susanna Edwards, of Biddiford, aforesaid, in the County aforesaid, Widow, taken the Tenth Day of July, Anno Dom. 1682.

THE said Examinant being brought before us, and accused for Practising of Witchcraft upon the Body of Grace Barnes, the Wife of John Barnes, of Biddiford aforesaid, Yeoman, was asked, how long since she had Discourse or Familiarity with the Devil; and says, That about Two Years ago she did meet with a Gentleman in a Field called the Parsonage Close, in the Town of Biddiford; and that his Apparel was black; whereupon the Gentleman drawing near to her, she made a Curtesie to him, as she used to do to Gentlemen.

    Being asked what, and who the Gentleman she spoke of was, she answered, it was the Devil; and confessed, that the Devil asked her if she was a poor Woman; to whom she answered, that she was. And then the Devil, in the Shape of the Gentleman, told her, That if the would grant him one Request, she should never want Meat, Drink, nor Cloaths: Upon which she said to the Gentleman, or Devil, in the Name of God what is it I shall have? And upon that the Gentleman vanished quite away from her. And she further confessed, That afterwards there was something in the Shape of a little Boy, which she thinks to be the Devil, came into her House, and lay with her, and that he sucked her at her Breast. She confesses, That she afterwards met him in a Place call'd Stambridge-Lane, in the Parish of Biddiford, leading towards Abbottisham, which is the next Parish to the West of Biddiford, and that there he sucked Blood out of her Breast; and on Sunday, which was the 16th of July Instant, she, together with Mary Trembles, of Biddiford, single Woman, did go into the House of John Barnes, of Biddiford, Yeoman, and that no Body did see them; and that they were in the same Room where Grace, the Wife of John Barnes was, and that there they did prick and pinch the said Grace Barnes with their Fingers, and put her to great Pain and Torment, so that she was almost dead.

And she confesseth, That this Day she pricked and tormented her again, shewing with her Fingers how she did it: and confesses also, That the Devil did entice her also to make an end of the said Grace Barnes, and that he told her that he would come again to her once more before she should go out of Town. She confesses, That she can go to any Place invisible, and yet her Body will be lying in her Bed; and further, she says, That the Devil hath appeared to her in the Shape of a Lion as she supposed. Being asked, whether she had done any Bodily Hurt to any other Person, besides the said Grace Barnes, she confesses, that she did prick and torment one Dorcas Coleman, the Wife of John Coleman, of Biddiford aforesaid, Mariner, and says, That she gave her self to the Devil when she met him in Stambridge-Lane, as aforesaid. And says, that the said Mary Trembles was a Servant to her, as she was to the Devil, or Gentleman aforesaid, as she called him.

Thomas Gist, Mayor,
John Davie, Alderman.
Examined with the Original,
whereof this is a true Copy.
John Hill, Town-Clark.

The Substance of the last Words and Confessions of Susanna Edwards, Temperance Lloyd, and Mary Trembles, at the Time and Place of their Execution.

MAry Trembles being asked what she had to say, as to the Crime she was to die for, said, She had already said as much as she could say, and could say no more. Being asked in what Shape the Devil came to her, she said in the Shape of a Lion once. Being asked whether he offered any Violence to her, she said, Not at all, but frightened her, and did nothing to her, and that she cried to God, and asked what he would have, and he vanished. Being asked whether he gave her any Gift, or whether she made him any Promise, she said, No. Being asked whether he had any of her Blood, she said, No. Being asked whether he made use of her Body in a Carnal Manner, she answered, Never in her Life. Being asked whether she had a Teat in her private Parts, she said she had none; but the Grand Jury said it was sworn to them. Mr. H---- asking, whether the Devil was not there with Susan, when he was in Prison with them, and under her Coats? Says he, The other told me she was there, but is now fled; and that the Devil was in the Way when I was going to Taunton with my Son, who is a Minister. Says he, Thou speaks now as a dying Woman, and as the Psalmist says, I will confess my Iniquities, and acknowledge all my Sin. We find that Mary Magdalen had Seven Devils, and she came to Christ and obtained Mercy; and if thou break thy League with the Devil, and make a Covenant with God, thou mayest also obtain Mercy. If thou hast any thing to speak, speak thy Mind. Says she, I have spoke the very Truth, and can speak no more; I desire they may come and confess as I have done.

Then Mr. H---- asked Temperance Lloyd, whether she had made any Contract with the Devil? She said, No. Being asked if he had ever any of her Blood, she said, No. Being asked where he appeared to her first, and in what Shape, she answered, In a woeful Shape. Being asked if he had any Carnal Knowledge of her, she said, Never. Being asked what he did when he came to her, she said, He bid her go and do Harm. Being asked whether she did so, she said, She did hurt a Woman, much against her Conscience, he carried her up to the Door, which was open, and the Woman's Name was Grace Thomas. Being asked, what Cause she had to do her Harm? What Malice she had against her? Or had she done her any Harm? She answered, She never did me any Harm, but the Devil beat me about the Head grievously, because I would not kill her, but I did bruise her after this Fashion, laying her two Hands to her Sides. Being asked whether she bruised her till the Blood came out of her Mouth, she said, Yes. Being asked how many she destroyed and hurt, she said, None but her. Being asked, If she ever hurt any Ships or Boats, she said, She never did. Being asked whether it was she or Susan bewitched the Children; she said, she sold Apples, and a Child took an Apple from her, and the Mother took the Apple from the Child, for which she was angry, but the Child died of the Small-Pox. Being asked whether she knew Mr. Lutteril or his Confederates, and whether they or she bewitched the Child; she said, No. Being asked how she came to hurt Mrs. Grace Thomas, and whether she came through the Key-Hole, or whether the Door was open; she said, The Devil led her up Stairs, and the Door was open, and that was all the Hurt she did. Being asked how she knew it was the Devil, she said, By his Eyes. Being asked whether she had no Discourse or Treaty with him, she said, No; he said she should go along with him to destroy a Woman, and she told him she would not. He said, he would make me; and then the Devil beat me about the Head. Being asked why she called not upon God, she answered, He would not let me do it. Being asked whether she never rid over an Arm of the Sea on a Cow; No, Master, said she, it was she, meaning Susan. When Temperance said it was Susan, she said she lied, and that she was the Cause of her coming to die; for she said, when she was first brought to Goal, If she was hanged, she would have me hanged too; she reported I should ride on a Cow before her, which I never did. Then says Mr. H. to Susan Edwards, Did you see the Shape of a Bullock? At the first of your Examination you said, it was like a short black Man, about the Length of your Arm. Says she, He was black, Sir. Being asked if she had any

Knowledge of the bewitching of Mr. Lutteril's Child, or whether she knew a Place called Taunton Burroughs; she said, No. Then Mr. H. said Prayers, and when Susan mounted the Ladder, she said, The Lord Jesus speed me, though my Sins be as red as Scarlet, the Lord Jesus can make them as white as Snow, the Lord help my Soul. Then she was Executed.

  Mary Trembles said, Lord Jesus receive my Soul, Lord Jesus speed me; and then was also Executed. Temperance Lloyd said, Jesus Christ speed me well; Lord forgive all my Sins; Lord Jesus Christ be merciful to my poor Soul. Then said Mr. Sheriff to her, You are looked upon as the Woman that hath debauched the other two; did you ever lie with Devils? She said, No. Did you not know of their coming to Goal? She said, No. Have you any thing to say to satisfy the World? Says she, I forgive them, as I desire the Lord Jesus to forgive me. The greatest thing I did was to Mrs. Grace Thomas, and I desire I may be sensible of it, and that the Lord Jesus may forgive me. The Devil met me in the Street, and bid me kill her, and because I would not, he beat me about the Head and Back. Says the Sheriff, In what Shape and Form was he? Said she, In Black, like a Bullock. How did you know you did it, says he? went you in at the Key-Hole, or the Door; she answered, at the Door. He asked her, Had she no. Discourse with the Devil? Never, said she, but this Day Six Weeks. Said he, You were charged about Twelve Years since, and did you never see the Devil but this Time. Yes, said she, once before. I was going for Brooms, and he came to me, and said,

  This poor Woman hath a great Burthen, and would have helped me; and I said, The Lord hath enabled me to carry it so far, and I hope I shall be able to carry it further. Being asked whether the Devil never promised her any thing, she said, No. Then, says he, you have served a bad Master, who gave you nothing. Well, consider you are just departing this World, Do you believe there is a God? She said, Yes. Do you believe in Jesus Christ? She said, Yes, and I pray Jesus Christ to pardon all my Sins, and then she was executed.

CHAP. XI.

Giving an Account of the Tryals of several Witches, and of a very strange Apparition.

BEfore we proceed to give an Account of the Trials of the Witches, we shall premise a brief Narrative of an Apparition, which appeared to a Gentleman in Boston, his Brother being just Murthered in London. The Second Day of May 1687, Mr. Joseph Beacon, as he lay in his Bed about five a-Clock in the Morning, had a Sight of his Brother, who was then in London, which is a Thousand Leagues distant from that Place, he appeared in a Bengal Gown, which he usually wore, with a Napkin tied about his Head; his Countenance was very pale, ghastly and deadly, with a bloody Wound on one side of his Forehead. Brother, says Joseph, being very much frightened. To which the Apparition answered again, Brother. Then Joseph asked him, What's the Matter Brother? How came you here? The Apparition answered, Brother, I have been most barbarously and injuriously Butchered, by a debauched drunken Fellow, to whom I never did any Wrong in my Life. Upon which he gave a particular Description of the Murther, adding the following Words, Brother, this Fellow changing his Name, is attempting to come over into New England, in the Foy or Wild, I would pray you upon the Arrival of these, to get an Order from the Governour, to seize the Person whom I have now described, and then do you Indict him for the Murther of me your Brother, I'll stand by you and prove the Indictment, and then vanished. Mr. Beacon was very much surprized at this Apparition, and then gave an Account of it to several Persons.

At that time Mr. Beacon had no Account of any thing being amiss with his Brother from England; but the next June after he heard, that the April before, his Brother going in haste to call a Coach for a Lady in the Night, met a Fellow in Drink, with his Doxy in his Hand, who thinking himself affronted with his hasty Passage, immediately ran into a Neighbouring Tavern, and fetched a Fire-Fork from the Fire-side, and wounded Beacon in the Skull with it, in the same Place where the Apparition shewed the Wound. He languished of this Wound, and died the Second of May, about Five a-Clock in the Morning, at London. He who murthered him was indeavouring to escape, as the Apparition declared, but the Friends of the Person deceased, seized him, and prosecuted him, though his Friends saved his Life.

Having premised this Relation, we shall proceed to the History of several Trials before Judge Hale.

Rose Callender and Anne Duny, were severally Indicted, for bewitching Elizabeth Durent, Anne Durent, Jane Booking, Susan Chandler, William Durent, Elizabeth and Deborah Pacy, the Evidence which convicted them, standing upon several particular Circumstances.

First, Anne Durent, Susan Chandler, and Elizabeth Pacy, when they came into the Hall to give Instructions for drawing the Bills of Indictment, fell into strange and violent Fits, being unable to give in their Depositions during the whole Assizes. William Durent being an Infant, his Mother swore, That Amy Duny looking after her Child one Day in her Absence, confessed at her Return, that she had given Suck to the Child, though she was an old Woman; and when Durent expressed her Displeasure, Duny went away with Discontent and Menaces.

The Night after, the Child fell into strange and sad Fits: wherein it continued several Weeks. And Dr. Jacob advising her to hang up the Child's Blanket in the Chimney-Corner all Day, and at Night when she went to put it on the Child, if she found any thing in it, to throw it into the Fire without Fear; At Night when she went to put the Child in it, there fell a great Toad out of it, which ran up and down the Hearth. A Boy catched it, and held it in the Fire with a Pair of Tongues, where it made a horrible Noise, and flashed like Gunpowder, with a Report like that of a Pistol. Upon which the Toad was no more to be seen. The next Day a Kinswoman of Duny's told the Deponent, That her Aunt was all grievously scorched with the Fire, and the Deponant going to her House, found her in such a Condition.

Duny told her, She might thank her for it, but she should live to see some of her Children dead, and her self go upon Crutches. But after the burning of the Toad the Child recoverd.

This Deponent further testify'd, That her Daughter Elizabeth, being about Ten Years of Age, was taken after the same manner with the former, and in her Fits complained very much of Amy Duny, and said, That she appeared to her, and afflicted her, One Day she found Amy Duny in her House, and thrusting her out of Doors, said, You need not be so angry, your Child will not live so long; and within Three Days the Child died. And this Deponent further added, That she her self, not long after, was taken with such a Lameness in one of her Legs, that she was forced to go upon Crutches, and she appeared in Court upon them. And what was very remarkable was, that immediately, as soon as the Jury brought Duny in guilty, Durent was restored to the Use of her Limbs, and went Home without her Crutches.

As for Elizabeth and Deborah Pacy, one Eleven, and the other Nine Years of Age, the eldest being in Court, was made utterly senseless, all the Time of the Trial, or at least Speechless, and by the Direction of the Judge Duny was brought privately to Elizabeth Pacy, and she touched her Hand; whereupon the Child, without seeing her, suddenly leaped up and flew upon the Prisoner. The younger was too ill to be brought to the Assizes. But Samuel Pacy their Father testify'd, That his Daughter, Deborah was taken with a sudden Lameness; and upon Amy Duny's grumbling, being denied something where this Child was then sitting, she was taken with a violent Pain in her Stomach, like the pricking of Pins; and shrieking dreadfully, like a Whelp, rather than a Rational Creature. The Physitians could not conjecture the Cause of the Distemper; but Amy Duny being a Woman of ill Fame, and the Child in Fits crying out of Amy Duny, affrighting her with the Apparition of her Person, the Deponent suspected her, and got her set in the Stocks. Whilst she was there, she was heard to say, by Two Witnesses, Mr. Pacy keeps a great Stir about his Child, but let him stay till he hath done as much by his Children as I have done by mine. And being asked what she had done to hers, she answered, She had been forced to open its Mouth with a Tap to give it Victuals.

The Deponent added, That within Two Days his Daughters Fits were such, that they could not preserve either Life or Breath without the Help of a Tap; and that the Children cried out of Amy Duny and of Rose Callender afflicting them with their Apparition.

The Childrens Fits were various; they would be sometimes lame on one Side, and sometimes on the other; sometimes very sore, and sometimes restored to their Limbs; and then Deaf, or Blind, or Dumb for a long Time together. Upon the Recovery of their Speech, they would cough extreamly, and with much Phlegm; they would bring up crooked Pins, and at one Time a Two-Penny Nail, with a very broad Head. Commonly at the End of every Fit they would cast up a Pin. When the Children read, they could not pronounce the Name of Lord, or Jesus, or Christ, but would fall into Fits, and say, Amy Duny says I must not use that Name. When they came to the Name of Satan, or Devil, they would clap ther Fingers upon the Book, crying out, This bites, but it makes me speak right well. The Children in their Fits would often cry out, There stands Amy Duny and Rose Callender; and they would afterwards say, That when these Witches appeared before them, they threatened them, That if they told of what they heard or saw, they would torment them more than ever they did.

Margaret Arnold, Sister to Mr. Pacy, witnessed, That the like Sufferings were upon the Children at her House, whither her Brother had removed them; and that sometimes the Children would see Things like Mice run about the House, and one of them suddenly snapped one of them with the Tongs, and threw it into the Fire, where it scrietched out like a Rat. Another Time a Thing like a Bee flew at the younger Child's Face, and the Child fell into a Fit, and presently vomited up a Two-Penny Nail with a broad Head, affirming, That the Bee brought this Nail, and thrust it into her Mouth. The Child would in like manner be assaulted with Flies, which brought crooked Pins into her, and made her first swallow them, and then vomit them. She one Day caught an invisible Mouse, and throwing it into the Fire, it flashed like Gunpowder. None besides the Child saw the Mouse, but every one saw the Flash. She also declared out of her Fits, That when she was in them, Amy Duny tempted her to destroy her self.

As for Anne Durant, her Father testify'd, That upon a Discontent of Rose Callender, his Daughter was taken with much Illness in her Stomach, and violent Pains, like the pricking of Pins, and then swooning Fits, from which recovering, she declared, she had seen the Apparition of Rose Callender, threatening to torment her; she likewise vomited up several Pins. The Maid was present at Court, but when Callender looked upon her, she fell into such Fits, that made her quite unfit to declare any Thing. Anne Baldwin deposed the same.

Jane Bocking, who was too weak to be at the Assizes, her Mother testify'd, That her Daughter having formerly been afflicted with Swooning Fits, and recovered of them, was now taken with a great Pain in her Stomach, and new Swooning Fits. That she took little Food, but every Day vomited crooked Pins. In her first Fits she would extend her Arms, and use Postures, as if she catched at some thing; and when her gripend Hands were stretched open by Force, they would find several Pins, several Ways crooked, strangely lodged there; she would also discourse with some Body invisibly present there, and casting abroad her Arms, she would often say, I will not have it; but at last, Then I will have it; and closing her Hand, which they presently after opened, a Lath Nail was found in it. But her great Complaints were, of being visited by Amy Duny and Rose Callender.

As for Susan Chandler, her Mother testify'd, That being at the Search of Rose Callender, they found on her Belly a Thing like a Teat, of an Inch long, which the said Rose ascribed to a Strain. But near her Privy-Parts they found Three more smaller than the former. At the End of the long Teat, there was a little Hole, which appeared as if newly sucked, and upon straining it, a white Milky Matter issued out. The Deponent further said, That her Daughter being one Day concerned at Rose Callender's taking her by the Hand, she fell very sick, and at Night cried out, That Rose Callender would come to Bed to her. Her Fits grew violent, and in the Intervals of them she declared, that she saw Rose Callender in them, and once having a great Dog with her. She also vomited up crooked Pins, and when she was brought to Court she fell into Fits. She recovered her self in some time, and was asked by the Court, whether she was in a Condition to take an Oath, and give Evidence, she answered, she could, but being swore, she fell into her Fits again, and Burn her! Burn her! were all the Words she could speak. Her Father gave the same Testimony with her Mother, as to all but the Search.

  Yet this Evidence was thought too little to convict the Prisoners, though Dr. Brown gave it as his Opinion that they were bewitched. And what was further observable, and worth our Notice was, that when the afflicted Persons were utterly deprived of all Sense in their Fits, yet upon the Touch of the accused, they would scrietch and fly up, but not at any other Person, except once, for which some Reason might be given.

  Next John Soam testify'd, That bringing Home his Hay in three Carts, one of the Carts wrenched the Window of Rose Callender's House, upon which she threatened him violently. The other two Carts passed by twice loaden that Day, but that which touched Callender's House, was twice or thrice overturned that Day. Having again loaded it, as they brought it out of the Gate from the Field, the Cart stuck so fast in the Gates Head, that they could not possibly get it through, but were forced to cut down the Post of the Gate to make the Cart pass through, though they could not perceive that the Cart touched the Gate Post on either Side. They afterwards with much ado got it Home to the Yard, but could not possibly get it near the Place where they should unload it, but were fain to unload it at a great Distance; and when they were tired, the Noses of them that came to assist them, would burst out a Bleeding, so that they were forced to give over till the next Morning, and then they unloaded without any Difficulty.

Robert Shermingham also testify'd, That the Axletree of his Cart happening to break, as it passed some part of Rose Callender's House, in her Anger she threaten'd him his Horses should suffer for it; and within a short Time all his Four Horses died, and he sustained several other Losses in a short Time by his Cattle dying, he was also taken with a Lameness in his Limbs, and so vexed with Lice of an extraordinary Number and Bigness, that no Art could hinder the swarming of them, till he burnt Two Suits of Cloaths.

As for Amy Duny, it was testify'd by one Richard Spencer, That he heard her say, That the Devil would not let her rest till she was revenged on the Wife of Cornelius Sandwell. And that Sandwell testify'd, That her Poultry died suddenly upon Amy Duny's threatening them, and that her Husband's Chimney fell quickly after Duny had spoke of such a Disaster. And a Firkin of Fish could not be kept from falling into the Water, upon suspitious Words of Duny's.

The Judge told the Jury, They were to enquire, first, Whether the Children were betwitched, and next, whether the Prisoners at the Bar were guilty of it. And that they ought not to condemn the Innocent, nor let the Guilty go free, both being an Abomination to the Lord.

The Jury in half an Hour brought them in guilty upon the several Indictments, which were Nineteen.

The next Morning, the Children with their Parents, came to the Lodgings of the Lord-Chief-Justice, and were in as good Health as ever they were in their Lives, being restored within half an Hour after the Witches were convicted.

The Witches were Executed, and confessed nothing, which needs not be wondered at, if we consider, and are of the Opinion of a Judicious Writer, who says, That the unpardonable Sin is most usually committed by Professors of the Christian Religion falling into Witchcraft.

The Conclusion.

HAving in this Work inserted no Relations but what are confirm'd by the best Authorities, we shall close this Volume, with an Account of a surprizing Apparition, in Relation to the Duke of Buckingham, as delivered and attested by the Authority of my Lord Clarendon in his History of the Rebellion and Civil Wars in England; in the following Words.

"There were many Stories scattered Abroad at that Time of several Prophecies and Predictions of the Duke's untimely End, and violent Death. Amongst the rest, there was one which was upon a better Foundation of Credit, than usually such Discourses are founded upon. There was an Officer in the King's Wardrobe in Windsor-Castle, of a good Reputation for Honesty and Discretion, and then about the Age of Fifty Years or more. This Man had in his Youth been bred in a School in a Parish where Sir George Villars, the Father of the Duke lived; and had been much cherished and obliged, in that Season of his Age by Sir George, whom afterwards he never saw. About six Months before the miserable End of the Duke of Buckingham, about Midnight, this Man being in his Bed at Windsor, where his Office was, and in very good Health; there appeared to him on the Side of his Bed, a Man of a very venerable Aspect, who drew the Curtains of his Bed, and fixing his Eyes upon him, asked him if he knew him. The poor Man half dead with Fear and Apprehension, being asked the second time, Whether he remembred him? and having in that time called into his Memory, the Presence of Sir George Villars and the very Cloaths he used to wear, in which at that time he seemed to be habited; He answer'd, That he thought him to be that Person. He reply'd, that he was in the right, that he was the same, and that he expected a Service from him; which was, that he should go from him to his Son the Duke of Buckingham, and tell him, that if he did not something to ingratiate himself with the People, or at least, to abate the extreme Malice they had against him, he would be suffered to live but a short time. After this Discourse he disappeared, and the poor Man if he had been at all Waking, slept very well till Morning, when he believed all this to be a Dream, and considered it no otherwise.

The next Night, or shortly after, the same Person appeared to him again in the same Place, and about the same Time of the Night, with an Aspect a little more severe than before, and asked him, Whether he had done as he had required him? And perceiving he had not, gave him very severe Reprehensions; and told him, he expected more Compliance from him; and, That if he did not perform his Commands, he should enjoy no Peace of Mind, but should be always pursued by him; Upon which he promised to obey him. But the next Morning, awaking out of a good Sleep, though he was exceedingly perplexed with the lively Representation of all Particulars to his Memory, he was willing still to perswade himself that he had only Dreamed: And considered that he was a Person at such a Distance from the Duke, that he knew not how to find any Admission to his Presence; much less, hoped to be believed in what he should say.

The same Person appear'd to him a Third time with a terrible Countenance, and bitterly reproaching him for not performing what he had promised to do. The Poor Man had by this time recovered his Courage to tell him, That in Truth he had deferred the Execution of his Commands, upon considering, how difficult a Thing it would be for him to get any Access to the Duke, having Acquaintance with no Person about him, and if he could obtain Admission to him, he should never be able to perswade him, that he was sent in such a Manner; but he should, at best, be thought to be mad, or to be set on and employ'd by his own, or the Malice of other Men, to abuse the Duke; and so he should be sure to be undone. The Person reply'd as he had done before, That he should never find Rest, till he should perform what he required; and therefore he were better to dispatch it. That the Accession to his Son was known to be very easy, and that few Men waited long for him; and for the gaining him Credit, he would tell him two or three Particulars, which he charged him never to mention to any Person living, but to the Duke himself;

and he should no sooner hear them, but he should believe all the rest he should say:" And so repeating his Threats he left him.

In the Morning, The Poor Man, more confirmed by the last Appearance, made his Journey to London, where the Court then was. He was very-well known to Sir Ralph Freeman, one of the Masters of Requests, who had married a Lady that was nearly allyed to the Duke, and was himself well received by him. To him this Man went: And though he did not acquaint him with all Particulars, he said enough to him to let him see, there was somewhat extraordinary in it; and the Knowledge he had of the Sobriety and Discretion of the Man made the more Impression on him. He desired that by his means he might be brought to the Duke to such a Place, and in such a Manner as should be thought fit, affirming, That he had much to fay to him, and of such a Nature, as would require much Privacy, and someTime and Patience in the Hearing. Sir Ralph promised he would speak first with the Duke of him, and then he should understand his Pleasure; and accordingly, the first Opportunity he acquainted him with the Reputation and Honesty of the Man, and then what he desired, and of all he knew of the Matter. The Duke, according to his usual Openness and Condescension, told him, That he was the next Day early to Hunt with the King; That his Horses should attend him at Lambeth-Bridge, where he would Land by Five a Clock in the Morning; and if the Man attended him there at that Hour, he would walk and speak with him as long as should be Necessary. Sir Ralph carried the Man with him the next Morning, and presented him to the Duke at his Landing, who received him Courteously, and walked aside in Conference near an Hour, none but his own Servants being at that Hour in that place, and they, and Sir Ralph at such a Distance, that they cou'd not hear a Word, though the Duke sometimes spoke with great Commotion, which Sir Ralph the more easily observed, and perceived, because he kept his Eyes always fixed upon the Duke, having procured the Conference on something he knew was extraordinary. And the Man told him in his Return over the Water, That when he mentioned those Particulars which were to gain him Credit, the Substance whereof he said he durst not impart to him, the Duke's Colour changed, and he Swore he could come to that Knowledge only by the Devil, for that those Particulars were known only to himself and to one Person more, who he vas sure would never speak of it.

The Duke pursued his Purpose of Hunting, but was observed to Ride all the Morning with great Pensiveness, and in deep Thoughts, without any Delight in he Exercise he was upon; and before the Morning was spent, left the Field, and alighted at his Mother's Lodgings at Whitehall; with whom he was shut up for the space of two or three Hours; The Noise of their Discourse frequently reaching the Ears of those who attended in the next Rooms; and when the Duke left her, his Countenance appeared full of Trouble, with a Mixture of Anger; a Countenance, that was never before observed in him, in any Conversation with her, towards whom he had a profound Reverence: And the Countess her self for though she was married to a private Gentleman, Sir Thomas Compton, she had been created Countess of Buckingham shortly after her Son had assumed that Title) was, at the Duke's leaving her, found overwhelmed in Tears, and in the highest Agony imaginable. Whatever there was of all this; 'tis a Notorious Truth, that when the News of the Duke's Murther (which happened within few Months after) was brought to his Mother, she seemed not in the least degree surprized; but received it as if she had foreseen it; nor did afterwards express such a Degree of Sorrow, as was expected from such a Mother, for the Loss of such a Son.

This Relation, as delivered by my Lord Clarendon, is looked upon to be the most Authentick; yet since there is another Account, which contains some Particulars not mention'd in this, and some of which are confirmed by Hints and Circumstances here intimated, and others only differ in the Manner of relating the same Story; for the sake of those material Circumstances and Particulars left out in this Account, we shall subjoin what is further related in respect of the Duke's Death.

Mr. Lilly speaking of the Death of the Duke of Buckingham, says, an aged Gentleman, Mr. Parker, having formerly belonged to the Duke or of great Acquaintance with the Duke's Father, and now retired, had a Dæmon appeared to him several times, in the Shape of Sir George Villers, the Duke's Father: This Dæmon walked several times in Parker's Bedchamber, without any Action of Terror, Noise, Hurt or Speech; but at last one Night broke out in these Words; Mr. Parker, I know you lov'd me formerly, and my Son George at this time very well; I would have you go from me (you know me very well to be his Father, old Sir George Villers of Leicesershire) and to acquaint him with these, and these Particulars, &c. And that he above all refrain the Company and Counsel of such and such, whom he then nominated, or else he will come to Destruction and that suddenly. Parker though a very discreet Man, partly imagined himself in a Dream all this time; and being unwilling to proceed upon no better Grounds, forbore Addressing himself to the Duke; for he conceived if he should acquaint the Duke with the Words of his Father, and the Manner of his Appearance to him (such Apparitions not being usual) he should be laughed at and thought to doat, in regard he was Aged. Some Nights past without further Trouble to the Old Man, but not very many Nights after, old Sir George Villers appeared again, walked quick and furiously in the Room; seemed angry with Parker, and at last said, Mr. Parker, I thought you had been my Friend so much, and loved my Son George so well, that you would have acquainted him with what I desired, but I know you have not done it; by all the Friendship that ever was betwixt you and me, and the great Respect you bear my Son, I desire You to deliver what I formerly commanded You, to my Son.

  The old Man seeing himself thus followed, promised the Dæmon he would; but first argued it thus, That the Duke was not easily to be spoke withal, and that he would account him a vain Man to come with such a Message from the Dead, nor did he conceive the Duke would give any Credit to him; to which the Dæmon thus answered; If he will not believe you have this

Discourse from me, tell him of such a Secret (and named it) which he knows none in the World ever knew but my self and him.

Mr. Parker being now well satisfied that he was not asleep, and that the Apparition was not a vain Delusion, took a sit Opportunity, and seriously acquainted the Duke with his Father's Words, and the Manner of his Apparition. The Duke heartily laugh'd at the Relation, which put old Parker to a stand; but at last he assumed Courage, and told the Duke, that he acquainted his Father's Ghost, with what he found now to be true, Viz. Scorn and Derision; but my Lord, says he, Your Father bid me acquaint you by this Token, and said it was such as none in the World but your two selves did yet know. Hereat the Duke was amazed, and much astonished, but took no Warning or Notice thereof; Keeping the same Company still; Advising with such Counsellors, and performing such Actions, as his Father by Parker Countermanded.

Shortly after, old Sir George Villers, in a very quiet but sorrowful Posture, appears again to Parker, and said; Mr. Parker, I know you delivered my Words to George, my Son, I thank you for so doing, but he slighted them: and now I only request this more at your hands, that once again you go to my Son, and tell him, that if he will not amend, and follow the Counsel I have given him, this Knife or Dagger (and with that he pulled a Knife or Dagger from under his Gown) shall end him; and do you, Mr. Parker, set your House in order; for you shall Die at such a Time.

Mr. Parker once more engaged, though very unwillingly, to acquaint the Duke with this last Message, and so did: But the Duke desired him to trouble him no more with such Messages and Dreams, and told him, that he was now an Old Man and doated; and within a Month after meeting Mr. Parker on Lambeth-Bridge, said, Now, Mr. Parker, What say you of your Dream? who only answered, Sir, I wish it may never have Success, &c. but within six Weeks after he was stabbed with a Knife, according to his Father's Admonition, and Mr. Parker died soon after he had seen the Dream or Vision performed.

To this remarkable History, we shall add a Relation of an Apparition from the Lord Bishop of Gloucester, delivered in these Words.

Sir Charles Lee, by his first Lady, had only one Daughter, of which she died in Childbirth; and when she was Dead, her Sister the Lady Everard, desired to have the Education of the Child, and she was by her very well educated, till she was marriageable; and a Match was concluded for her with Sir William Perkins, but was then prevented in an extraordinary manner. Upon a Thursday Night, she thinking she saw a Light in her Chamber after she was in Bed, Knocked for her Maid, who presently came to her, and she asked her, Why she left the Candle burning in her Chamber? The Maid said she left none, and there was none but what she brought with her at that time. Then she said it was the Fire, but her Maid told her that was quite out; and said, she believed it was only a Dream; whereupon she said it might be so, and composed her self again to Sleep: But about Two a Clock she was awakened again, and saw the Apparition of a little Woman, between her Curtain and her Pillow, who told her she was her Mother, that she was happy, and that by Twelve of the Clock, that Day, she should be with her: Whereupon she knocked again for her Maid, called for her Clothes, and when she was Dress'd, went into her Closet, and came not out again till Nine, and then brought out with her a Letter sealed to her Father; brought it to her Aunt, the Lady Everard; told her what had happened, and desired that as soon as she was Dead, it might be sent to him: But the Lady thought she was suddenly fallen Mad; and thereupon presently sent away to Chelmsford, for a Physician and Surgeon, who both came immediately; but the Physician could discern no Indication of what the Lady imagined, or of any Indisposition of her Body, not withstanding the Lady would needs have her let Blood, which was done accordingly: And when the Young Woman had patiently let them do what they would do with her, she desired that the Chaplain might be called to read Prayers; and when Prayers were ended, she took her Gittar and Psalm-Book, and sat down upon a Chair without Arms, and

Played and Sang so Melodiously and Admirably, that her Musick-Master, who was then there, admired at it; and near the Stroke of Twelve, she rose and sat her self down in a great Chair with Arms, and presently fetching a strong Breathing or two, immediately expired, and was so suddenly cold, as was much wondered at by the Physician and Surgeon. She died at Waltham in Essex, three Miles from Chelmsford; and the Letter was sent to Sir Charles at his House in Warwickshire; but he was so afflicted with the Death of his Daughter, that he came not till the was Buried; but when he came, caused her to be taken up, and to be Buried by her Mother at Edminton, as she desired in her Letter. This was about the Year 1662, or 63. And this Relation the Lord Bishop of Gloucester had from Sir Charles Lee himself.

FINIS.

A Compleat History OF MAGICK, SORCERY, AND WITCHCRAFT; CONTAINING,

I. The TRYALS of several WITCHES at Salem in New-England.
II. A Narrative of many Surprizing and Amazing Sorceries, and Witchcrafts practised in Scotland. With the Learned Arguments of Lawyers on both sides, at the TRYALS of Seven WITCHES, and the Remarkable Passages which happen'd at their Execution.
III. The Surrey DEMONIACK. With all the Testimonies and Informations taken upon Oath relating thereunto.

by
Richard Boulton
1716

VOLUME II.

CHAP. I.

Containing an Account of some Tryals of Witches, at a Court of Oyer and Terminer, held in Salem, in New-England.

THE first History we shall give an Account of, in this Second Part of the History of Witchcraft, is, the Tryal of one G. B. who was Indicted for Witchcraft, and in the Prosecution of the Charge against him, he was accused by five or six Persons bewitched, as the Author of their Miseries; he was accused by eight of the confessing Witches, as being a chief Actor at some of their hellish Rendezvouses, and one who had a Promise of being a King in Satan's Kingdom, which was now going to be erected in New-England. He was accused by nine Persons for extraordinary Lifting, and such extraordinary Things done by Strength, as could not be performed without diabolical Assistance. He was accused for other such likethings, by thirty Persons who testified against him, nor were these thought to be half of what might have been brought against him. However they were thought sufficient to convict him of Witchcraft, by the Judge who directed in that Case.

The Court being sensible, that the Testimonies of the Parties bewitched used to be esteemed as Suspicions or Presumptions against one indicted for Witchcraft, the Testimonies of several Persons were heard, who were notoriously bewitched, and every Day tortured by invisible Hands, and charging the Spectres or Apparitions of G. B. to be concerned in their Torments. At the Examination of this G. B. the Persons bewitched were most grievously handled, with preternatural Effects which could not be counterfeited, all ascribing what happened to them to the Endeavours of G. B. to kill them. One of the bewitched Persons upon Tryal confessed, That in all her Agonies, a little black haired Man came to her, saying his Name was B. bidding her set her Hand to a Book which he shewed her, and boasting that he was a Conjurer above the ordinary Rank of Witches. He often persecuted her with the Offer of that Book, saying, she should be well, and need fear no Body if she would but sign it; but he often inflicted cruel Pains and Sufferings upon her because she refused it.

    The Testimonies of the other Sufferers concurred with this, and it was remarkable, that whereas biting was one of the Ways, which Witches used to torment the Sufferers; when they cried out of G. B. biting them, the print of Teeth would he seen on the Flesh of the Complainers, and just such a Set of Teeth as G. B's would then appear upon them, which could be distinguished from those of other Men. Others of them testified, that in their Torments G. B. tempted them to go to a Sacrament, to which they perceived him, with the Sound of a Trumper, summoning other Witches, who quickly after the Sound would come from all Quarters unto the Rendezvous. One of them falling into a Trance, affirmed that G. B. had carried her away into a very high Mountain, where he shewed her Mighty and Glorious Kingdoms, and said, he would give her them all, if she would write in his Book; but she told him, they were none of his to give, and refused his Proposals, enduring a great deal of Torment for that Refusal.

    It cost the Court a great deal of Trouble to hear the Testimonies of the Sufferers; for when they were going to give if their Depositions, they would for a long time be taken with Fits, that made them incapable of saying any thing. The Chief Judge asked the Prisoner, who he thought hindered the Witnesses from giving their Testimonies; and he answered, he supposed it was the Devil. That Honourable Person replied, How comes the Devil to be so loth to have any Testimony born against you? which cast him into very great Confusion.

But further, It hath been very usual for the People bewitched to be entertained with the Apparitions of Ghosts of murdered People, at the same time that the Spectres of the Witches troubled them; and these Ghosts always frighted the Beholders more than all the other spectral Representations; and when they shewed themselves, they always cried out of being murthered by the Witchcrafts or other Violences of the Persons who were present in Spectre. And we are further to consider, that once or twice these Apparitions have Been seen by others, at the same time that they have appeared to the bewitched; and these Apparitions have seldom been seen, but when something unusual or unsuspected hath attended the Death of the Party thus appearing; some who have been accused by these Apparitions accosting of the bewitched People, who had never heard a Word of any such Persons ever being in the World, have upon a fair Examination, freely and fully confessed the Murthers of those very Persons, though these also did not know how the Apparitions had complained of them. Accordingly several of the bewitched had given in their Testimony, that they had been troubled with the Apparitions of two Women, who said they were G B's two Wives, and that he had been the Death of them, and that the Magistrates must be told of it, before whom, if B. upon his Tryal denied it, they did not know but that they should appear again in Court.

Now G. B. had been Infamous, for the barbarous Usage of his two late Wives; all the Country over; besides it was testified, that the Spectre of G. B. threatning of the Sufferers told them, that besides others, he had killed Mrs. Lawson and her Daughter Anne. And it was observed, that these were the Wife and Daughter of one, whom this G. B. might have a prejudice towards, being serviceable at Salem Village, from whence himself had, in ill times removed some Years before; and that when they died, which was long since, there were some odd Circumstances about them, which made some of the Attendants there suspect something of Witchcraft, though none imagined from whence it should come.

G. B. being now upon his Tryal, one of the bewitched Persons was seized with Horror by the Ghosts of B's two deceased Wives, then appearing before him, and crying for Vengeance against him. Upon which several of the bewitched Persons were successively called in, who not knowing what the former had seen or said, concurred in their Horror of the Apparition, which each affirmed he had before him. But he, though much concerned, absolutely denied that he saw any thing of it, nor was it any Part of his Conviction.

Judicious Persons have allowed it, as a strong Evidence in the Convicting of Witches, when Persons are impeached by other Notorious Witches, to be as ill as themselves, especially if the Persons have been much noted for neglecting the Worship of God. Now as there might have been Testimonies enough of G. B's Antipathy to Prayer, and the other Ordinances of God, though by his Profession, singularly obliged to it; so there now come in against the Prisoner the Testimonies of several Persons, who confessed their having been horrible Witches, and ever since their Confessions, had been themselves terribly tormented by the Devils and other Witches, as much as the other Sufferers, and undergone the Pains of many Deaths for their Confessions. These now testified, that G. B. had been at Witch-meetings with them, and that he was the Person that had seduced and compelled them into the Snares of Witchcraft. That he promised them fine Cloaths for doing it, that he brought Poppets to them and Thorns to stick into those Poppets for the afflicting of other Persons; and that he exhorted them with the rest of the Crew to bewitch all Salem Village, but to do it gradually if they would prevail in what they did.

When the Lancashire Witches were condemned, I don't remember there was any considerable further Evidence than that of the bewitched. with that of some that confessed; but there were other Things against G. B. to render what had been already produced more credible. It is reckoned amongst the Convictions of a Witch, by a famous Divine, That the Testimony of the Party bewitched, whether pining or dying, together with the joint Oaths of sufficient Persons, that have seen certain prodigious Pranks or Feats wrought by the Party accused, were sufficient; and it appeared, that G. B. had ensnared himself by several Instances, which he had formerly given of his preternatural Strength, which were now produced against him; for though he was a very puny Man, yet he had often done Things beyond the Strength of a Giant. A Gun of about seven Foot Barrel, and so heavy, that Strong Men could not steadily hold it out with both Hands, as appeared by the Testimonies of several Persons of Credit and Honour, he made nothing of taking it up behind the Lock, with one Hand, and holding it out like a Pistol, at Arm's Length; but G. B. in his Vindication, said that an Indian was there and held it out at the same time; whereas none of the Spectators ever saw any such Indian, but supposed, the Black Man (which the Witches call the Devil, and they commonly say resembles an Indian) might afford him Assistance. Evidence was likewise brought in, that he made nothing of taking up a whole Barrel filled with Malasses or Cider, in very disadvantagious Postures, and carrying them through the Difficultest Places out of a Canoo to the Shoar.

Two other Witnesses testified, that G. B. only putting the Fore-finger of his Right-hand into the Muzzle of a heavy Gun, or a Fouling-piece about six or seven Foot Barrel, lifted up the Gun and held it out at Arm's Length, which the Deponents thought a Strong Man could not with both Hands lift up, and hold out at the Butt-end as usual. One of these Witnesses was over-perswaded by some People, to be out of the way upon G. B's Tryal, but he came afterwards with sorrow for his withdrawing, and gave his Testimony.

Several Witnesses likewise came in, whose Testimonies related to the Domestick Affairs of G. B. which had a very hard Aspect upon him, and not only proved him a very ill Man, but also confirmed the Belief of the Character which had already been given.

It was also testified, that keeping his two successive Wives in a strange Kind of Slavery, he would when he came home from abroad, pretend to tell the Talk which any had with them; that he had brought them to the point of Death by his hard dealing with them, and then made the People about him to promise that in case Death should happen, they would say nothing of it: that he used all the means he could to make his Wives to Write, Sign, Swear and Seal a Covenant, never to reveal any of his Secrets; That his Wives had privately complained to the Neighbours about frightful Apparitions of evil Spirits, with which their House was sometimes infested, and that many such Things have been whispered amongst the Neighbourhood; there were also some other Testimonies relating to the Death of People, whereby the Consciences of an impartial Jury were convinced that G. B. had bewitched the Persons mentioned in the Complaints.

One Mr. Ruck, Brother-in-Law to this G. B. testified that G. B. and himself, and his Sister G.B's Wife, going out for two or three Miles to gather Strawberries, Ruck with his Sister rode home very softly, with G. B. in their Company on foot, who stepped aside a little into the Bushes, upon which they stopped a little, and hallowed for him, but he not answering they went homewards, and quickened their Pace without expecting to see him in a considerable time; yet when they were got home almost, to their great Astonishment, they found him on Foot with them, having a Basket of Strawberries. G. B then immediately fell to chide his Wife, for what she had been speaking to her Brother of him on the Road, which when they wondered at, he told them he knew their Thoughts. Ruck being startled at that, made some Reply, intimating, that the Devil himself did not know so far; but G. B. made answer, My God makes known your Thoughts to me.

The Prisoner now at the Bar had nothing to answer unto what was now witnessed against him, that was worth considering, only he said, Ruck and his Wife left a Man with him, when they left him, which Ruck now affirmed to be false; and when the Court asked him, what the Man's Name was, his Countenance was much altered, nor could he say who it was. But the Court began to think, that he then stepped aside, that by the Assistance of the Black-Man he might put on his Invisibility, and in that Fascinating Mist, gratify his own Jealous Humour to know what they said of him; which Trick of rendering themselves invisible, Witches pretend to, and which is often Demonstrated that they do perform.

But further, as faltring, faulty, inconstant and contrary Answers, upon judicial and deliberate Examination, are counted unlucky Symptoms of Guilt, in all Crimes and especially Witchcraft; there never was a Person more eminent for them than G. B. both at his Examination, and on his Tryal; his Contradictions and Falsehoods, showing, that he had very little to say, having alledg'd some things which he could not prove, reflecting on the Reputation of some of the Witnesses; only he gave in a Paper to the Jury, wherein though he had many times before granted, not only that there are Witches, but also that the present Sufferings of the Country are the Effects of Horrible Witchcraft, yet he now endeavoured to evince, That there neither are, nor ever were Witches, that having made a Compact with the Devil, can send a Devil to torment other People at a Distance. This Paper was transcribed out of Acly, which the Court presently knew as soon as they heard it, but he denied it, and said a Gentleman gave it him in Writing. The Jury brought him in Guilty, but when he came to Die, he utterly denied the Fact, of which he had been convicted.

The Tryal of Bridget Bishop, alias Oliver, at the Court of Oyer and Terminer, held at Salem.

SHE was Indicted for Bewitching several Persons in the Neighbourhood. The Indictment being drawn up according to the Form in such Cases made use of, and she pleading not guilty, several Persons were brought in, who had long undergone many kind of Miseries, which were preternaturally inflicted, and generally ascribed to a horrible Witchcraft. There was little occasion to prove the Witchcraft, it being Evident and Notorious to all the Beholders; yet to fix it on the Prisoner at the Bar, the first Thing made use of was the Testimony of the bewitched, several of which testified, that the Shape of the Prisoner oftentimes very grievously pinched them, choaked them, bit them and afflicted them, urging them to write their Names in a Book, which the said Spectre called Ours. One of them further testified, that it was the Shape of this Prisoner, with another, which one Day took her from her Wheel, and carried her to the River Side, and threatned to drown her, if she did not sign to the Book mentioned, which notwithstanding she refused. Others also testified, that the said Shape did in her Threats boast to them, that she had been the Death of sundry Persons, which she then named, and that she had ridden a Man whom she then named. Another testified, the Apparition of the Ghosts unto the Spectre of Bishop cried out, You murthered us, The Matter of Fact giving sufficient Suspicion of the Truth of it.

It was also testified, that at the Examination of the Prisoner before the Magistrates, the bewitched were extremely tortured. If she did but cast her Eyes on them, they were presently struck down, and in such a manner that there could be no Deceit in the Matter; but as soon as she touched them with her Hand, when they lay in their Swoons, they would immediately Revive, and not upon the Touch of any one else. Besides upon some particular Actions of her Body, as the shaking of her Head, or the turning of her Eyes, they presently and painfully fell into the like Postures. And many of the like Accidents now fell out whilst she was at the Bar; one at the same time testifying, that she said, she could not be troubled to see the Afflicted thus tormented. There was Testimony likewise brought in, that a Man striking once at a Place where a bewitched Person said the Shape of this Bishop stood, the bewitched cried out, that he had tore her Coat in a Place then particularly mentioned, and the Woman's Coat was found to be torn in the same Place.

Further, one Deliverance Hobbs, who had confessed her self to be a Witch, was now tormented by the Spectres for confessing. And she now testify'd, That this Bishop tempted her to sign the Book again, and to deny what she had confessed, and affirmed, That it was the Shape of this Prisoner that whipped her with Iron-Rods to compel her thereunto; and also, that this Bishop was at a general Meeting of the Witches in a Field at Salem Village, and there partook of a Diabolical Sacrament in Bread and Wine there administred. And to render it further unquestionable, that the Prisoner at the Bar was the Person truly charged in this Witchcraft, several Evidences of other Performances of Witchcraft by her, were produc'd. First John Cook testify'd, That above five or six Years ago, one Morning about Sun-rise, he was assaulted in his Chamber by the Shape of this Prisoner, which looked on him, grinned at him, and very much hurt him with a Blow on one Side of the Head; and that on the same Day, about Noon, the same Shape walked about in the Room where he was, and an Apple strangely flew out of his Hand into his Mother's Lap six or eight Foot from him.

Samuel Grey testify'd, That about Fourteen Years agoe, he waked in the Night, and saw the Room where he lay full of Light; and that he then saw a Woman plainly between the Cradle and Bed-side, which looked upon him; but when he rose, it vanished, though he found all the Doors fast. Looking out at the Entry Door, he saw the same Woman in the same Garb again, and said in God's Name, what do you come for? He went to Bed and had he same Woman assaulting him again. The Child in the Cradle gave a great Scrietch, and the Woman disappeared. It was long before the Child could be quieted, and though it were a very likely thriving Child, yet from this Time it pined away, and after several Months died in a sad Condition. He knew not Bishop nor her Name, but when he saw her after this, he knew by her Countenance and Apparel, and all Circumstances, that it was the Apparition of this Bishop which had thus troubled him.

John Bly and his Wife testify'd, That he bought a Sow of Edward Bishop, the Husband of the Prisoner, and was to pay the Price agreed unto another Person. This Prisoner being angry that she was hindred from fingring the Money, quarrelled with Bly. Soon after which the Sow was taken with strange Fits, Jumping, Leaping, and knocking her Head against the Fence; she seemed blind and deaf, and would neither eat nor be sucked; whereupon a Neighbour said, she believed the Creature was over-looked, and sundry other Circumstances concurred, which made the Deponents believe that Bishop had bewitched it.

Richard Coman testify'd, That eight Years ago, as he lay awake in his Bed, with a Light burning in the Room, he was annoyed with the Apparition of this Bishop, and of two more that were Strangers to him, who came and oppressed him so, that he could neither stir himself; nor wake any one else, and that he was the Night after molested in the like manner, the said Bishop taking him by the Throat, and pulling him almost out of the Bed. His Kinsman for this Reason offer'd to lodge with him, and that Night, as they were awake, discoursing together, this Coman was once more visited by the Guests which had formerly been so troublesome, his Kinsman at the same time being struck Speechless, and unable to move Hand or Foot. He had laid his Sword by him, which these unhappy Spectres strove to wrest from him, only he held too fast for them. He then grew able to call the People of the House, but although they heard him, yet they had not Power to speak or stir until at last one of the People crying out what is the matter, the Spectres all vanished.

Samuel Shattock testify'd, That Bishop often came to his House upon such frivolous and foolish Errands, that they suspected she came with a mischievous Purpose; whereupon presently his eldest Child, which was of a promising Health and

Strength, as any Child of his Age, began to droop exceedingly, and the oftner Bishop came to the House, the Child grew worse. As the Child would stand at the Door, he would be bruised and thrown against the Stones by an invisible Hand, and likewise knock his Face against the Sides of the House, and bruise it after a miserable Manner. Afterwards Bishop would bring him Things to dye, which he could not imagine the Use of, and when she paid him a Piece of Money, the Purse and Money were unaccountably conveighed out of a Locked-Box, and never seen any more. The Child was immediately upon that taken with terrible Fits, which his Friends thought he would have dy'd off. Indeed he did almost nothing but Cry and Sleep for several Months together, and at last his Understanding was quite taken away. Amongst other Symptoms of an Enchantment upon him, one was, that there was a Board in the Garden, on which he would walk, and all the Inventions in the World would never fetch him off. About seventeen or eighteen Years after, there came a Stranger to Shattock's House, who seeing the Child, said, This poor Child is bewitched, and you have a Neighbour not living far off who is a Witch. He added, Your Neighbour hath had a falling out with your Wife, and she said in her Heart, Your Wife is a proud Woman, and she would bring down her Pride in this Child. He then remembered, that Bishop had parted from his Wife in muttering and menacing Words, a little before the Child was taken ill. The above-mentioned Stranger would needs carry the bewitched Boy with him, to Bishop's House, on Pretence of buying a Pot of Cyder. The Woman entertained him in a furious Manner, and flew also upon the Boy, scratching his Face till the Blood came, and saying, Thou Rogue, what dost thou bring this Fellow here to plague me? Now, it seems, the Man had said before he went, that he would fetch Blood of her. Ever after the Boy was followed with grievous Fits, which the Doctors themselves generally ascribed to Witchcraft, and wherein he would be thrown still into the Fire or Water, if he was not constantly looked after, and it was really thought that Bishop was the Cause of it.

John Londer testify'd, That upon some little Controversie with Bishop about her Fowls, going well to Bed, he awaked in the Night by Moon-light, and saw clearly the Likeness of this Woman grievously oppressing him, in which miserable Condition she held him, unable to help himself, till near Day. He told Bishop of this, but she denied it, and threatned him very much. Quickly after this, being at Home on a Lord's-Day, with the Doors shut about him, he saw a black Pig approach him, at which, he going to kick, it vanished away. Immediately after, sitting down, he saw a black Thing jump in at the Window, and come and stand before him. The Body was like that of a Monkey, the Feet like a Cock's, but the Face much like a Man's; he being so much frightned that he could not speak, this Monster spoke to him, and said, I am a Messenger sent unto you, for I understand that you are in some Trouble of Mind, and if you will be ruled by me, you shall want for nothing in this World. Whereupon he endeavoured to clap his Hands upon it, but he could feel no Substance, and it jumped out of the Window again, but immediately came in by the Porch, though the Doors were shut, and said, You had better take my Counsel. He then struck at it with a Stick, but the Arm with which he struck was presently disabled, and it vanished away. He presently went out at the back Door, and spy'd this Bishop in her Orchard, going towards her House, but he had no Power to set one Foot forwards towards her; whereupon returning into the House, he was immediately accosted by the Monster he had seen before, which Gobling was now going to fly at him, whereat he cried out, The whole Armour of God be between thee and me; whereupon it sprung back, and flew over the Apple-Tree, shaking many Apples off the Tree as it flew over. At this Leap it flung Dirt with its Feet up against the Man's Breast, upon which he was then struck dumb, and so continued for three Days together. Upon producing of this Testimony, Bishop denied that she knew this Deponent; yet their two Orchards joined together, and they often had their little Quarrels for two Years together.

William Stacy testify'd, That receiving Money of this Bishop, for Work done by him, he was gone but about three Rods from her, and looking for his Money, found it unaccountably gone from him. Sometime after Bishop asked him, whether his Father would grind her Grist for her? He demanded why? She answered, Because Folks count me a Witch. He answered, No Question but he will grind it for you. Being then gone about six Rods from her, with a small Load in his Cart, suddenly the Off-Wheel of his Cart stumped, and sunk down into a Hole, upon plain Ground, so that the Deponent was forced to get Help to recover the Wheel; but stepping back to look for the Hole, which might occasion this Disaster, there was none at all to be found. Some time after he was waked in the Night, but it seemed as light as Day, and he perfectly saw the Shape of this Bishop in the Room, troubling him; but upon her going out, all was dark again. He charged Bishop afterwards with it, and she denied it not, but was very angry.

Quickly after, this Deponent having been threatned by Bishop, as he was in a dark Night a going to the Barn, he was very suddenly taken or lifted from the Ground, and thrown against a Stone-Wall. After that he was again hoisted up, and thrown down a Bank at the End of his House. After this, again passing by this Bishop, his Horse with a small Load, striving to draw, all his Geer slew in Pieces, and the Cart fell down; and this Deponent going then to life a Bag of Corn of two. Bushels, could not move it with all his Strength.

This Deponent was ready to testify several other Pranks, played by this Bishop. He also testify'd, That he believed that the said Bishop was the Cause of his Daughter Priscilla's Death, giving very good Reasons for that Suspicion.

To confirm all, John Bly, and William Bly testify'd, that being employ'd by Bridget Bishop to help to take down the Cellar Wall of the old House, wherein she formerly lived, in the Holes of the old Wall, they found several Poppets made up of Rags and Hogs Bristles, with headless Pins in them, the Points being outward, of which she could give no reasonable or tolerable Account to the Court.

One Thing that made against the Prisoner was, her being evidently convicted of gross lying in the Court, several Times whilst she was making her Plea. Besides this, a Jury Woman found a Preternatural Teat upon her Body; and upon a second Search, within three or four Hours, there was no such Thing to be found. There was also another Account of other People whom this Woman had afflicted, and there might have been many more, had there been occasion for them.

There was one thing more which was very strange, with which the Court was newly entertained. As this Woman was under a Guard, passing by the great and spacious Meeting-House of Salem, she gave a Look towards the House, and immediately a Dæmon invisibly entring the Meeting-House, tore down a Part of it, so that though there was no Person to be seen there, yet the People, at that Noise, running in, found a Board which was strongly fastened with several Nails, removed to another part of the House.

The Tryal of Susanna Martin, at the Court of Oyer and Terminer, held by Adjournment at Salem.

Susanna Martin pleading Not guilty to the Indictment of Witchcraft which was brought in against her, the Evidences of several People were produc'd, who were sensibly and grievously bewitched, all complaining of the Prisoner at the Bar, as the Cause of all their Miseries. And now, as well as in the other Trials, an extraordinary Endeavour by Witchcraft, with cruel and frequent Fits, was made use of to prevent the poor Sufferers from making their Complaints, which the Court was forced to sustain with a great deal of Patience and Time, before they could give in their Evidence.

There was also an Account given of what passed at her Examination before the Magistrates, the Cast of her Eye then striking the afflicted down to the Ground, whether they saw that Cast of her Eye or no; and amongst other Passages, these following were remarkable betwixt the Person examined and the Magistrate.

Magistrate. Pray, what ails these People?
Susan. Martin. I don't know.
Mag. But what do you think ails them?
Martin. I don't desire to pass my Judgment upon it.
Mag. Don't you think they are bewitched?
Martin. No, I don't think they are.
Mag. Tell us your Thoughts about them then.
Martin. No, my Thoughts are my own, when they are in, but when they are out, they are another's. Their Master
Mag. Their Master? Who do you think is their Master?
Martin. If they be dealing in the Black Art, you may know as well as I.
Mag. Well; what have you done towards this?
Martin. Nothing at all.
Mag. Why; it is you or your Appearance.
Martin. I cannot help it.

Mag. Is it not your Master? How comes your Appearance to hurt these?

Martin. How do I know? He that appeared in the Shape of Samuel, a glorify'd Saint, may appear in any one's Shape.

It was then also noted in her, as in others like her, that if the afflicted went to approach her, they were flung down to the Ground; and when she was asked the Reason of it, she said, I cannot tell; it may be, the Devil bears me more Malice than another.

The Court was encouraged and excited by these Things, to enquire further into the Conversation of the Prisoner, and to examine what might occur, to render these Accusations further credible. Upon which, John Allen of Salisbury testify'd. That he refusing, because of the Weakness of his Oxen, to cart some Staves at the Request of this Martin, she was displeased at it, and said, It had been as good that he had, for his Oxen should never do him much more Service. Upon which this Deponent said, Doest thou threaten me, thou old Witch? I will throw thee into the Brook, to avoid which she flew over the Bridge and escaped. As he was going Home, one of his Oxen tired, so that he was forced to unyoke him, that he might get him Home. He then put his Oxen, with many more, upon Salisbury Beach, where Cattle used to get Flesh. In a few Days all the Oxen upon the Beach were found, by their Tracks, to have run into the Mouth of Mermack River, and not returned; but the next Day they were found ashoar upon Plum Island. They that sought them used all imaginable Gentleness, but they would still run away with Violence, which seemed wholly Diabolical, till they came near Merimack River, where they ran right into the Sea, swimming as far as they could be seen. One of them then swam back again, with a Swiftness amazing to the Beholders, who stood ready to receive him, and help up his tired Carcass; but the Beast ran furiously up into the Island, and from thence through the Marches, up into Newbury Town, and so up into the Woods, and after a while was found near Amesbury, so that of fourteen good Oxen, there was only this saved; the rest were all cast up, some in one Place, and some in another, drowned.

John Atkinson testify'd, That he exchanged a Cow with a Son of Susan. Martin's, whereat she muttered, and was unwilling he should have it. Going to receive this Cow, though he hamstringed her, and haltered her, she of a tame Creature grew so mad, that they could scarce get her along. She broke all the Ropes that were fasten'd to her; and though she was tied fast to a Tree, yet she made her Escape, and gave them such further Trouble, that they could ascribe it to no other Cause but Witchcraft.

Bernard Peach testify'd, That being in Bed on the Lord's Day at Night, he heard a scrabling at the Window, where he saw Susanna Martin come in, and jump down upon the Floor. She took hold of this Deponent's Feet, and drawing his Body up into a Heap, she lay upon him near two Hours, in all which Time he could neither speak nor stir. At length, when he could begin to move, he laid hold on her Hand, and pulling it up to his Mouth, he bit three of her Fingers, as he judged, to the Bone, whereupon she went from the Chamber, down the Stairs, out at the Door. This Deponent, upon this, called to the People of the House, to tell them what had happened, and he himself followed her. The People saw her not, but there being a Bucket at the Left-Hand of the Door, there was a Drop of Blood found upon it, and several more Drops of Blood found, upon the Snow newly fallen abroad. There was likewise the Print of her two Feet just without the Threshold, but no Sign of any Footsteps farther.

Another time this Deponent was desired by the Prisoner to come to a Husking of Corn at her House, and said, If he did not come, it were better that he did! He did not go, but the Night following, Susanna Martin and another came towards him. One of them said, Here he is! But he having a Quarter-staff, made a Blow at them. The Roof of the Barn broke his Blow, but following them to the Window, he made another Blow at them, and struck them down, yet they got up, and went out, and he saw no more of them. About this Time there was a Rumour about the Town, that Martin had a broken Head, but the Deponent could say nothing to that. The said Peach also testify'd the bewitching the Cattle to Death upon Martin's Discontents.

Robert Downer testify'd, That this Prisoner being some Years ago prosecuted at Court for a Witch, he then said to her, He believed she was a Witch; at which she was much dissatisfy'd, and said, That some She Devil would shortly fetch him away; which Words were heard by others as well as himself. The Night following, as he lay in his Bed, there came in at the Window the Likeness of a Cat, which flew upon him, took fast hold of his Throat, lay on him a considerable Time, and almost killed him. At last he remembred what Susanna Martin had threaten'd the Day before, and with much striving he cried out; Avoid, thou She Devil, in the Name of God, the Father, the Son, and the Holy Ghost, avoid! Whereupon it left him, leaped on the Floor, and flew out at the Window.

There also came in several Witnesses, who testify'd, That before Downer ever spoke a Word of this Accident, Susanna Martin and the Family had related how this Downer had been handled.

John Kembal testify'd, That Susanna Martin, upon a causeless Disgust had threatned him about a Cow of his, That she should never do him any more good, which came to pass accordingly. For soon after the Cow was found stark dead on the Ground, without any Distemper to be found upon her. After which several of his Cattle died very strange Deaths, losing in one Spring the value of thirty Pounds. But the said John Kembal had a further Testimony to give against the Prisoner, which was very admirable.

Being desirous to furnish himself with a Dog, he applied himself to buy one of this Martin, who had a Bitch with Whelps in her House. But she not letting him have his Choice, he said, He would supply himself at one Blezdal's. Having marked a Puppy which he liked at Blezdal's, he met George Martin, the Husband of the Prisoner, going by, who asked him, whether he would not have one of his Wife's Puppies, and he answered, No. The same Day one Edmund Elliot, being at Martin's House, heard George

Martin relate, where this Kembal had been, and what he had said. Upon which Susauna Martin reply'd, If I live I'll give him Puppies enough Within a few Days after, this Kembal coming out of the Woods, there arose a little black Cloud in the N. W. and Kembal immediately felt a Force up on him, which made him not able to avoid running upon the Stumps of Trees that were before him, though he had a broad plain Cart-way before him; and though he had his Ax upon his Shoulder to make his Falls the more dangerous, he could not forbear going out of his Way to tumble over them. When he came below the Meeting-house there appeared to him a little Thing like a Puppy of a darkish Colour, which shot backwards and forwards between his Legs. He had the Courage to use all possible Endeavours to cut it with his Ax, but he could not hit it: The Puppy gave a Jump from him, and went, as it seemed to him into the Ground. Going a little farther, there appeared to him a little black Puppy somewhat bigger than the first, but as black as a Coal; its Motion were quicker than those of his Ax; it flew at his Belly, and then at his Throat, and then over him Shoulders, first one way, and then another. His Hear now began to fail him, and he thought the Do would have tore his Throat out. But he recovert himself, and called upon God in his Distress, an naming the Name of Jesus Christ, it vanished a way at once. The Deponent spoke not one Word of these Accidents, for fear of affirghting his Wife but the next Morning Edward Elliot going into Matin's House, this Woman asked him where Kembal was. He answered, at Home in Bed, for ought he knew. She reply'd, They say he was frighted last Night. Elliot asked with what? She answered with Puppies. Elliot asked where she heard of it for he had heard nothing of it? She reply'd, about the Town. Although Kembal had mentioned the Matter to no Creature living.

    William Brown testify'd, That heaven having blessed him with a most Pious and Prudent Wife, this Wife of his one Day met with this Susanna Martin, but when she came near to her, Martin vanished out of Sight, and left her extreamly frighted. After which time, the said Martin often appeared to her, giving her no little Trouble; and when she did come, she was visited with Birds, which sorely pecked and pricked her, and sometimes a Bunch as big as a Pullet's Egg would rise in her Throat, ready to choak her, till she cry'd out, Witch, thou shan't choak me. Whilst this good Woman was in this Extremity, the Church appointed a Day of Prayer on her behalf, whereupon her Trouble ceased, she saw not Martin as formerly, and the Church instead of their Fast, gave Thanks for her Delivery. But a considerable Time after, she being summoned to give in some Evidence at the Court against this Martin, quickly upon it, Martin came behind her, whilst she was Milking her Cow, and said unto her, For thy defaming me at Court, I will make thee the most miserable Creature in the World.

Soon after this, she fell into a strange Kind of Distemper, and became horribly Frantick, and incapable of any reasonable Action, the Physitians declaring, That her Distemper was preternatural, and that some Devil had certainly bewitched her, and in this Condition she now remained.

Sarah Atkinson testify'd, That Susanna Martin came from Amesbury to their House at Newbury, in an Extraordinary Season, when it was not fit to travail, she came as she said to Atkinson, all that long Way on Foot. She bragged and shewed how dry she was, nor could it be perceived, that so much as the Soles of her Feet were wet. Atkinson was amazed at it, and professed, That she should her self have been wet up to the Knees, if she had then come so far; but Martin reply'd, She scorned to be drabbled. It was noted upon her Trial, that this Testimony cast her into an extraordinary Confusion.

John Pressy testify'd, That being one Evening most unaccountably bewildred near a Field of Martin's, and several Times, as one under an Enchantment, returning to the Place he had left, at length he saw a marvellous Light, about the Bigness of half a Bushel, near two Rod out of the Way. He went and struck at it with a Stick, and laid it on with all his Might. He gave it above forty Blows, and felt it a palpable Substance, but going from it his Heels were struck up, and he was laid with his Back on the Ground, sliding, as he thought, into a Pit, from whence he recovered, by taking hold on a Bush, though afterwards he could find no such Pit in the Place. Having after his Recovery gone five or six Rod, he saw Susanna Martin standing on his Left Hand, as the Light had done before, but they changed no Words with one another. He could scarce find his House in his Return, but at length he got Home extremely affrighted. The next Day it was upon Enquiry understood, That Martin was in a miserable Condition, by Pains and Hurts that were upon her.

It was further testify'd by this Deponent. That after he had given some Evidence against this Susanna Martin, many Years ago, she gave him foul Words about it, and said he should never prosper more; particularly, that he should never have any more than two Cows; that though he was never so likely to have more, yet he should never have them. And that from that very Day to this, for 20 Years together, he could never exceed that Number, but some strange Thing or other still prevented him having any more.

Jervis Ring testify'd, That about seven Years ago, he was oftentimes grievously oppressed in the Night, but saw not who troubled him, till at the last, he lying perfectly awake, plainly saw Susanna Martin approach him. She came to him, and forcibly bit him by the Finger, so that the Print of the Bite is now, though so long after, to be seen upon him.

Besides all these Evidences, there was a most wonderful Account of one Joseph Ring produc'd on this Occasion.

This Man hath been strangely carried about by Dæmons, from one Witch-meeting to another, for near two Years together, and for one quarter of this Time they have made him, and keep him dumb, though he is now able again to speak. There was one T. H. who having, as it is judged, a Design of engaging this Joseph Ring in a Snare of Devilism, contrived a way to bring this Ring two Shillings in Debt to him.

Afterwards this poor Man would be visited with unknown Shapes, and this T. H. sometimes amongst them, which would force him away with them to unknown Places, where he saw Meetings, Feastings, and Dancings; and after his Return, wherein they hurried him along through the Air, he gave Demonstrations to the Neighbours, that he really had been so transported. When he was brought unto these Hellish Meetings, one of the first Things they did to him, was to give him a knock on the Back, upon which he continued as if bound with Chains, uncapable of stirring out of the Place, till they released him. He related, That there often came to him a Man who presented to him a Book, to which he would have him set his Hand; promising that he should then have what he would, and presenting him with all the delightful Things, Persons and Places that he could imagine. But he refusing to subscribe, the Business would end with dreadful Shapes, Noises, and Scrietches, which almost scared him out of his Wits. Once with the Book there was a Pen offered him, and an Inkhorn with Liquor in it, which seemed like Blood, but he never touched it. This Man now affirmed, That he saw the Prisoner at several of those hellish Rendevouzes.

And here it is to be noted, That this Woman was one of the most impudent, scurrilous, wicked Creatures in the World, and discovered her self to be such through the whole Course of her Trial; yet when she was asked, what she had to say for her self, her chief Plea was, That she had led a most virtuous and holy Life.

The Trial of Elizabeth How, at the Court of Oyer and Terminer, held at Salem.

Elizabeth How then pleading not guilty to the Indictment of Witchcraft, which she was charged with, the Court according to the usual Proceedings of Courts in England, began with hearing the Depositions of several afflicted Persons, who were grievously tormented by evident and sensible Witchcraft, all complaining of the Prisoner as the Cause of their Trouble. It was also found, that the Sufferer was not able to bear her Look; as likewise, that in their greatest Swoons, they distinguished her Touch from other Peoples, by which they were raised out of them. There were other Testimonies of People, whom this How troubled nine or ten Years ago.

It hath been usual for bewitched Persons, at the same Time that the Spectres representing the Witches troubled them, to be visited with the Apparitions of Ghosts, pretending to have been murthered by the Witches then represented; and sometimes the Confessions of the Witches afterwards acknowledged those Murthers, which those Apparitions charged them with, though they had never heard what Informations had been given by the Sufferers. There were such Apparitions of Ghosts testify'd by some of the present Sufferers, and the Ghosts affirmed, That this How had murthered them, which things were suspected but not proved.

This How had made some Attempts of joining to the Church of Ipswich several Years ago, but she was denied an Admission into that Society, partly through a Suspicion of Witchcraft then urged against her. And there now came in Testimonies of preternatural Mischiefs, presently befalling some who had been Instrumental in hindering her from entering into the Communion she endeavoured to intrude her self into.

There was a particular Deposition of Joseph Stafford, That his Wife had receiv'd an extream Aversion to this How on the Reports of her Witchcrafts; but How one Day taking her by the Hand, and saying, I believe you are not ignorant of the great

Scandal I lie under by an evil Report raised upon me, she immediately, and without Perswasion, like one enchanted, began to take this Woman's Part. How being sometime after proposed, as desirous to be admitted to the Table of the Lord, some of the pious Brethren were dissatisfy'd about her. The Elders appointed a Meeting to hear Matters objected against her, and no Arguments in the World would hinder this Good-wife Stafford from going to the Lecture. She promised indeed with much ado, That she would not go to the Church-Meeting, yet she could not refrain going there also. How's Affairs were there so examined, that she came off rather guilty than cleared; nevertheless, Good-Wife Stafford could not forbear taking her by the Hand, and saying, Though you are condemned before Men, you are justify'd before God; she was quickly taken in a very strange manner, ranting, raving, raging, and crying out, Goody How must come into the Church; she is a precious Saint, and though she be condemned before Men, she is justify'd before God; so she continued for the Space of two or three Hours, and then fell into a Trance. But coming to her self, she cried out, Ha! I was mistaken, repeating again the same Words; and being asked by the Standers by wherein; she said, I thought Goody How had been a precious Saint of God, but now I see she is a Witch; she hath bewitched me and my Child, and we shall never be well till we have a Testimony for her, that she may be taken into the Church. And How said afterwards, That she was very sorry to see Stafford mentioned at the Church-meeting. Stafford after this declared her self to be afflicted by the Shape of How, and from that Shape she endured many Miseries.

  John How, Brother to the Husband of the Prisoner, testify'd, That he refusing to accompany the Prisoner to her Examination, as she desired, immediately some of his Cattle were bewitched to Death, leaping three or four Foot high, turning about, falling and dying at once; and going to cut off an Ear for a Use, which might perhaps as well have been omitted, the Hand wherein he held his Knife was taken very numb, and continued so, being full of Pain, for several Days, and not very well at this present Time; and he suspected the Prisoner to be the Cause of it.

Nehemiah Abbot testify'd, That unusual and mischievous Accidents would befal his Cattle, whenever he had any Difference with the Prisoner. Once particularly she wished his Ox choaked, and within a little while that Ox was choaked, with a Turnep in his Throat. At another Time, refusing to lend his Horse at the Request of her Daughter, the Horse was in a preternatural Manner abused. And several other odd Things of that kind were testify'd.

There came in Testimony, That one Goodwife Sherwin, upon some Difference with How was bewitched, and that she died, charging this How with having a Hand in her Death. And that other People had their Barrels of Drink unaccountably mischieved, spoiled and spilled, upon displeasing of her.

The Things in themselves were trivial, but there being such a Course of them, it made them more considered. Amongst other Things Martha Wood gave her Testimony, that a little after her Father had been employed in gathering an Account of How's Conversation, they frequently lost great Quantities of Drink out of their Vessels, in such a manner as they could ascribe to nothing but Witchcraft. As also that How giving her some Apples, when she had eaten of them, she was taken with a very strange kind of a Maze, so that she knew not what she said or did.

There was likewise a Heap of Depositions, That one Isaac Cummings refusing to lend his Mare to the Husband of this How, the Mare was within a Day or two taken in a strange Condition. The Beast seemed much abused, being bruised as if she had been running over the Rocks, and marked where the Bridle went, as if burnt with a red hot Bridle. Moreover, one using a Pipe of Tobacco for the Cure of the Beast, a blew Flame issued out of her, took hold of her Hair, and not only spread and burnt on her, but it also flew upwards towards the Roof of the Barn, and had like to have set the Barn on Fire, and the Mare died very suddenly.

Timothy Pearly and his Wife testified, not only that unaccountable Mischiefs befel their Cattle, upon their having Differences with this Prisoner, but also that they had a Daughter destroyed by Witchcrafts, which Daughter charged How as the Cause of her Afflictions; and it was observed, that she would be strucken down whenever How was mentioned. She was frequently in danger of being thrown into the Fire, and into the Water in her strange Fits. Though her Father had corrected her for charging How with bewitching her, yet as was testified by others also, she said she was sure of it, and must die standing to it. Accordingly she charged How to her very Death, and said, Though How could afflict and torment her Body, yet she could not hurt her Soul. And that the Truth of this Matter would appear, when she should be dead and gone.

Francis Lane testified, That being hired by the Husband of this How to get him a Parcel of Posts and Rails, this Lane hired John Pearly to assist him. This Prisoner then told Lane that she believed the Posts and Rails would not do, because John Pearly helped him; but if he had got them alone without John Pearly's Help, they might have done well enough. When James How came to receive his Posts and Rails of Lane, How taking them up by the Ends, though good and sound, yet they unaccountably broke off, so that Lane was forced to get thirty or forty more. And this Prisoner being informed of it, she said, she told him so before, because Pearly helped about them.

Afterwards there came in the Confessions of several other Witches who were penitent, and affirmed this How, to be one of those, who with them had been baptized by the Devil, in the River at Newbury-Falls. Before which he made them kneel down there before the Brink of the River and worship him.

The Tryal of Martha Carrier, at the Court of Oyer and Terminer, held at Salem by Adjournment.

Martha Carrier was Indicted for bewitching several Persons, according to the form usual in such Cases, pleading Not Guilty to her Indictment. There were first brought in a considerable Number of bewitched Persons, who not only made the Court sensible of the horrid Witchcraft committed upon them; but also deposed, That it was Martha Carrier, or her Shape, that grievously tormented them, by biting, pricking, pinching and choaking of them. It was further deposed, That while this Carrier was upon her Examination before the Magistrates, the poor People were so tormented, that every one expected their very Death upon the Spot, but that upon the binding of Carrier they were eased. Moreover the Look of Carrier laid the afflicted People for Dead, and her Touch, if her Eye was off them, raised them again; which Things appeared also upon her Tryal. And it was testified, That upon the mentioning of some having their Necks almost twisted round by the Shape of this Carrier, she replied, It's no Matter though their Necks had been twisted quite off.

Before the Tryal of this Prisoner, several of her own Children had frankly and freely confessed, not only that they were Witches themselves, but that this their Mother had made them so. This Confession they made with great Shows of Repentance, and with much Demonstration of Truth. They related Place, Time and Occasion; they gave an Account of Journies, Meetings and Misthiefs by them performed, and were very credible in what they said. Nevertheless this Evidence was not produced against the Prisoner at the Bar, in as much as there was other Evidence enough to proceed upon.

Benjamin Abbot gave his Testimony, That last March was Twelve Months, this Carrier was very angry with him, upon laying out some Land near her Husband's. Her Expressions in this Anger were, That she would stick as close to Abbot as the Bark stuck to the Tree; and that he should repent of it e're seven

Years came to an end, so that Dr. Prescot should never cure him. These Words were heard by others besides Abbot himself, who also heard her say, she would hold his Nose as close to the Grindstone as ever it was held since his Name was Abbot. Presently after this he was taken with a Swelling in his Foot, and then with a Pain in his Side, and exceedingly tormented. It bred to a Sore, which was launced by Dr. Prescot, and several Gallons of Corruption ran out of it. For six Weeks it continued very bad, and then another Sore bred in the Groin, which was also launced by Dr. Prescot. Another Sore then bred in his Groin, which was also cut, and put him to very great Misery: He was brought to Death's Door, and so continued till Carrier was taken, and carried away to the Constable, from which time every Day he began to mend, and so grew better every Day, and is well ever since.

Sarah Abbot also his Wife testified, That her Husband was not only all this while afflicted in his Body, but also that strange and extraordinary and unaccountable Calamities befell his Cattle, their Death being such as they could guess at no Natural Reason for.

Allin Toothaker testified, That Richard the Son of Martha Carrier, having some Difference with him, pulled him down by the Hair of the Head. When he rose again he was going to strike at Richard Carrier, but fell down flat upon his back to the Ground, and had not Power to stir Hand or Foot, till he told Carrier he yielded, and then he saw the Shape of Martha Carrier go off his Breast.

This Toothaker had received a Wound in the Wars, and he now testified, That Martha Carrier told him, he should never be cured. Just before the apprehending of Carrier he could thrust a Knitting Needle into his Wound four Inches deep, but presently after her being seized, he was thoroughly healed.

He further testified, That when Carrier and he sometimes were at Variance she would clap her Hands at him, and say he should get nothing by it, whereupon he several times lost his Cattle by strange Deaths, whereof no Natural Causes could be given. John Roger also testified, That upon the Threatning

Words of this malicious Carrier, his Cattle would be strangely bewitched, as then was more particularly described.

Samuel Preston testified, That about two Years ago, having some Difference with Martha Carrier, he lost a Cow in a strange preternatural unusual Manner, and about a Month after this the said Carrier, having again some Difference with him, she told him, he had lately lost a Cow, and it should not be long before he lost another, which accordingly came to pass; for he had a thriving and well kept Cow, which without any known Cause quickly fell down and died.

Phebe Chandler testified, That about a Fortnight before the Apprehension of Martha Carrier, on a Lord's Day, whilst the Psalm was singing in the Church, this Carrier then took her by the Shoulder, and shaking her, asked where she lived: she made her no Answer, though Carrier, who lived next Door to her Father's House, could not but know where she lived, and who she was. Quickly after this as she was several times crossing the Fields, she heard a Voice, that she took to be Martha Carrier's, and it seemed as if it were over her Head. The Voice told her, she should within two or three Days be poisoned; accordingly within such a little time, one half of her Right Hand was greatly swelled, and very painful, as also part of her Face, which she could give no Account how it came. It continued very bad for some Days; and several times since she hath had a very great Pain in her Breast, and been so seized in her Leggs, that she hath hardly been able to go. She added, That lately going well to the House of God, Richard, the Son of Martha Garrier, looked very earnestly upon her, and immediately her Hand which had formerly been poisoned, began to pain her very much, and she had a strange burning at her Stomach, but was then struck Deaf, so that she could not hear any of the Prayer or Singing till the two or three last Words of the Psalm.

One Foster, who confessed her own Share in the Witchcraft, for which the Prisoner stood indicted, affirmed, That she had seen the Prisoner at some of their Witch-meetings, and that it was this Carrier who perswaded her to be a Witch. She confessed that the Devil carried them on a Pole to a Witch-meeting, but the Pole broke, and she hanging about Carrier's Neck they both fell down, and she received a Hurt by the fall, whereof she was not then recovered.

One Lacy, who likewise confessed her Share in the Witchcraft, now testified, That she and the Prisoner were once bodily present at a Witch meeting, in Salem Village; and that she knew the Prisoner to be a Witch, and to have been at a Diabolical Sacrament; and that the Prisoner was the undoing of her and her Children, by enticeing them into the Devil's Snare.

Another Lacy, who also confessed her Share in this Witchcraft, also testified, That the Prisoner was at the Witch-meeting in Salem Village, where they had Bread and Wine administred to them.

In the time of this Prisoner's Tryal, one Susanna Shelden, in open Court, had her Hands unaccountably tied together with a Wheel-band, so fast, that without cutting, it could not be loosed: It was done by a Spectre, and the Sufferer affirmed it was the Prisoner's.

It is to be noted, That this Hag, Martha Carrier, was the Person, of whom the Confessions of the Witches, and of her own Children amongst the rest, agreed, That the Devil promised her, that she should be Queen of Hell.

CHAP. II.

Containing an Account of several Remarkable Passages and Curiosities, which attended the Witchcraft practised in this Country.

Amongst the Curiosities remarkable in the Practice of Witchcraft and Sorcery, it is very observable, what impious and impudent Imitation of Divine Things, is apishly affected by the Devil in several respects, in which the Confessions of Witches and the Afflictions of Sufferers have given us Information.

The Reverend Mr. John Higginson gave Occasion to this Reflection, that the Indians who came to settle about Mexico, were, in their Progress to that Settlement, under the Conduct of the Devil; strangely emulating what the Blessed God did to Israel in the Wilderness.

Acasto tells us, That the Devil in their Idol Vitzlipultzli governed that mighty Nation. He commanded them to leave their Country, promising them to make them Lords over all the Provinces possessed by six other Nations of Indians, and give them a Land abounding with all pretious Things. They went forth, carrying their Idol with them in a Coffer of Reeds, supported by four of their Principal Priests, with whom he still discoursed in secret, revealing to them the Successes, and Accidents of their Way. He advised them when to march and when to stay, and without his Command they moved not. The first Thing they did, wherever they came, was to erect a Tabernacle for their false God, which they set always in the Midst of their Camp, and they placed the Ark upon an Altar. When they, tired with Pains, talked of proceeding no further in their Journey, than a certain pleasant Stage at which they were arrived; this Devil in one Night, horribly killed them that started this Talk, by pulling out their Hearts. And so they passed on till they came to Mexico.

The Devil which then imitated what was in the Church in the Old Testament, now amongst us, would imitate the Affairs of the Church in the New. The Witches say, That they imitate the Manner of Congregational Churches, and that they have a Baptism and a Supper, and Officers amongst them, abominably resembling those of our Lord.

But there are several other Things, besides these, which shew their gross and abominable Imitations, as their knocking down with a Look; their making the Afflicted rise; their Transportation through the Air; their travelling in Spirit, whilst their Body is cast into a Trance; their causing Cattle to run mad and perish; their entring their Names in a Book; their coming together from all Parts at the Sound of a Trumpet; their appearing sometimes cloathed with Light or Fire; their covering of themselves and their Instruments with Invisibility. Together with a Blasphemous Imitation of certain things recorded about our Saviour and his Prophets, or the Saints in the Kingdom of God.

Another Thing remarkable in Witchcraft is, besides rendring themselves and their Tools invisible, the Method and Skill of applying the plastick Power, or Spirit of the World to unlawful purposes, by means of a Confederacy with evil Spirits.

How Witches come by this Power, or how Spirits are able to put it in Practice, we cannot pretend to understand. One Person who was of the Number of the bewitched, was cruelly assaulted by a Spectre, which she said run at her with a Spindle, tho' no body else in the Room could see either the Spectre or the Spindle. At last in her Misery, giving a snatch at the Spectre, she pulled the Spindle away, and it was no sooner got into her Hand, but the other People then present beheld, that it was indeed a real proper Iron Spindle belonging to a Person they knew, which though locked up very safe, was nevertheless unaccountably stole away by Dæmons to do further Mischief.

Another was haunted with a most abusive Spectre, which came to her, she said, with a Sheet about her. After she had undergone a great deal of Teazing, by the Annoyance of the Spectre, she gave a violent Snatch at the Sheet that was upon it, and tore off a Corner of it, which was presently visible in her

Hand to the rest in the Room. Her Father who was then holding of her, catched that he might hold what his Daughter had so strangely seized, but the unseen Spectre had like to have pulled his Hand off, by endeavouring to wrest it from him; however he still held it, and kept it a considerable Time.

A Young Man delaying to procure Testimonials for his Parents, who being under Confinement on Suspicion of Witchcraft, required him to do that Service for them, was quickly pursued with odd Inconveniences. But once particularly, an Officer going to put his Brand on the Horns of some Cows belonging to these People which though he had seized for some of their Debts, yet he was willing to leave in their Possession, for the Subsistence of the poor Family; this Young Man helped in holding the Cows to be thus branded. The Three first Cows he held well enough; but when the hot Brand was put upon the fourth, he winched and shrunk at such a rate that he could hold the Cow no longer. Being afterwards examined about it, he confessed, That at that very Instant when the Brand entered the Cows Horn, exactly the like Burning Brand was clapped upon his own Thigh, where he hath shewn the lasting Marks of it to such as asked to see them.

Another Thing worthy our Notice is, That the Execution of some that have lately died, hath been immediately attended with a strange Deliverance, of some that had lain for many Years in a sad Condition, under they knew not whose evil Hands; and many of the Self-murthers committed here, have been the Effects of Cruel and Bloody Witchcraft, by the Power of which, and the Force of the Devil, many poor People have been driven into Despair, their Minds being puzzled with such Buzzes of Atheism and Blasphemy, as have made them even run distracted with Terrors; and some have been bowed down under such a Spirit of Infirmity, who have wonderfully recovered upon the Death of the Witches.

One Whetford, particularly, Ten Years ago, challenging Bridget Bishop with stealing of a Spoon, Bishop threatned her very dreadfully; and presently after Whetford being in her Bed in the Night, was visited by Bishop with one Parker, who making the Room light at their coming in, they discoursed of several Mischiefs they would inflict upon her. At last they pulled her out, and carried her to the Sea-side to drown her; but she calling upon God, they left her, though not without Expressions of Fury. From that very Time this Whetford was quite spoiled, and grew a froward, crazed Sort of a Woman, a Vexation to her self and all about her, and several Ways unreasonable. She lay in this Distraction till those Women were apprehended by Authority, and then she began to mend, and upon their Execution was presently and perfectly recovered from the ten Years Madness that had been upon her.

To this we shall add an Extract of a Letter written to the Honourable Samuel Sewel, Esq; by Mr. Putman.

THE last Night my Daughter Anne was grievously tormented by Witches, threatening that she should be pressed to Death before Giles Cory. But through the Goodness of a gracious God, the had at last a little Respite. Whereupon there appeared unto her, a Man in a Winding-Sheet, who told her, That Giles Cory had murthered him, by pressing him to Death with his Feet, but that the Devil then appeared to him, and covenanted with him, and promised him he should not be hanged. The Apparition said, God harden'd his Heart, that he should not hearken to the Advice of the Court, and so die an easie Death, because, as it said, It must be done to him as he hath done to me. The Apparition also said, That Giles Cory was carried to the Court for this, and that the Jury had found the Murther, and that her Father knew the Man, and the Thing was done before she was born. Now, Sir, this is not a little strange to us, that no Body should remember these Things all the while that Giles Cory was in Prison, and so often before the Court. For all People now remember very well, and the Records of the Court also mention it, That about seventeen Years ago Giles Cory kept a Man in his House that was almost a natural Fool, which Man dy'd suddenly. A Jury was impannelled upon him, amongst whom was Dr. Zerobabel Endicot, who found the

Man bruised to Death, and having Clodders of Blood about his Heart. The Jury, whereof several are yet alive, brought in the Man murthered; but, as if some Enchantment had hindered the Prosecution of the Matter, the Court proceeded not against Giles Cory, though it cost him a great deal of Money to get off.

To these we shall add some parallel and remarkable Passages relating to Witchcraft in Sweden.

In the Year 1669, at Mobra in Sweden, the Devils, by the Help of Witches, committed a most horrible Outrage. Amongst other Instances of Hellish Tyranny there exercised, one was, That Hundreds of their Children were usually in the Night fetched from their Lodgings to a Diabolical Rendevous, at a Place they call Blockula, where the Monsters that so conveighted them, tempted them all manner of Ways to associate with them. Nay, the Growth of Witchcraft was so great, that Persons of Quality were forced to send their Children into other Countries to avoid it. And though the Inhabitants had earnestly sought God by Prayer, yet the Affliction continued. Whereupon Judges had a special Commission to find and root out the Hellish Crew, since another Country in the Kingdom, which had been so molested, was delivered upon the Execution of the Witches.

The Examination was begun with a Day of Humiliation appointed by Authority. Whereupon the Commissioners consulting how they might resist this Growth of Witchcraft, the suffering Children were first examined, and though they were questioned one by one apart, yet their Declarations all agreed. The Witches accused in these Declarations were then examined, and though at the first they obstinately denied, yet at length many of them ingenuously confessed the Truth of what the Children said, owning with Tears, that the Devil, whom they call'd Locyta, had stopped their Mouths, but he being now gone from them, they could no longer conceal the Business. The Things by them acknowledged, wonderfully agreed with what other Witches in other Places had confessed.

They confessed, That they used to call upon the Devil, who thereupon would carry them away over the Tops of Houses, to a green Meadow, where they gave themselves to him, only one of them said, That sometimes the Devil only took away her Strength, leaving her Body on the Ground, but that she went at other Times in Body too.

Their Manner was to come into the Chambers of. People, and fetch away their Children upon Beasts of the Devil's providing, promising fine Cloaths, and other fine Things to them, to inveagle them. They said they never had Power to do thus but of late, but now the Devil did plague and beat them, if they did not gratifie him in this Piece of Mischief. They said they made use of all Sorts of Instruments in their journeys; of Men, of Beasts, of Posts; the Men they commonly laid asleep at the Place they rode them to; and if the Children mentioned the Names of the Persons that stole them away, they were miserably scourged for it, until some of them were killed. The Judges found the Marks of the Lashes on some of them, but the Witches said they would quickly vanish. Moreover, the Children would be in strange Fits, after they were brought Home from these strange Transportations.

The first Thing they said they were to do at Blockula, was to give themselves to the Devil, and vow that they would serve him. Hereupon they cut their Fingers, and with Blood writ their Names in his Book. And he also caused them to be baptized by such Priests as he had in this horrid Company. In some of them the Mark of the cut Finger was to be found; they said, That the Devil gave Meat and Drink, as to them, so to the Children they brought with them; that afterwards their Custom was to dance before him, and to Swear and Curse most horribly. They said, That the Devil shewed them a great frightful Dragon, telling them, If they confessed any Thing, he would let loose that great Devil upon them. They added, That the Devil had a great Church, and that when the Judges were coming, he told them, He would kill them all, and that some of them had attempted to kill them, but could not.

Some of the Children talked much of a white Angel, which used to forbid them what the Devil bid them do, and assured them, That these Doings would not last long, but that what had been done was permitted for the Wickedness of the People. This white Angel would sometimes rescue the Children from going in with the Witches.

The Witches confessed many Mischiefs done by them, declaring with what Kind of enchanted Tools they did their Mischiefs. They thought especially to kill the Minister of Elfdula, but could not. But some of them said, That such as they wounded would be recovered, upon, or before their Execution.

The Judges would fain have had them shew some of their Tricks, but they unanimously declared, That since they had confessed all, they found all their Witchcraft gone, and the Devil then appeared very terrible to them, threatening them with an Iron Fork to thrust them into a burning Pit, if they persisted in their Confession.

There was no less than Threescore and ten Witches discovered in one Village, three and twenty of which freely confessing their Crimes, were condemned to die. The rest (one pretending she was with Child) were sent to Fabluna, where most of them were afterwards executed. Fifteen Children, who confessed themselves engaged in this Witchery, died as the rest. Six and thirty of them between Nine and Sixteen Years of Age, who had been less guilty, were forced to run the Gantlet, and to be lashed on their Hands once a Week, for a Year together. Twenty more, who had less Inclination to these Infernal Enterprizes, were lashed with Rods upon their Hands, for three Sundays together at the Church-Door. The Number of the seduced Children was about Three Hundred. This Course, together with the Weekly Prayers in all the Churches through the Kingdom, issued in the Deliverance of the Kingdom.

CHAP. III.

Containing an Account of strange Apparitions, or the Ghosts of King James; with a Conference betwixt the Ghosts of that good King, the Marquess Hamilton, and George Eglisham's, Doctor of Physick, to which appeared the Ghost of the Duke of Buckingham, concerning the Death and Poysoning of King James, and the rest of them.

THis Account being published in a Dialogue, and so short that it admits of no Contraction or Alteration, without representing it different from the Original, we shall insert it here in the same Words.

     King James. Do'st thou know me, Buckingham; if our Spirits or Ghosts retain any Knowledge of Mortal Actions, let us discourse together.

     Buckingham. Honour hath not now transported me to forget your Majesty; I know you to be the Umbra or Shade of my Sovereign King James, to whom Buckingham was once so great a Favourite; but what Ghost is that, which bears you Company, his pale Looks shew him to be some Scholar.

     King James. It is the changed Shadow of George Eglisham, for ten Years together my Doctor of Physick, who in the Discharge of his Place was ever to me most faithful; this other is his and my old Friend Marquess Hamilton.

Buckingham. My Liege, I cannot discourse as long as they are present, they behold me with such threatening Looks, and your Majesty hath a disturbed Brow, as if you were offended with your Servant Buckingham.

     King James. I and the Marquess Hamilton have just Cause to frown, and to be offended. Hast thou not been our most ungrateful Murtherers.

     Buck. Who, I my Liegcy. What Act of mine could make you suspect, that I could do a Deed so full of Horror, produce a

Witness to my Face, before you condemn me upon bare Suspicion.

  King James. My Dr. Eglisham will prove it to thy Face; and if thou hast but any Sense of Goodness, shall make thy pale Ghost blush, ungrateful Buckingham.

Buckingham. I defie all such Votes and false Accusations; If I had been so wicked, why was not I when living brought to Trial, and sacrificed to Justice?

  King James. A Petition was drawn by my Dr. George Eglisham, wherein he most lovingly amplify'd the Ingratitude of thee my Favourite Buckingham, in Poisoning me his Sovereign, which he then presented to my Son King Charles, and to the Parliament, (for he had vowed to revenge our Deaths) but they taking no Course for the Examination of the Guiltiness, by Reason of thy Plot which dissolved that Parliament, Dr. Eglisham was fain to go over into Holland to avoid the Fury of thy Malice.

  Marq. Hamilton. Nay, he discovered thee Georg Villers, Duke of Buckingham, to have commited two Eminent Murthers, namely, of the King's Majesty, and of me the Lord Marquess Hamilton, for all thy Subtlety in thy Poisoning Art, God hath or Earth Manifested thee to be the Author of our Deaths.

  Buckingham. Were we living thou durst not use this Language, thy Words are false; who dare appear to prove what thou did'st speak?

  Dr. Eglisham. I Dr. Eglisham, as I did once accuse thee unto the King and Parliament, and to the whole World, so I affirm again, that thou did'st poyson King James and Marquess Hamilton; and first I will prove the Murther of Marquess Hamilton, who died first.

  Buckingham. I stand without all Fear, and dare thee, base Doctor, to speak even all thy Malice can invent against me.

  Dr. Eglisham. Then know, Buckingham, that being raised from mean Blood to Honour, and therefore extream proud, thou had'st an Ambition to match thy Niece with the Marquess's eldest Son, and the Bride should have had Fifty thousand Pounds for her Portion. Buckingham. But what is this to the Matter of

Poysoning the Marquess. Eglisham. Yes, thy Niece being unequal in Degree to the Marquess's Son, the Marquess thrice refused the Offer of such a Marriage, but at last, hoping some Way might be found to annul it before it should be confirmed, he yielded unto the King's Desire of the Match, and at Greenwich, before the King, it was concluded; and you, Buckingham, caused your Niece to be laid in Bed with the Marquess's Son, in the King's Chamber, the Bride being unfit, and not Marriageable. Afterwards, the Marquess having sent his Son into France to prevent the Confirmation of the Marriage and your Niece growing Marriageable, and the Confirmation of the Marriage, by you desired, the Marquess answered her, since the Motion, which caused a deadly Quarrel betwixt you and the Marquess, often reconciled, and often breaking out again.

Buckingham. It may be I was offended, but I sought no base Revenge.

Eglisham. That shall appear hereafter. The Marquess of Hamilton, after this Quarrel happened betwixt you, fell Sick, and you, whom King James knew to be vindicative, had occasioned this his Sickness, and afterwards his Death by Poyson.

Marq. I could not endure that thou should come near me, Buckingham, in my Sickness.

Buckingham. But I was still desirous to visit you in your Sickness, though this Urinal-Observer, Dr. Eglisham kept me away.

Eglisham. I knew your Visitation proceeded from Dissimulation, but to hasten to the end of my Accusation, you Buckingham, and my Lord Denby, would not all the Time of his Sickness suffer his Son to come near him, least my Lord Marquess should advise him not to marry Buckingham's Niece. Matters being thus suspiciously carry'd, my Lord Marquess deceased, and you Buckingham would have him buried that Night in Westminster Church. When he was dead, his Body was swell'd to a strange and monstrous Proportion. I desired his Body might be viewed by Physicians, but you Buckingham being guilty, endeavoured to hinder it; but view him they did, and all the

Physicians acknowledged that he was poisoned; and after he was dead, you Buckingham sent my Lord Marquess's Son out of Town, made a dissembling Shew of Mourning for his Death, and a Noise was spread of Poisoning Buckingham's Adversaries, and the Poison-Monger, or Mountebank, was graced by Buckingham; all which are sufficient Grounds to prove you guilty of Marquess Hamilton's Death. Now I will also declare thee to be a Traitor in Poisoning my Sovereign King James.

Buckingham. Speak what thou canst, and add more Lyes to this Relation, I will not answer thee until the End.

King James. Was Buckingham the Author of my Death? I would have thought those Heavenly Essences called Angels might have been sooner corrupted than Buckingham. Was he my Poisoner?

Eglish. He was, my Liege, for Buckingham being advertised that your Majesty had by Letters Intelligence of his bad Behaviour in Spain, and that your Affection towards him was by that grown somewhat colder, Buckingham after his coming from Spain, said, That the King being grown old, it was fit he should resign all Government and let the Prince be crowned.

King James. Didst thou desire the Death of thy aged Prince? I could not have lived long by Nature's Course, Must Poison needs dispatch me? But proceed Eglisham, give us the Circumstances briefly how, and what manner I was poisoned by Buckingham.

Eglisham. Then thus my Liege, Your Highness being sick of an Ague, and in the Spring, which is no deadly Disease, Buckingham when your Doctors of Physick were at Dinner, on the Monday before your Death, offered you a White Powder to take, you refused it, but after his much Importunity took it, and thereupon you grew extream Sick, crying out against that White Powder and the Countess of Buckingham. Buckingham's Mother applied a Plaister to the King's Heart and Breast, whereby all the Physitians said that he was poisoned; but Buckingham threatned the Physitians and quarrelled with them, and Buckingham's Mother fell down on her Knees, and desired Justice against those that had said that her Son and She had poisoned Your Majesty. Poisoned me! said you, and with that you turned your self, King James swooned and died.

Buckingham as before made a dissembling Shew, that he was so sorry for the King's Death, which was nothing so, for he was not moved at all, either in his Sickness, nor after his Death. To conclude, the Dead Body of King James, like as Marquess Hamilton's swelled up, their Hair came off, their nails became loose, now therefore upon these Proofs in the Presence of the King and Marquess confess thy self Guilty, for Buckingham thou wert both a Murderer and a Traytor.

King James. Buckingham, What canst thou alledge for thy self, Did not I end many Differences and Jealousies betwixt my Son Charles and thee, and compose many Fractions? Did not I, when ill Language issued from thee, so that Blows were struck and Swords drawn in my Presence to the hazard of thy Life, cry, Save my George, save my George: Did not I love thee as if thou hadst been my only Son? Made thee from low Degree Rise so fast, that thy sudden growth in Honour was envied at Court? Hadst thou poisoned some other Man, thy Soul had not been half so black or foul; thou might have been compelled to it by Envy, or transported by some cruel Passion, or urged by jealous Fears to make away thy Enemy; but to kill him that was thy Gracious Prince, whose Favour had created thee Duke, and gave thee Honours far above Desert, it was the highest Step of base Ingratitude. O Buckingham, go and lament thy Sins, and here to ease thy troubled Mind confess unto me, Didst thou Poison thy Master King James, shew me why and for what Reason thou didst it.

Buck. First your Majesty began to decline your wonted Affection to me, and likewise to be very jealous of all my Actions and Sayings. Secondly, your Majesty was stricken in Years, and grew intemperate and a Burthen to your self and your People, and they sick of an old Government and desiring a new Change. Thirdly, had I not undertaken it, I could not have stood a Favourite to a succeeding King, nor been so eminent in Court.

King James. Who were Actors besides thy self in this Hellish Plot?

Buck. Many more besides my self whom I dare not reveal as yet, but Time shall produce them, and their foul Actions. Sir, I desire your Pardon, I did contrive your Death by Poison, but I have paid full Justice for it since; my Conscience hath been my Judge and my Executioner.

King James. Let Princes learn from thee, never to trust a Favourite; But what dost thou answer to the Poisoning of Marquess Hamilton?

Buck. This Dr. Eglisham hath spoke all Truth, and proved by many Circumstances that I procured his Death by Poison; I know that I am guilty, but cannot more be punished; Furies of Conscience torment my Soul, and I have no hopes of ease until you seal my Pardon, and say you can forgive me, for I George Duke of Buckingham poisoned King James and Marquess Hamilton.

Eglisham. And lastly, for fear that I George Eglisham should discover you as I have now done to be the Poisoner, I was sought to be murthered, but I fled into Holland; and there by your Appointment I was stabbed and killed.

Buck. I do acknowledge, that my mortal Hatred unto thee was great, and I acknowledge my self guilty of thy Death too, Dr. Eglisham.

King James. Then Buckingham thou was to me an ingrateful Traytor.

Marq. Hamilton. To me a cunning and dissembling Poisoner.

Buck. I suffer for it now, for Heaven is just; farewell, I'll go and weep for Grief.

CHAP. IV.

Containing a Narrative of the Sorceries and Witchcrafts, exercised by the Devil and his Instruments upon Mrs. Christian Shaw, Daughter of Mr. John Shaw of Bargarran, in the County of Rensrew, in the West of Scotland; shewing the Journal of her Sufferings as it was exhibited and proved by the voluntary Confession of some of the Witches, and other unquestionable Evidence, before the Commissioners appointed by the Privy Council of Scotland to enquire into the same; Collected from Records. Together with Reflections upon Witchcraft in General, and the Learned Arguments of Lawyers on both sides, at the Tryal of seven of those Witches, who were Condemned, and some Passages which happened at their Execution.

About the End of August, One Thousand six hundred and Ninety six, Christian Shaw, Daughter to John Shaw of Bargarran, Gent. in the Parish of Erskine and County of Renfrew, a smart, lively, and well inclined Girl, about Eleven Years of Age, perceiving one of the Maids of the House named Catherine Campbel, to steal some Milk, she told her Mother of it, upon which the said Maid (being a Young Woman of a proud and revengeful Temper, and much addicted to Cursing, Swearing and Purloining) did, in a mighty Rage, imprecate the Curse of God three times upon the Child; and at the same time thrice uttered these horrid Words, The Devil drag your Soul through Hell. This was done on Monday, August 17, in presence of several Witnesses, who afterwards gave Evidence of it.

On the Friday following being the Twenty first of August, about Sun-rising, one Agnes Naismith, an old ignorant Woman, of a malicious Disposition, addicted to Threatnings (which sometimes were observed to be followed with fatal Events) came to Bargarran's House, where finding Christian Shaw in the Court with her Younger Sister, she asked how the Lady and the young Child did, and how old the Young sucking Child was? To which Christian replied, What do I know? Then Agnes asked, How she her self did, and how old she was? to which she answered, That she was well, and in the Eleventh Year of her Age.

On the Saturday Night after, being the Twenty second of August, the said Christian Shaw went to Bed in good Health, but as soon as she fell asleep, began to struggle and cry, Help, Help; and then suddenly got up, and flew over the Top of the Bed where she lay, to the great Astonishment of her Parents and the rest in the Room, which was with so much force, that probably her Brains might have been dashed out, if a Woman providentially standing by, had not broke the Force of the Child's Motion. She was afterwards laid in another Bed, and remained stiff and insensible as if she had been dead, for the Space of half an Hour, and for Forty eight Hours after could not sleep, crying out of violent Pains throughout her whole Body, and no sooner began to sleep or turn drowsie, but seemed greatly afrighted, crying still, Help, help.

After this a Pain fixed in her Left-side, and her Body was often so bent and stiff, that she stood like a Bow on her Neck and Feet at once, and continued without being able to speak for Eight Days, excepting some very short Intervals; during which Time she had scarce half an Hour's Intermission together, the Fits taking her suddenly, and coming on and going off with a Swoon or short Deliquium, but she appeared perfectly well and sensible betwixt whiles.

About the Middle of September her Fits returned, in a Manner different from the former, wherein she seemed to fight and struggle with something that was invisible to the Spectators; and her Actions appeared as if she had been defending her self from some who were assaulting her, or endeavouring to hurt her, and that with such Force, that four strong Men were scarce able to hold her; and when any of the People present touched any Part of her Body, she cried out with such Vehemence, as if they had been killing her, but could not speak.

When she was seized with those Fits, her Parents sent to Pasly, for John White an Apothecary, and afterwards for Dr. Johnston, who ordered her to be let Blood, and applied several

Things to her without any discernible Effect. All the while she had these latter Fits, she was afflicted with extraordinary Risings and Fallings in her Belly, like the Motion of a Pair of Bellows, and with such strange movings of her Body, as made the Bed to shake under her.

Some Days after she was able to speak, during her Fits, and cried, That Catherine Campbel and Agnes Naismith were cutting her Side and other Parts of her Body, which were at that time violently tormented. And when the Fit was over she still asserted, that she had seen those Persons doing the Things which she complained of in her Fits; (it being observable that in the Intervals she was as well and sensible as ever) and could not believe but that other Persons present, saw them as well as she. In this Condition she continued without any considerable Variation, either as to the Fits or Intervals for about a Month.

After this she was carried to Glasgow, where Dr. Brisbane an able Physitian, ordered Mr. Henry Marshal an Apothecary to prepare Medicines for her; so that having staid in Glasgow about ten Days, she was brought home to her Father, and had about a Fortnight's Intermission. But then her Fits returned, and with this Difference, that she knew when they were coming by a Pain in her Left-side. In these Fits her Throat was prodigiously drawn down towards her Breast, and her Tongue back into her Throat, her whole Body becoming stiff and extended as a dead Corps, without Sense or Motion; and sometimes her Tongue was drawn out of her Mouth over her Chin, to a wonderful Length, her Teeth closing so fast upon it, that those about her were forced to thrust something betwixt to save her Tongue. And it was often observed, that her Tongue was thus tortured when she attempted to pray. In this Condition she was for some time, with sensible Intervals, in which she had perfect Health, and could give a full Account of what she was heard to express whilst she was in her Fits. Her Parents resolved to carry her again to Glasgow, for the greater Conveniency of being under the Doctor's Inspection and Care, and for the further Discovering the Nature of her Distemper, and making use of the most probable natural

Medicines. But being on her Way thither, in her Grandmother's House at Northban, she thrust of spit out of her Mouth Parcels of Hair, some curled, some platted, some knotted, of different Colours and in considerable Quantities. And thus she continued to do, with several fainting Fits every Quarter of an Hour, both in her passage to Glascow, November 12. and after she arrived there, for the Space of three Days; then from Monday to Thursday following, she put out of her Mouth Coal-cinders, about the Bigness of Chesnuts, some of them so hot, that they could scarcely be handled, as Dr. Brisbane witnesses in his Attestation. Then for the Space of two Days in her Swooning Fits, there came out of her Mouth great Numbers of Straws, by one at a time, folded up, but when out, returned to their natural Shape; and it was observable, that in one of them there was a Pin. After this Bones of several Shapes and Sizes issued out of her Mouth, and then some small Sticks of Candle-sir (a sort of Fir in that Country which burns like a Candle) one of them about three or four Inches long; which when any of them attempted to pull out, they found them either held by her Teeth fixed upon them, or forceably drawn back into her Throat, particularly Archibald Bannatine of Helle Junior, observing a Bone in her Mouth like that of a Duck's Leg, and trying to pull it out, he declared he found something drawing it back into her Throat, so that it required a great deal of Strength to pull it out. It is to be observed, that hitherto she knew not how these Things were brought into her Mouth, and when they were pulled out, she immediately recovered of her Fit for that time. After this there came out of her Mouth some Quantity of Hay, intermixed with Dung as if it had been taken out of a Dunghill, which stunk so, that the Girl could not endure the Taste and smell of it, but was forced to wash her Mouth with Water. Then for a Day's Space, she put out of her Mouth a great Quantity of Feathers of Wild Fowl; after that a Stone, which in Judgment of Beholders, had been passed by some Person in a Fit of the Stone, with some small white Stones, and a whole Nutgall (with which they use to dye Cloaths and make Ink) also Lumps of Candle-grease and Eggshells; of all which there were many Witnesses.

When the Sticks abovementioned came out of her Mouth, she foretold that she was to be grievously tormented with sore Fits that Night, which accordingly fell out; for a little after she fell into a Swoon, wherein she had no Use of her Senses, and though the Spectators called to her aloud and moved her Body, and Mr. Bannatine abovenamed gave her a severe Pinch in the Arm, she was not sensible of it. After she recovered from the Swoon, but continuing in the Fit, she began to talk to Gat herine Campbel after this manner, Thou fits there with a Stick in thy Hand to put into my Mouth, but through God's Strength thou shalt not get Leave. Thou art permitted to torment me, but I trust in God, thou shalt never get my Life, though it is my Life thou designest. And calling for a Bible and Candle said, Come near me Kate, and I will let thee see where a Godly Man was given up to Satan to be tormented, but God kept his Life in his own Hand; and so I trust in God, thou shalt never get my Life, and all that thou shalt be permitted to do unto me, I hope through God's Mercy, shall turn to my Advantage. This Man was robbed of all, and tormented in Body, and had nothing left him but an ill Wife. Come near me Kate, and I will read it to thee; and reading that Passage of Job, when she came to the Place where she said, Curse God and die, the Damsel considering these Words a little, said, O! what a Wife was this, that'bid her Husband curse God and die! She who should have been a Comfort to him in his Trouble, turned a Cross to him. Then, after reading the Chapter through to the End, she looked towards the Feet of the Bed, and said, Now Kate, what thinks thou of that? Thou seest, for all the Power the Devil got over Job, he gained no Ground on him, and I hope he shall gain as little on me. Thy Master, the Devil deceives thee, he is a bad Master whom thou servest, and thou shalt find it to thy Sorrow, except thou repentest; there is no Repentance after Death. I'll let thee see Kate, there is no Repentance in Hell. And looking over the Book, and citing Luke Chap. 16. near the latter End, and reading the same said, Kate, thou seest there is no

Repentance in Hell, for the Rich Man besought Abraham to testifie to his five Brethren, that they come not to the Place of Torment where he was; but repent and turn to the Lord; for there was no getting out if once they came there. Now Kate, thou hearest this, what think'st thou of it? I'll let thee hear another Place which should piece thy Heart. And turning over the Book, she said she would read about Adam and Eve; thou knowest Kate, the Serpent (the Devil thy Master) thought to have ruined Mankind in the Beginning, his Malice was so great at that Blessed-State, wherein they were, seeing himself cast down from all Hopes of Mercy, he used all Means possible to subvert their. Happiness, by suggesting to them fair Promises, and a Prospect of Advantage in causing them to eat of that forbidden Fruit, and were made subject to God's Curse for ever. But God did not suffer them to remain in this Condition, but of his Infinite Mercy shewed to them a better Way, whereby they might have Eternal Life, by revealing to them that blessed Promise, The Seed of the Woman shall bruise the Head of the Serpent. Now Kate, what think'st thou of that Promise? But observe this, thou wilt get no Advantage by it, it is not made to thee, who hast renounced God's Service and listed thy self under the Devil; thou art his Slave; I know thou deniest this; but I know thou art a Hypocrite; for I remember when thou wast in my Mother's House, thou boughtest a Catechism, with a Pretence to learn to read, to cloak thy Sin. Wilt thou hear me, knowest thou the Reward of the Hypocrite? I'll let the hear it; I remember Mr. William Gillies, was Lecturing the other Day, upon the 23d of Matthew, where many a Woe is pronouced against the Hypocrite; Eight dreadful Woes Kate, and some of them belongs to thee; but I'll tell thee more, knowest thou the Reward of the Hypocrite, they shall be cast into the Lake that burns for ever, that's their Portion; Dost thou hear this now? Thou turnest thy Back to me, when I am telling thee the Truth; If I were reading a Story Book, or telling a Tale to thee, thou wouldst hear that. Remember it will be thy Portion too, if thou do not repent and confess and seek Mercy. Again, turning over the Book, she read about Pilate; saying, Pilate he made a

Shew of cleansing himself from Christ's Blood, he washed his Hands and declared himself innocent; but for all his washing, he had a foul Heart, he would not lose his Office for the saving of Christ's Life; he knew well enough that Christ was an innocent Person, but he preferred his Honour before Christ; therefore to please the Jews, and to quench the Struggling in his Conscience, he washed his Hands, and then delivered Christ to be crucified by them. Thus she continued for more than two Hours Space, reasoning at this rate, and exhorting her to repent, quoting many Places in Scripture, in the Revelations and the Evangelists. And when any one offered to take her Bible from her, she uttered dreadful Shrieks and Out-cries; saying, She would never part with her Bible as long as she lived, she would keep it in spite of all the Devils.

Before we pass from this it will be necessary to give the Reader notice of some few Things worthy Observation; as, First, That while she called for her Bible and a Candle, she neither heard nor saw any of those Persons, who were then a actually and discernibly present in the Room with her, and that Catherine Campbel, to whom she directed her Speech, was not discernibly present to any Body but her self. And the Pinch Mr. Bannatine gave her in her insensible Fit, she complained of afterwards, but knew not how she came by it, nor did she blame any of her Tormenters for it. Secondly, That these Words set down as spoke by her, were the very same both for Words and Order, as nearly as they could be gathered and remembered by the Hearers, without any Addition of their own. Thirdly, That although she was a Girl of a pregnant Spirit above her Age, knew more of the Scriptures and had a good Understanding, above what might be expected of one of her Years, of the fundamental Principles of Religion; yet we doubt not but in so strong a Combat, the Lord did by his good Spirit graciously afford her a more than ordinary Measure of Assistance.

Some time after the Trash above mentioned issued out of her Mouth she fell into extream violent Fits, with lamentable Outcries, four Persons being hardly able to hinder her from climbing up the Walls of the Chamber, or from doing her self Hurt; in the mean time she had no Power to speak, her Back and the rest of her Body was grievously pained, and in this Condition she continued four or five Days with the usual Intervals. During which she declared, That four Men, Alexander and James Anderson, and other two (of whom she gave particular and exact Marks, but knew not their Names) were tormenting her. It was observed that many of those she named were known to be Persons of ill Fame, as were these two Persons last mentioned. It is also remarkable, that for sometime she knew not the Name of the said, Alexander Anderson, till one Day he came a begging to the Door of the House where she was, then immediately she cried out, That was he whom she had seen amongst the Crew.

After this she fell into other Fits, wherein she saw the Persons before named with some others, and heard and saw several Things that pass'd amongst them. Particularly she sometimes foretold when she was to have the Fits, and how often she should have them, which fell out accordingly.

About the eighth of December being brought home from Glascow, and having had six or seven Days Respite from her Fits, she fell into a frightful and terrible Relapse; the Occasion whereof she declared to be, her seeing the Devil in prodigious and horrid Shapes, threatning to devour her, she would fall down dead and become stiff, with all the Parts of her Body stretched out, like a Corps without Sense or Motion; these Fits came suddenly without her Knowledge, and she did as suddenly recover and grow perfectly well; and they usually came on her when she offered to pray. Sometimes she knew when the other Fits were a coming; how long they would continue, and when they would return. In which Fits her Eyes altered strangely, and turned in her Head, to the Admiration of the Beholders, with a continual Pain about her Heart; sometimes her Joints were contracted together, and her Forehead drawn forcibly about towards her Shoulders; these Fits she took by falling into a Swoon, and would instantly recover in the same manner.

During this time her Fits altered again, as to their Times of coming and Continuance, in which time she sometimes endeavoured to bite her own Fingers, or any thing else that came in her way; she did the like when she saw the Persons before mentioned, or any one of them about her; she would point out to the People about her where they were, but they could not see them; and sometimes she declared, that she had Hold of them by their Cloaths. Particularly the Seventeenth of December, being in a severe Fit, she cried out of several Persons that were tormenting her, and being in the Bed, grasped with her Hands towards the Foot of it, and cried out, that she had catched hold of the Sleeves of one G. P's Jerkin or Jacket, which was as she said, ragged at the Elbows; and at that very time, her Mother and Aunt heard the Sound of the rending or tearing of a Cloth, but saw nothing, only they found in each of the Girl's Hands a bit of Red Cloth, which looked as if it had been torn off of a Garment, of which kind of Cloth there was none in the Room, nor in any Part of the House. At the same time she told them, there was such a one among the Crew going to pinch her Tongue, which was thereupon instantly pulled back into her Throat, and she lay Dumb for a considerable time. Sometime after her Recovery from her Fits, she told that she heard several Things spoke by her Tormentors, but durst not make them known, because they threatned to torment her more if she did; and accordingly, when her Mother, or others prevailed with her to tell them any thing, she was instantly tormented. She added, That her Tormentors appeared to her with Lights, and strange sorts of Candles, which were frightful to look on.

Thus she continued till the first of January, in such Fits as were before mentioned, with some Alterations, and had likewise other swooning Fits, wherein she continued for Two or Three Hours together, sometimes more, sometimes less, with very short Intervals, in which Fits she did not complain much of Pain, but had a great Palpitation in her Breast, and sometimes strange and unaccountable Motions in other Parts of her Body, which continued, in a greater or less degree, during the whole time of the Fit, wherein she was light-headed, and not so solid in her Mind as at other times; though in the Intervals of these, as of all other Fits, she was composed enough; and these Fits, as all the rest, came suddenly on, and went as suddenly off by a Swoon.

    Before we proceed any further, it is fit to observe, First, That Agnes Naismith, before mentioned, being brought by the Parents a second time to see the Girl, did (without being desired) pray that the Lord God of Heaven and Earth might send the Damsel her Health, and discover the Truth. After which the Child declared, that though the said Agnes had formerly been very troublesome to her, yet from that time forwards, she did no more appear to her, as her Tormenter; but as she thought defended her from the Fury of the rest. Secondly, That Catherine Campbel before-mentioned, could by no means be prevailed on to pray for the Damsel; but on the contrary, cursed them and all the Family of Bargarran, and particularly the Girl, and all that belonged to her, with this grievous Imprecation, The Devil let her never grow better, nor any concerned in her, be in a better Condition than she was in, for what they had done to her: Which Words she spoke before several credible Witnesses. Thirdly, That Bargarran having prevailed with the Under Sheriff, to Imprison the said Catherine Campbel, she never after appeared to the Child, (though formerly she was one of her most violent Tormenters) except once or twice, when it was found upon Enquiry, that she was not in the Prison, but either in the Jaylor's House, or when she had Liberty to go to Church. Fourthly, That at the same time when the Child voided at her Mouth the Hair and other Trash above-mentioned, Catherine Campbel being taken into Custody, there was found in her Pocket a Ball of Hair of several Colours, which being thrown into the Fire, the Child from that time forward vomited no more Hair; she declared, that she heard her Tormenters say, That Catherine Campbel made the Ball, of the Hair cut off of Christian's Head, when the Trouble was first inflicted on her.

    Upon the first of January, about Ten a Clock at Night she swooned, and fell into Fits different from the former; so that after her Swooning was over she lay still, as if she had been dead;

yet at the same time she was heard talking mournfully with a low Voice, and repeating several Stories in Metre, which they thought to be an Account of the Rise and Progress of her own Troubles, and thus she continued, naming several of the fore-mentioned Persons at times, till her Parents and others offered to rouze her, by touching and moving her Body; whereupon she uttered horrid Schreetches, and cried as if she had been pierced through with Swords, and assaulted for her Life. After this she fell a Singing, Leaping and Dancing for a long time, Laughing with a loud Voice in an unusual manner, tearing down the Hangings of the Bed, and pulling off her Head-Cloaths, in which Extravagancies she acted with such Force and Strength, that her Father and the Minister, though joining with their whole Strength, could not hinder her from Dancing and Leaping. But after Prayer, the Minister finding her composed, enquired if she remembered what she had done, in the time of the Fit; to which she answered, That she distinctly remembered her Miscarriages, and particularly her Singing and Dancing; adding, that the Witches inclosed her in a Ring; and that their Dancing and Singing about her, was the Occasion of her Dancing, which she then gladly performed with the rest. For some Days after, she had Fits much after the same manner, with some small Variation: In one of them she tore off her Head-Cloaths, and would have stripped her self of all her Cloaths, if she had been permitted.

  About the Eleventh of January, she fell into Fits different from the former, in which she was carried away from her Parents, and others that were about her with a sudden Flight; and the first time, to their great Amazement, through the Chamber and Hall, down a long winding Stairs towards the Tower-Gate, with such a swift and unaccountable Motion, that it was not in the Power of any to prevent her; her Feet did not touch the Ground, so far as any Body was able to discern, and as she went she was heard to laugh in an unusual manner: But by Divine Providence the Gate being shut, her Motion was stopped, till such time as one of the Family could overtake her, who endeavouring to carry her back, she immediately fell down, and became as stiff as a dead Corps, and being brought back to her Chamber, lay so for a considerable time, Upon her Recovery she declared, That there were about Nine or Ten Persons who carried her away as if she had been in a Swing, wherein she then took Pleasure, her Feet not at all touching the Ground to her Apprehension.

The Night following she was suddenly carried away as before, from her Parents and others, thro' the Chamber and Hall, and Sixteen large Steps of a winding Stair toward the Top of the House, where she met with Apparitions of strange and unaccountable Things; but was carried down again as she thought in a Swing, by six Women and four Men towards the Gate, where she was found, and thence carried up as formerly, with all the Parts of her Body distended, and stiff like one dead. She lay so for some time, and when recovered, declared, That both then and before, she had endeavoured to open the Gate, and that those she saw about her helped her, with a design to get her to the Court and drown her in the Well, which she heard them say, they intended to do, and that then the World would believe she had drowned her self. It is observable, that in one of these Fits afterwards, she was stopped at the Gate, though it was not bolted or locked; yet the Providence of God ordered it so, that neither she nor her Tormenters could open it, so that they left her there as usual.

Before we proceed further, it is fit to take Notice, That as soon as the Girl's Affliction was observed to be extraordinary and preternatural, there was (besides former private Prayers and Fasts by the Family) at the Desire of the Parents and Minister of the Parish, and by the Presbytery's special Order, a Minister or two appointed to meet one Day every Week to join with the Family, the Minister of the Parish and other good Christians in the Neighbourhood in Fasting and Prayer. And on the Twelfth of January, it being the Turn of Mr. Patrick Simson, a Neighbouring Minister to be there; when he came, he found the Minister of the Parish, and the other, who was to join with him, absent upon necessary Occasions, yet resolved to carry on the Work with Three Elders, and some other good People that were present.

When he first saw the Girl, he found her under some lesser Fits, which came and went off quickly; she was sober and quiet in the time of Prayer, but when they sung the Ninety third Psalm, she fell into a very severe Fit of longer continuance, first laughing, then making a Noise like Singing; after that pulling her Head-Cloaths over her Face, and turning so outragious at the last in her Motions, that her Father could scarce hold her till the Fit abated. After her Fit she was quiet and composed all the Time of Prayer; and whilst the Minister lectured on the Ninth of Mark, from v. 14 to the 30th, was very attentive, carefully looking for the Scriptures quoted, and so continued till the religious Exercise ended, and sometimes after, when she acquainted the Company that she had something to tell, which she heard some amongst her Tormenters say, but durst not reveal it; upon which the Minister and her Mother urged her to be free, and not obey the Devil; but before she got a Sentence fully pronounced, in her Mother's Ear, she fell into a violent Fit, so that her Mother and others could scarce hold her, till the Violence of it began to abate, and then her. Mother told the Company, that she was speaking of a Meeting, and a Feast her Tormenters had spoken of in Bargarran's Orchard, but was able to say no more. After her Recovery her Mother desired her to tell the rest of it, and she began again to whisper in her Ear; but could not get one Word uttered, till she was seized again with another Fit, as violent as the former; whereupon the Minister desired them to forbear troubling her any further. But it was observed afterwards, that Elizabeth Anderson, James Lindsay, and Thomas Lindsay, Three of those that tormented her, confessed that they and others had a Meeting in the Orchard at that time, though neither of them knew what the Girl had said, or what the others had confessed concerning it.

  A little after this, she was again suddenly carried from them down a Pair of Stairs, which goes off from the Corner of the Chamber to a Cellar, just below it, where her Brother and Sister were providentially gone before, to bring some Drink, with a lighted Candle, which she soon put out: But they crying, and holding her by the Head-Cloaths, quickly discovered to the rest where she was. Upon which Mr. Alexander King, Minister of Bonnil, made haste down Stairs, where her Brother and Sister had lost their Hold of her; but Mr. King having got Hold of her again, kept her in his Arms till another Candle was brought, and endeavouring to bring her up Stairs, declared that he perceived something forcibly drawing her downwards; but still keeping his Hold, she fell as one dead upon the Stairs, and being carried up and laid in Bed, she lay so for a considerable time. When recovered from her Fit, she declared, That the Occasion of her going forcibly down Stairs, was, that the Crew had suggested to her whilst she was light-headed, that the Devil was in the Meal-Chest in the Cellar, and that if she would go down and put out the Candle, she might force him out of it. When some Fits of this kind were ready to seize her, she now and then gave Notice thereof to those that were present, and earnestly desired their Help to prevent her Motion, which usually proved to be of good Effect, wherein the Divine Mercy is toward her much to be observed.

When she was in these flying Fits, she used to utter horrid Shrieks and Cries, not like those of Rational Creatures; and Three or Four Nights together, when she was asleep in Bed, there were heard Shrieks and Cries of the same kind in the Court, when none of the Family was without Doors, which very much frighted those that heard them, because they exactly resembled the Shrieks and Cries the Girl used to utter when she was in her Fits; and in one of her Intervals, hearing the Family talk of those Cries and Shrieks, and affirming they were uttered by some Wild Beast or another, she told them they were mistaken, for it was Margaret, and two other of the Name of Margats, called by their Crew their Moggi's, that made those Shrieks, the Devil having promised them at that time to carry her out of the House, that they might drown her in the Well, where there were Eighten more waiting for her.

After this she fell into fretting and angry Fits, in which she was cross to all those about her, nothing they said or did proving to her Satisfaction; but when restored to a right Composure of Mind, she declared that her Tormenters still suggested to her, and advised her to go to such and such remote Places of the House alone, and bring with her a String or Cravat, or some such Thing, promising her Almonds and other sweet things, and bid her bring her Apron with her to hold them in; and accordingly when she was seized again with Fits of this Nature, she did resolutely endeavour to repair to those Places with a String, Cravat and Apron, and would suffer none to be in her Company, which put her Parents, and others under a necessity of detaining her by force, and being thus prevented she would Shriek and Cry hideously.

On Thursday, the Fourteenth of January, at Night a young Girl appeared to her with a scabbed Face; amongst the rest of her Tormenters, telling her she was to come to the House to Morrow about Ten a Clock, and forbidding her to reveal it.

The next Day in the Afternoon the Young Girl earnestly enquired of her Mother and the rest of the Family, what Beggars had come to the Gate that Day, and of what Countenance and Visage they were of? But not knowing her Design in such a Question, they gave no heed to it; yet she still insisting on it, and being in Company with her Mother and another Gentlewoman, about Four a Clock at Night she said to them, She thought she might tell them something (the time being now past) that she was forbidden to reveal; but as she began to tell it, she presently fell a crying, that she was tormented through her whole Body, however recovering from her Fit, she went on and told them, that a scabbed Faced Lass appeared to her Yester-night, and was to be at the Gate at Ten a Clock, upon which the Servants being asked, what fort of Beggars had been at the Gate that Day, they declared that amongst others, there had been a Beggar-Woman at the Door and a Young Lass with her, who had Scabbs on her Face, and received their Alms.

January the Sixteenth and Seventeenth, when recovered of her Swooning Fits, she voided at her Mouth a great Number of Pins, which she declared J. P. and a Gentlewoman, who had been always one of her most violent Tormentors, had forced into her Mouth.

January the Twenty First, her Fits altered again, after this manner; she would fall into them with heavy Sighs and Groans, and hideous Out-cries, telling those about her, that Cats, Ravens, Owls, and Horses were destroying her, and pressing her down in the Bed. And at the same time her Mother and another Gentlewoman being in the Room with her, declared, that immediately after they had taken the Girl out of the Bed in this Condition, they saw something moving under the Bed-Cloaths as big as a Cat.

The same Morning, in the Intervals of her Fits, she said, She heard her Tormentors whisper amongst themselves, and suggest to one another, naming J. P. the Andersons, and others, that the Devil had promised and engaged to them, to carry her out at the Hall Window, to the end they might drown her in the Well which was in the Court, and then they said the World would believe she had destroyed her self; and the same Day, and several Days after, when seized with her grievous Fits, she attempted with such force to get out of the Window, that the Spectators with their whole force could scarce prevent her.

About this Time, nothing in the World would so discompose her as religious Exercises, if there were any Discourses of God or Christ, or any of the Things which are not seen, and are eternal, she would be cast into most grievous Agonies; and when she tried, in her milder Fits, to read any Portion of Scripture, repeat any of the Psalms, or answer any Question of the Catechisms, (which she could do exactly well at other Times) she was suddenly struck dumb, and lay as dead; her Mouth opened to such a Wideness, that her Jaws seemed to be out of Joynt, and presently they would clap together again with incredible Force. The same happened to her Shoulderblade, her Elbow and Wrists. She would at other Times lie in a benumbed Condition, and drawn together as if she had been tied Neck and Heels with Ropes; and on a sudden would, with such Force and Violence, be pulled up, and tear all about her, that it was as much as One or

Two could do to hold her in their Arms: But when Ministers and other good Christians (seeing her in such intollerable Anguish) made serious Application by Prayer to God on her Behalf, she had Respite from her grievous Fits of this Kind, and was commonly free from them, during most of the Time of Prayer, though seized by them before. Usually when Ministers began to pray, she made great Disturbance by idle loud Talk, Whistling, Singing and Roaring, to drown the Voice of the Person praying; particularly, January the Twenty second, she was more turbulent than at other Times, and continued some Space after the Minister began to pray, Singing and making a hideous Noise, fetching furious Blows with her Fist, and Kicks with her Foot at the Minister, uttering reproachful Talk to him, and calling him Dog, &c. yet being composed, and her Fits over before Prayer was ended, the Minister, when he had done, finding her sober, and in a right Composure of Mind, enquired why she had made such Disturbance? She reply'd, she was forced to do it by the Hellish Crew about her, and that she thought that they were none of her own Words that she uttered.

January the Twenty-fourth, she said that some Things, relating both to her self and others, had been suggested to her by her Tormenters, but that they had threatned to torment her, if she should offer to make them known: And accordingly, as she offered to express her Mind, she was cast into two grievous Fits, in which she cried out with violent Pains, all the Parts of her Body becoming stiff, and extended like a Corps; her Head was twisted round, and if any Body offered by Force to obstruct such dangerous Motions, she would roar out exceedingly. Sometimes her Neck-bone seemed to be dislocated, and yet suddenly became so stiff, that there was no moving of it; and when those grievous Agonies were over, she again tried to express her Mind in Writing, but to no Purpose, for she was instantly cast into two other severe Fits, in which she was struck dumb, deaf and blind, and her Tongue drawn to a prodigious Length over ooher Chin: And when the Fits were over she declared, That the Andersons, J. P. the Gentlewoman, and J. D. with the Rest of the Hellish Crew, some of whom she could not name, had been tormenting her in her Fits, and that there had been Fifteen of them about the House all that Night, but that now they were all gone but One, who was to stay about the House 'till her Fits were over: And accordingly her Brother and Sister declared, That they saw in the Morning a Woman in the Garden, with a red Coat about her Head, sitting at the Root of an Apple-tree; But Bargarran, with most of the Servants, being abroad, that Matter was not further searched into.

That same Day, about Six at Night, she was seized with a Variety of grievous Fits, in which sometimes she lay wholly senseless and breathless, with her Belly swelled like a Drum, her Eyes were pulled into her Head, so far, that the Spectators thought she would never have used them more. Sometimes when she was tying her own Neck-cloaths, her enchanted Hands would tie them so strait, that she had certainly strangled her self, if the Standers by had not prevented her; sometimes she offered, with Violence, to throw her self into the Fire, and several Times she struck furiously at her nearest Relations. In her Fits she would hold Discourse with her Tormenters, ask Questions concerning her self and others, and receive Answers from them, which none but her self could hear.

She reasoned particularly with One of them after this Manner. O, what ailed thee to be a Witch? Thou say'st it was but three Nights since thou wast a Witch. O if thou would'st repent, it may be God would give thee Repentance, if thou would'st seek it and confess: If thou would'st desire me, I would do what I could, for the Devil is an ill Master to serve, he is a Lyar from the Beginning; he promises, but he cannot perform. Then calling for her Bible, she said, I'll let thee see where he promised to our first Parents, that they should not die, and reading the Passage, said, Now thou seest he is a Lyar; for by breaking the Commandment, they were made liable to Death here, and Death everlasting; O that's an uncouth Word, long Eternity, never to have an End; had not God, of his Infinite Mercy, ordained some to Eternal Life, through Jesus Christ. The Devil makes thee believe thou wilt get great Riches by serving him; but come near, and having expressed that Word, she lost the Use of her Speech, her Tongue being drawn back into her Throat; yet beckening with her Hand to the Spectre to come near her, and turning over the Book, kept her Eye upon that Passage of Scripture, Job xxvii. 18. and pointing with her Finger at the Place, and shaking her Head she turned over the Book again, and recovering Speech, said, I'll let thee see where God bids us seek and we shall find; and reading over the Place, she said, It is God that gives us every good Gift; we have nothing of our own; I submit to his Will, though I never be better; for God can make all my Trouble turn to my Advantage, according to his Word; Rom. viii. 28. which Place she then read, and thus continued Reasoning for the Space of an Hour.

Sometimes she cried out of a violent Pain, by Reason of furious Blows and Strokes received from the Hands of her Tormenters, the Noise of which those who stood by heard distinctly, though they perceived not the Hands that gave them. One Night, sitting with her Parents and others, she tried out, something was Wounding her Thigh; upon which her Mother presently puting her Hand into the Girl's Pocket, found her Folding-knife open, which had been folded when put into her Pocket; but her Uncle not believing it, again put up the Knife, and leaving it folded in her Pocket, on a sudden she cried out as before that the Knife was Cutting her Thigh, being unfolded by the Help of J. P. and others; upon which her Uncle searching her Pocket, found the Knife opened as before: This happened twice or thrice to the Admiration of the Beholders, who took special Notice, that neither her self, nor any other visible Hand opened it.

Jan. the 25th she was again seized with her swooring Fits, with this remarkable Variation; her Throat was sometimes prodigiously extended, and sometimes as strangely contracted, so that she appeared in palpable Danger of being choaked; and through the Violence of Pain in her Throat, and Difficulty of Breathing, struggled with her Feet and Hands, as if some Body had been actually strangling her, and she could neither speak nor cry out to any. With these kind of Fits she was frequently seized for several Days, and in the Intervals declared, that the forementioned Persons, and others, (whom she could not then name) were strangling her; and that the Occasion of her not having Power to speak or cry in the Fit, was a Ball in her Throat, which also was visible to the Spectators, for they clearly discerned a Bunch in her Throat (whilst in the Fit) as big as a Pullet's Egg, which had almost choak'd her.

Sometimes she was kept from eating her Meat, having her Teeth close together when she carried any Meat to her Mouth. Also she was several Times kept from Drinking when at Meat; no sooner tasting the Drink, but she was in Danger of being choaked. Sometimes she held the Cup so hard, betwixt her Teeth, that it was not in the Power of those that were with her to unloose it: And when any Thing had fallen out amiss in the Place where she was, as the Falling and Breaking of a Cup, any Body receiving Harm, or the like, she would fall a Laughing, and rejoyce extreamly, which was far from her Temper at other Times.

February the First, she attempted to tell some Things she had been forbidden by her Tormenters, upon which she was grievously tormented. At the Beginning of her Fits she would look odly; sometimes towards the Chimney, sometimes towards other Places of the Room, but could not always tell what she saw; yet commonly she would name such and such Persons, who, she said, were then come to cast her into Fits. And when any desired her to cry to the Lord Jesus for Help, her Teeth were instantly set close, her Eyes twisted almost round, and she was thrown upon the Floor in the Posture of one that had been some Days laid out for dead; and on a sudden she would recover again, and weep bitterly to think what had befallen her. That same Day, when her Fits were over, she said, she perceived it was by Means of a Charm, that such Restraints were laid upon her, that she could not tell what the Witches had forbidden her to make known; but the Charm might be found out, as she said, by searching beneath the Bed where she lay; and having quickly done it her self, she found (to the Apprehension of the Spectators) an Egg-shell open in the End, which being thrown into the Fire melted like Wax, without any Noise, which Egg-shells make, when thrown into the Fire.

After this, she said, she should not now be handled so severely, upon Trying to make known what the Witches had forbidden her, only her Tongue would be drawn back into her Throat, which accordingly happened. She likewise informed her Friends of many Things she had not Liberty to do before the Charm was found out; particularly, that the Tormenters had often sollicited her to become a Witch her self, and promised her great Riches, and perfect Health, to perswade her to it: Which Temptation, through the Infinite Mercy of God, she still refused, Reasoning with them after this Manner: The Devil promises what he cannot perform; and granting he could fulfil his Promises, yet I am sure, from the Scriptures, that Hell, and the Wrath of God, will be the final Reward of all such as yield to his Wickedness; to which she received this Reply, which none but her self could hear; Hell, and the Wrath of God, was not so formidable as it was represented. She also said, that the Witches had importunately urged her to give her Consent to the Taking away the Life of her young Sifter, who was at that Time upon her Mother's Breast; which Temptation also, she was, through the Grace of God, enabled to resist. She told her Parents likewise, that there had been a Charm also laid upon the Top of the House where her young Sister was, (the Child having been sent out to Nursing, by reason of the continual Affliction of the Family) and that the Charm had been placed there by Pinched Moggy, who by that designed the Taking away of her Sister's Life, and that this was the Cause why she had so often, for some Weeks before, desired her Mother to bring home her Sister, constantly affirming that the Child would daily decay as long as she stayed there: Whereupon, her Parents observing the Decay of the Infant, even to Skin and Bone, they brought her Home, where she recovered. The Girl being asked how she came to the Knowledge of these Things, reply'd, that something speaking distinctly, as it were over her Head, had suggested there and other Things of that Nature to her.

February the Second, being in the Chamber with her Mother and others, she was suddenly struck with a great Fear and Consternation, and fell a Trembling upon the Sight of one John Lindsay of Barclock, Talking with her Father in the Hall. She told her Mother, the aforesaid Lindsay had been always: one of her most violent Tormenters, and that she had been threatned with extreame Tortures, if she should offer to name him; whereupon she was desired to go towards the Place where he was, and touch some Part of his Body unknown to him; which having done, with some Aversion, she was instantly seized with extream Tortures all over her Body. Upon this Lindsay was examined, but giving no satisfactory Answer, was desired to take the Girl by the Hand, which being unwillingly prevailed with to do, she was immediately, upon his Touch, cast into intollerable Pain; her Eyes almost twisted round, all the Parts of her Body becoming stiff, upon which she fell down in the Posture of one that had been, for some Days, dead; and after got up of a sudden, and began to tear her Cloaths, threw her self, with Violence, upon him; and when her Fits were over, the Standers by also took her by the Hand, but no such Effects followed.

About Six at Night there came an old Highland Man to Bargarran, who calling himself weary Traveller, said, He desired to lodge there that Night; but the Servants refusing him Lodgings, gave him something by way of Alms. At this Time the Girl, being in the Chamber with her Mother and another Gentlewoman, said, to her best Apprehension, there was one of the wicked Crew in or about the House at that Time; upon which the Mother made Haste, with her Daughter, down Stairs towards the Kitchin; and finding, unexpectedly, the Highland Fellow there, whom the Girl, accused as one of her Tormenters, she desired him to take her Daughter by the Hand; which he being urged to do, the Girl immediately, upon his Touch, was grievously tormented in all the Parts of her Body; whereupon Bargarran gave Orders to secure him.

The next Morning, the Minister being come to visit the Girl, he called for the Highland Fellow, and having examined him about this Mattes, without any satisfactory Answer, he brought the Child out of the Chamber, covering her Face, and almost her whole body with his Cloak, and giving Signs to the Highland Man to touch her in this Posture, as he had ordered him before, without the Girl's Knowledge, which he did with a great Aversion, and the Girl not knowing of it, was instantly cast into intolerable Agonies, yet others afterwards touching her no such Event followed. When her Fits was over, she desired the Highland Man to allow her the Liberty to discover the Persons that haunted and molested her, whom he had forbidden her to make known. Upon which the. Old Fellow looking upon her with an angry Countenance, her Mouth was instantly stopped, and her Teeth-set; but being desired by those present to speak her Mind freely, whether he would or not; at last, she replied, That she was afraid to do it. And when by the Importunity of the Lairds of Dargarvel and Porterfield of Filwood, and some other Gentlemen there present, she tried to declare her Mind, she was seized with her Fits again.

Before this time, the lamentable Case of the afflicted Girl and Family had been represented to his Majesty's most Honourable Privy Council, who upon serious Application made to them, granted a Commission to a Noble Lord, and some Worthy Gentlemen to make Enquiry into the Matter.

By Virtue of this Commission some suspected Persons were seized, particularly on the Fourth of February Alexander Anderson (an Ignorant, Irreligious Fellow, who had been always of evil Fame, and accused by the afflicted Girl) was by a special Order from the Commissioner of Enquiry apprehended and committed to Prison; as also Elizabeth Anderson his Daughter, upon strong Presumptions of Witchcraft; for the other Year Jean Fulton her Grandmother, an Old scandalous Woman, being cited before the Kirk Session, and accused for cursing, and imprecating upon several Persons, which had been followed with fatal Events; the forementioned Elizabeth Anderson, her Grand Child, who lived in the House with her, declared before the Session, she had frequently seen the Devil in Company with her Grand-mother, in the Likeness of a small Black Man, and that he usually vanished on a suddain, when any Body came to the Door.

Upon this Presumption was the said Elizabeth Auderson seized with her Father, and committed to Custody; but at first denied any Manner of Accession to the Sin of Witchcraft, till afterwards being seriously importuned by two Gentlemen in Prison, before she came to Bargarran's, she confessed her Guilt; and that she had been at several Meetings with the Devil and Witches; and amongst others she accused her own Father, and the fore-mentioned Highland Fellow, to have been active Instruments in the Girl's Trouble; and before she was confronted with him, gave exact Marks of this Highland Man, though she knew not his Name, yet when she saw him did accuse him, and affirmed he was the Person she spoke of.

February the 5th, a Quotum of the Commissioners being met at Bargarran, and the Persons then accused by Elizabeth Anderson, to have been at Meetings with the Devil, and active Instruments of the Girl's Trouble, viz. Alexander Anderson her Father, Agnes Naismith, Margaret Fulton, James Lindsay, alias Curat, Catharine Cainphel, were all of them confronted, with Christian Shaw, before the Lord Blantyre, and the rest of the Commissioners, and several other Gentlemen of Note and Ministers, and accused by her as her Tormenters. And they having all severally touched her in the Presence of the Commissioners, she was at each of their Touches, seized with severe Fits, and cast into intollerable Agonies: Others then present did also touch her in the same manner, but no such Effect followed: And it was remarkable, That when Catharine Campbel touched the Girl, she was immediately seized with more grievous Fits, and cast into more intolerable Torments, than upon the Touch of the other accused Persons; whereat Campbel her self being daunted and confounded, though she had formerly declined to bless her, expressed these Words, The Lord of Heaven and Earth bless thee, and save both the Soul and Body; after which, the Girl, when the Fits were over, in which she had lain a most pitiful Spectacle, declared she was now loosed, and that she might freely touch any of the accused Persons, or they her, after this, without Trouble, which upon Trial, happened accordingly. And being asked how she came by that Knowledge, answered as formerly in the like Case, That something speaking distinctly as it were over her Head, suggested this to her, and likewise usually gave her the Knowledge of the Names of her Tormenters, and Places in which they lived.

February the 6th, The Girl being seized with severe Fits, something was seen in her Mouth like Pieces of Orange-Pills, which were invisibly conveighed thither: She seemed in her Agonies to chew them, and having got them down her Throat, she sell down as if she had been choaked, struggling with her Feet and Hands, and at the last Gasp, her Throat swelling in a prodigious manner, to the Terror of the Spectators When she recovered, she was light-headed for sometime, and would say, O, it was a very sweet Orange-Pill, which I got from the Gentlewoman; declaring also, that there had been others there, particularly Margaret L. or Pinch'd Moggi, whose Sirname she had neither Power nor Liberty to express; nor durst she offer to do it, lest she should be tormented as she was threatened, and always happened, when she tried to do it, either by speaking or writing, as appeared the Day before in the Presence of the Commissioners.

About this time Thomas Lindsay, a Young Boy, not yet Twelve Years of Age, was seized, upon strong Presumptions of Witchcraft; he had said before several credible Persons, that the Devil was his Father, and if he pleased he could fly in the likeness of a Crow, up to the Top of a Ship's Mast, he sometimes caused a Plough to stand, and the Horses to break their Yokes, upon the pronouncing of some Words, and turning himself about, from the Right Hand to the Left, contrary to the Natural Course of the Sun. This he would do when any Body desired him for a Half-Penny.

Upon these and the like Presumptions he was apprehended, and at the first continued most obstinate in Denial, yet afterwards confessed to the Minister, at his own House, before credible Witnesses, his Contract with the Devil, and that he had received the insensible Mark from him, which is visible upon his Body; as also that he had been at several Meetings with the Devil and Witches, where he said his Brother James and others were present, and particularly those who had been accused by Anderson. This he confessed with some others of the like kind, before he was committed to Custody.

After this Bargarran made diligent search for James Lindsay, Eldest Brother to Thomas, he having been all along accused by the afflicted Girl, as one of her Tormenters, by the Name of the Gleid, or Squint-Eyed Elf, (the rest of her Tormenters having called him so, because of his Squint-Eyes) when he was brought to the Place, he did at first obstinately deny his Guilt; yet at length by the Endeavours of Mr. Patrick Simpson, a Neighbouring Minister, he ingenuously confessed it, and agreed in every material Circumstance with the other two, though he knew not what they had confessed, he having neither seen them before his Confession, nor had any Occasion of Information in Conference with others, being immediately brought thither from the Prison of Glascow, where he had been shut up some Weeks before as a Vagabond, in order to be sent to Foreign Plantations.

A more particular Account of what all of them confessed, and acknowledged before the Commissioners for Enquiry, we have for further Satisfaction subjoined to this Narrative; with an Abstract of the Report made by the Commissioners to the Lords of his Majesties most Honourable Privy Council, concerning the whole Matter.

February the 11th, There was, by the Presbyterie's Appointment a Publick Fast, kept on the Girl's Account in the Church of Erskine, in which Mr. Turner, Minister of the Place, began with Prayer; Expounding, Rev. 12. from v. 7, to 13. Mr. James Hutchison, Minister at Killellin, took the next Turn of

Prayer, and Preached on the I. Pet. 5. 8. and Mr. Simpson concluded the Work, preaching on Mat. 17. 20, 21. The Girl was present all Day, and before she came to Church that Morning, told, That whilst she was in one of her Fits the Night before, she heard the Devil speaking of that Publick Fast, and what Ministers were to be there, and that the Old Man Mr. James Hutchison should stumble, and his Peruke fall off as he went up to the Pulpit, and all the People should laugh at him, and he should break his Neck going home. And when she came out of the Church, she said, The Devil was a Liar, for no such Thing fell out as he had threatned. She was all Day very quiet in Church, though troubled with some of her light Fits, during which, some Spectres appeared, as she said afterwards.

About Six at Night, there were present in the Chamber with the Girl, Mr. Simpson with his Wife, the Lady Northbarr and others, discoursing and conferring about her Case; and whilst they were thus conferring together, she told them, she would gladly make some Things known, if she durst for her Tormenters; and afterwards attempting to do it was seized with a violent Fit, in which she leaped strait up, and appeared as if she had been choaked, so that it was as much as one or two could do to hold her fast in their Arms. And when the Fit was over, Mr. Simpson going about Family Worship, Expounded the 110th Psalm, and speaking of the limited Power of the Adversaries of our Lord Jesus Christ, from the latter part of v. 1. She was suddenly seized with another violent Fit, and some Blood issued from her Mouth, which raised Grounds of Fear and Jealousie in the Minds of the Spectators, as to the Occasion of it; yet they could not get her Mouth opened, her Teeth being close set. And in the Interval of the Fit, being asked, If she found any Thing in her Mouth that had been the Occasion of that Blood, she replied, she found nothing, nor knew the Cause of it; but opening her Mouth, they found one of her Double-Teeth newly drawn; but though Search was made for the same, it could not be found. After this the Minister proceeded upon the same Subject, but was again interrupted by her renewed Fits, yet closed the Exercise with

Prayer; after this she was taken to Bed, without any further Trouble that Night.

February the 12th, Margaret Laing, and her Daughter, Martha Semple, being accused by the Three that had confessed, and accused by the Girl to have been active Instruments in her Trouble, came of their own accord to Barragarran's House, and before they came up Stairs, the Girl said, she was now bound up, and could not accuse Margaret Laing to her Face. Accordingly the Girl's Mother having desired some of those who were sitting by her to feel her Body, they found her so Stiff and Inflexible, that there was no moving of it, and immediately again found some Parts of her Body contracted and drawn hard as if by Cords; after this, Margaret Laing, and her Daughter going up to the Chamber to the Girl, in the Presence of the Minister and others, desired the Girl to come to her, for she would do her no Harm, and laying her Arms about her, spoke very fairly to her, and asked her, If ever she had seen her or her Daughter amongst her other Tormenters; to which the Girl did positively reply, She had frequently seen her Daughter, but declined, through Fear to accuse her self, saying faintly, no; after which Margaret and her Daughter returning into the Hall, and the Minister asking her why she said so, since she had accused her before, she answered, You must take my Meaning to be otherwise, upon which she was seized with a severe Fit, and after her Recovery being urged again to speak her Mind freely, Whether Margaret Laing was one of her Tormenters or not; the Child trying to say Yes, and having half pronounced the Word, was cast into inexpressible Anguish; and again in the Interval of her Fit, she tried to express the same Word, and saying only the Word Tint (that is, lost) was suddenly seized with another Fit; and when the Fit was over, and the Child returned to the Chamber, Margaret Laing, who was sitting near the Hall Door, spoke these Words after, The Lord bless thee, and drive the Devil out of thee. A little after this Margaret going down Stairs, the Girl came to the Hall and said, her Bonds were now loosed, and that she could accuse Margaret Laing to her Face, and declared the Occasion of being so restrained while Margaret was present, was, her letting fall a Parcel of Hair at the Hall Door as she came in, being a Charm made by her for that end, which occasioned her also to mention the Word Tint in her former Fit. And accordingly a Parcel of Hair had been found at the Hall Door, after Margaret Laing had gone strait from the Hall to the Chamber, which was immediately cast into the Fire and burnt. And it is remarkable, that it could be attested, that there was no Hair, or any other Thing before Margaret Laing came in; and the Girl being asked, how she knew Margaret Laing had laid the forementioned Charm upon her, she answered, that something speaking distinctly to her as it were over her Head, informed her so.

About Eight at Night she was very severely handled in her Fits, much after the former manner; and while she was in her swooning Fits, a Pin was seen in her Mouth, with which she seemed almost choaked, but by Divine Providence it was got out, though with much Difficulty. After this she was somewhat composed, and did not much complain of Pain, but was distinctly heard to discourse with some invisible Creatures about her, and the Replies given by her, and heard by those that took care of her, gave them ground to conclude she was tempted to set her Hand to a Paper then presented her, with Promises that upon yielding to it, she should never be troubled no more; as also that she should have some Sweet-Meats, a Glass of Sack, and a handsome Coat with Silver-Lace; she was also distinctly heard to say, resisting the Tempter, Thou art a filthy Sow; should I obey thee, this was not the End of my Creation, but to glorify God and enjoy him for ever; and thou promisest what thou cannot perform. Art thou angry at me for saying, thou Sow? What should I call thee but a filthy Sow? Art thou not the filthy Devil, for as brave as thou art with thy Silver and Gold Lace? Wouldst thou have me renounce my Baptism? Dost thou promise to give me brave Men in Marriage and fine Cloaths, and perfect Health if I should consent to it? Dost thou say my Baptism will do me no Good, because thou sayest he was not a sufficient Minister that baptised me? Thou art a Liar, I will be content to die if ever I renounce my Baptism; O! through the Grace of God I'll never do it.

And thus she continued Reasoning, being both blind and deaf, for the Space of two hours, and when she came to her self, did declare it was the Devil, who first presented himself, tempting her in the Shape of a Sow, to renounce her Baptism, as is hinted, and that he chid her when she called him Sow; and immediately appeared to her in the Shape of a brave Gentleman, having Gold and Silver-Lace on his Cloaths, still urging her to renounce her Baptism; which Temptation thro' the special Assistance of the Grace of God she effectually resisted. She also said, That it had been suggested to her by the Spirit, speaking to her as formerly over her Head, after the Combat with the Tempter was past, that one of her Tormenters would be at the House to Morrow.

February the 13th, She was seized with a severe Fit about Twelve a Clock at Noon, in which she continued above two Hours, both deaf and dumb; those in the Room with her cried to her aloud, and pinched her Hands and other Parts of her Body, but all to no purpose. And in this Posture she was hurried to and fro with Violence through the Room; and when any Body offered to hinder the dangerous and violent Motion, she seemed to be in, she roared exceedingly. Sometimes she would desire her Father and Mother, and others to come and take her home (supposing her self not to be in her Father's House) when she was in this deplorable Condition, Margaret Roger who lived in the Neighbourhood, came to the House of Bargarran, enquiring for the Lady; and coming up Stairs, the Girl's Parents remembring she had said the Night before, that one of her Tormenters was to come that Day to the House, brought Margaret Roger to the Chamber where she was, and as soon as she entered the Door, the Girl though she could discern none of the People who were present with her, nor answer them when they cried to her, yet presently saw her, and ran towards her, crying, Moggi, Moggi, Where hast thou been? Wilt thou take me with thee, for my Father and Mother have left me. The Spectators being astonished at this, caused Margaret to speak to the Child, which she having done, the Girl distinctly spoke and answered her every Word. After this, the Three that had confessed were also brought to the Chamber where the Girl was, and as soon as they entered the Door, she ran also to them laughing, as if she had been overjoyed, answering them when they spoke to her; and Margaret Roger, being confronted with them, they declared that she had been at Meetings with the Devil and Witches in Bargarran's Orchard, consulting and contriving the Child's Ruin.

The Lord's Day following, being February the 14th, After some short Intervals, she was again seized with her Fits, in which she said Margaret Laing and her Daughter, Martha Semple, were tormenting her, and cutting her Throat; which Words, through Violence of Pain, and Difficulty of Breathing, she expressed with a low and scarce audible Voice; and upon naming. Margaret Laing and her Daughter, she was tossed and tormented in all the Parts of her Body, being caused sometimes to stand upon her Head and Feet at once; sometimes her Belly swelling like a Drum, and suddainly falling again; and sometimes her Head and other Parts of her Body were like to be shaken in Pieces, so that they that beheld her feared she would never speak more. And when the Fit was over, she declared, Margaret Laing said to her, whilst in the Fit, That she would give her a Tosty (which signifies hot and severe Handling) for naming her.

At this time she was seldom free of her light-headed Fits, which for the most part were all the Respite and Ease she had from the inexpressible Agonies which she endured, in her more grievous Fits, unless when asleep. And whilst she was in these Fits, no Body could perswade her to pray; yet when in a right Composure of Mind, she would weep bitterly at the Remembrance of this, expressing her Tears, lest it might be an Evidence that God would forsake her.

February the 18th, About Two in the Afternoon, she being in a light-headed Fit, said the Devil now appeared to her in the Shape of a Man; whereupon being struck in great Fear and Consternation, she was desired to pray with an audible Voice, The Lord rebuke thee Satan, which trying to do, she presently lost the Power of her Speech, her Teeth being set, and her Tongue drawn back into her Throat; and attempting it again, she was immediately seized with another severe Fit, in which her Eyes being twisted almost round, she fell down as one dead, struggling with her Feet and Hands, and getting up again suddainly, was hurried violently to and fro through the Room, deaf and blind, yet was speaking with some invisible Creature about her, saying, With the Lord's Strength thou shalt neither put Straw nor Sticks into my Mouth. After this she cried in a pitiful Manner, The Bee hath stung me; then presently sitting down, and untying her Stockings, put her Hand to that Part which had been nipped or pinched; upon which the Spectators visibly discerned the lively Marks of Nails of Fingers, deeply imprinted on that same Part of her Leg. When she came to her self, she declared that something spoke to her, as if it were over her Head, and told her it was M. M. in a Neighbouring Parish (naming the Place) that had appeared to her, and pinched her Leg in the Likeness of a Bee.

She likewise declared, That the forementioned M. M. soon after this had been suggested to her, appeared in her own Shape and Likeness, as she used to be at other times. Shortly after this, being being still affected with her light Fit, she whispered in her Mother's Ear, the Devil was now appearing to her again in the Shape of a Gentleman. And being instantly seized with her light Fit, in which she was both blind and deaf, she was distinctly heard, arguing after this Manner; Thou thinkst to tempt me to be a Witch, but through God's Strength thou shalt never be the better: I charge thee in the Name of God to be gone, and thy Papers too; in the Lord's Strength I'll not fear thee: I'll stand here, and see if thou can come one Step nearer me, I think thou fearest me, more than I fear thee. Then turning her self again, she was hurried to and fro with Violence through the Room, as formerly, saying, She was bitten or pinched very much in the Hands with Teeth, and nipped with Fingers above Twenty four times, which occasioned her to shriek horridly, and cry out every time she received them, shewing and pointing with her. Finger to those Parts of her Arm and Leg which had been pinched and bitten; but neither saw nor heard any about her. And accordingly the Spectators visibly discerned the evident Marks of the Teeth and Nails of Fingers upon her Arms and Legs. In this Posture the Girl continued, from Two to Five in the Afternoon, and when her Miseries were over, she said, M. M. told her in the Fit, that Margaret Laing, then in Custody, had ordered her to handle her after that Manner, and that Margaret Laing had a Commanding Power over her.

On Friday and Saturday, the 19th and 20th of February, she was frequently seized with the forementioned Fits, and violently bitten, pinched and nipped in her Hands, Neck, and other Parts of her Body; so that the Marks of Nails of Fingers and Teeth, with the Spittle and Slabber of a Mouth thereupon were evidently seen by the Spectators. When she was seized with her blind and deaf Fits, a crooked Fellow appeared to her, having his two Feet deformed, his two Knees turning inward towards one another, and the fore-parts of his Feet outwards, so that the broad side of his Foot moved foremost; and upon the appearing of this Fellow, her Feet were put in the same Posture, during the time he tormented her. It is to be observed, that there is a Fellow in one of the neighbouring Parishes, whose Feet are exactly deformed in this manner, who hath been along time of Evil Fame, and accused by those that confessed to have been at Meetings with the Devil, and the rest of the Crew in Bargarran's Orchard.

Saturday, Feb. the 20th, The whole Family being gone to Bed, they had left a great Quantity of Peets or Turf by the Hall Chimney, which the next Morning they saw burnt to Ashes, though there had been no Fire in the Chimney nor near them, so that the Plaister and Stones of the Wall where the Peets or Turf lay, were in a great part turned to Rubbish, by the Violence of the Fire, but no other Damage followed, the Hall Floor being laid with Stone, and the Peets lying within the Brace of a large Chimney.

February the 27th, The Chamber Fire having been covered with Ashes in the Chimney when the Family went to Bed, the next Morning, though a good Quantity of Ashes had been left, yet they found all swept away, and no Appearance of Ashes or Fire at all, though none in the Family had been there after the Fire was covered.

In Fits of this Kind she continued for several Days after, naming the forementioned crooked Fellow, J. R. and M. A. two Women that lived in the Neighbouring Parishes, which two latter were accused (by the Three that confessed) to be amongst her Tormenters, and particularly upon the Lord's Day, Feb. the 12th, and the Monday following the said J. R appearing to her, sadly vexed her, telling her she was commissioned so to do, the Gentlewoman M. M. having a Pain in her Head at that time, and so not able to come forth. In relation to which it is worthy Observation, that the Girl declared M. M. to have appeared about two Days after, with her Head bound up with a Hand kerchief, in which Posture she did not formerly appear.

On Thursday, February the 25th, She continued in her former Fits, weeping bitterly and complaining of a Pain in both her Sides, she also told in the Intervals of her Fits, that she was that Night to be in very grievous and severe Fits, her Tormenters being resolved to choak her, by putting Pins in her Mouth, which (though she emptied her self of all that were in her Cloaths) not withstanding came to pass accordingly. In those Fits she was both blind and deaf, leaping up and down in an extraordinary manner, and thus continued for some Days, voiding out of her Mouth, a great Quantity of small broken Pins, which she declared J. R. had forced into the same.

Upon the Lord's Day, being the last of February, about Five a Clock in the Afternoon, she fell into severe Fits, attended with loud laughing, leaping, and running with Violence to and fro, and afterwards wept very much, crying out of Pain, and that a little Highland Man (whom she knew to be such by his Habit and Speech) was now breaking her Leg; which (because of Pain) she scarce could get told in the Fit, and putting her Hand to the Part of her Leg affected, the Spectators untying her Stocking, distinctly observed, a severe Bruise on her Shin-bone, which when touched, did so pain her, that she shrieked and cried horridly, and when recovered declared, that the little Highland Fellow had given her that Bruise. After this she voided at her Mouth a crooked Pin, which she said the Highland Fellow had forced into her Mouth, and designed to choak her.

The first Eight Days of Marth, she continued in her former Fits, with little Variation, voiding at her Mouth a great Number of small Pins, and often fainted and fell dead upon the Ground suddainly, struggling with her Feet and Hands; by all which her natural Spirits were much weakened and exhausted; sometimes also she attempted to go into the Fire. About this time when Ministers and other Christians met in the Family for Prayer, she used at the Beginning of the Work to make great Disturbance, particularly March 2. which Day being set a-part for Fasting and Prayer, she was for some time very composed, till suddainly a strong Blast of Wind forced open the Windows of the Room; upon which she was instantly seized with a violent Fit, whilst the Minister was supplicating God that she might be delivered from Satan's Bonds. In this Fit she was both blind and deaf to all, except her Tormenters, and was hurried with Violence to and fro in the Room; sometimes falling down as one Dead, sometimes singing and making a hideous Noise; sometimes naming M. M. and others, who she said, were there present and tormenting her, and named the particular Places of the Room where she saw them standing and sitting. And when recovered from the Fit, she told that a Gentlewoman and a little Highland Fellow came in with the Blast of Wind which forced open the Windows. This falling out upon the Tuesday, she continued in the light Fit without any intermission till the Sabbath after, not being seized with any of her severe Fits; and having gone to Church the next Lord's Day following, was perfectly well for most part of the Day; yet affirmed she saw Janet Wigh and others in one of the Windows of the Church, though invisible to all others.

Tuesday, being March the 9th, Her Mother and Margaret Campbel her Cousin took the Girl to walk with them in the Orchard; and returning back to the House, her Mother entered the Tower-Gate first, with the Girl at her back, and Margaret Campbel tarrying a little while at the Gate, her Mother went into the Kitchin, supposing they had both been with her, whereas the Girl was suddainly carried away in a flight up Stairs, with so swift a Motion and so unaccountably, that her Absence was not in the least suspected, but her Mother turning about and missing her, cried, where is Christian and Margaret Campbel? and instantly running up Stairs to look for the Girl heard a Noise, and following the same, found her leaping and dancing upon one of the Stairs, being seized with Fits, out of which being recovered, she told, that J. P. had carried her away from her Mother's back, as she entered the Kitchin-Door (her Feet not touching the Ground to her Apprehension) with a Design to strangle her in a high Wardrobe, with Ropes, on which they used to dry Linnen, but that the said J. P. could carry her no further than the Place where they found her, and therefore left her in such a violent Fit.

Upon the Lord's Day after, being the 14th of March, her Fits altered; her Mouth and Nose were prodigiously distorted, and by that means her Face was strangely and horribly deformed. That same Day, being at Church in the Forenoon, her Glove falling from her, was again put into her Hand by some invisible Agent, to the Amazement of the Beholders. To which we may add here, which is worthy our Observation, that all this while an invisible Being haunted her upon all Occasions, suggesting many Things to her, both concerning her self and others, yet was never heard, by any but her self. The same Day betwixt Sermons, she foretold that she was to be violently tormented in the Afternoon, which accordingly came to pass; and in her Fits she named one J. K. a Woman living in the Neighbourhood, whom she said she had seen in the Church. As also that she was Master of these kind of Fits, she was now afflicted with, asserting withal, That if the said J. K. were not sent for, she would grow worse and worse, which her Parents finding to be true, sent in the Evening for the said J. K. Threatning her, that if the Girl was any further troubled with her, that she should be apprehended as others had been; after which, the Girl being in the mean time in a very severe Fit, the forementioned J. K. prayed, though not desired, that God might send the Girl her Health; upon which the Girl was no more troubled with these kind of Fits, but instantly recovered, by falling into a Swoon, as she used to do before her Recovery out of any of her Fits.

Tuesday, March the 16th, She was again seized with her other Fits, all the Parts of her Body being Stiff; and sometimes she was heard conversing with the Gentlewoman (as she called her) vindicating her self of what the Gentlewoman alledged against her, viz. That she had accused some innocent Persons as her Tormenters: To which the Girl directly answered, That she was a Liar, saying, It was you your self, and no other, mentioned ever any such Thing.

Thus she continued till Friday afterwards, being never free of the light Fits, and now and then also falling into Swoons, and appeared to be almost choaked, by means of some Charms and Inchantments invisibly conveighed into her Mouth; which to the Apprehension of the Spectators, were like pieces of Chesnuts, Orange-Pills, Whites of Eggs, or such like, all which were distinctly observed, when she opened her Mouth occasionally in the Fit, and when the Spectators tried to get them out, she kept her Mouth and Teeth so close, that no Body could open it. And when recovered out of the Fit, she told, that J. M. a Woman in the Neighbourhood, had put them in her Mouth.

Upon Friday, March the 19th, She was violently tormented with severe Fits, in which her Neck was distorted, and bended back like a Bow towards her Heels, she struggling with her Feet and Hands, and was sometimes stiff, blind and deaf, and voided at her Mouth a great Number of small Pins, which she said the forementioned J. M. had put there. About Six a Clock that same Night, being violently tormented, she fell a crying, that if the Gentlewoman was not apprehended that Night, it would be in vain to apprehend her to Morrow; for, said she, I have much to suffer at her Hands betwixt Twelve and One a Clock in the Morning. After this she lifting up her Eye-lids with her Hands, and looking upwards, said, What art thou that tells me, that the

Sheriff and my Father are coming here this Night? After which, the Sheriff, her Father, and James Guthry, Macer to the Justiciary Court, instantly came up Stairs, to the Amazement of those that remembred what the Girl had just said. The Girl continued afterwards blind and deaf, yet was heard in the Presence of the Sheriff, &c. discoursing with some invisible Being near her, saying, Is the Sheriff come, is he near me? and stretching forth her Hand to feel if any Body was near her, the Sheriff put his Hand in hers; notwithstanding which, she said to the invisible Being she discoursed with; I cannot feel the Sheriff, how can he be present here? Or how can I have him by the Hand, as thou sayest, since I feel it not? Thou sayest he hath Brown Cloaths, Red Plush-Breeches, with black Stripes, a flowered Muslin Cravat, and an Embroidered Sword-belt; Thou sayest there is an Old Grey-Haired Man with him, having a Ring upon his Hand, but I can neither see nor feel any of them; Is this their Errand indeed? The Girl being asked, how she came to the Knowledge of these strange Things, replied as formely in the like Case, That something speaking distinctly, as over her Head, suggested them to her. It is very observable, that the Persons aforesaid had that same Afternoon got an Order from the Commissioners of Justiciary, to apprehend the same Gentlewoman, and were so far on their way to put it in Execution against the next Morning; but being Witnesses to the Girl's Trouble, and hearing what she had told, viz. That a Delay in that Matter would prove exceeding dangerous to her, they went strait on, on their Journey to the Gentlewoman's House, and put their Warrant in Execution, that same Night. The Girl continued to be violently tormented, sometimes lying with her Neck, and other Parts of her Body upon the Ground, as if they had been disjointed, and sometimes endeavouring to throw her self into the Fire. About Ten a Clock, her Father, who had not gone with the Sheriff, began to read in the Bible, and she repeated the Words after him, though blind and deaf, which made the Spectators apprehend, that she had the Sense of hearing in those Fits, at least when the Word of God was read. To find out the Truth of which, her Father ceased from reading, yet she continued to repeat the following Verses of the Chapter, tho' none in the Room was reading, and she her self had no Book, but was heard to say to some invisible Being; Wilt thou teach me a Part of the Old Testament as well as the New. She continued in her Fit, and said to the People that were present; now it is Twelve a Clock, O! it is now past Twelve; sometimes lying as one dead thro' the Violence of the Pain, and Decay of her Natural Spirits; sometimes again recovering, she endeavoured to express something, but could not. A great Quantity of crooked Pins issued out of her Mouth, and her Body being prodigiously distorted with Pain, she complained of that Pain very grievously. Thus she continued till half an Hour past Twelve at Night, when suddainly she recovered, to the Admiration of the Beholders, telling them, she might now go to Bed, being told by some invisible Informer, That the Sheriff and the other Gentleman the Macer had now entered the Gentlewoman's House, and accordingly going to Bed, she was no further disturbed that Night. It is worthy of Remark here, that the Sheriff and Macer, at their Return declared, that it was just about that Time they entered the Gentlewoman's House, which the Girl mentioned.

Saturday, March the 20th, About Ten a Clock in the Forenoon, she was suddainly seized with Fits, falling down as dead, with her Eyes closed, and sometimes again opening and turning in her Head; she neither saw nor heard any about her, but was hurried with Violence to and fro through the Room, crying out with a loud Voice when any one offered to hinder her Motion. Being in this Posture, and deprived of her Senses, James Linasay, one of the Three that had confessed, was brought into the Room, and no sooner entered into the Room but was perceived by her, and she ran towards him Smiling, and saying, Jamy, Where hast thou been this long time? How is it with thee? and answered him distinctly to every Word he said, though at the same time she neither heard nor saw any other in the Room, nor could she converse with them, which was tried by several Experiments for that purpose, particularly a Tobacco-Box being held before her Eyes by one of the Company, she did not see it, but as soon as it was put into the Hand of James Lindsay. She asked him where he had got that Box? She continuing in this Condition, the Sheriff and her Father being present, thought fit to confront M. M. who was now come, to try if the Girl would see or hear her, as she had done James Lindsay, which accordingly they did. And as soon as M. M. entered the Door, the Girl (tho' still in her Fit) presently smiled and said, I see the Gentlewoman now; though she had never seen her personally before, but only by the Spectre in her Fits. She likewise heard when she spoke to her, and answered distinctly to some Questions proposed by her, such as, When it was she had seen her tormenting her? To which she answered, She had seen her the other Night in her Fits; and further challenged her why she had restrained her from making known the Highland Woman's Name? adding, Thou pretendest thou knowest not what I say, Thou knowest well enough. Upon which the Gentlewoman, suddainly, without being desired, prayed, That the Lord might send the Girl her Health, saying, Lord help thee poor foolish Child, and rebuke the Devil. Which Words were no sooner expressed, but the Girl fell down as dead, and being carried to another Room, forthwith recovered of her blind, deaf, and light-headed Fit, became perfectly well, and continued so for some Time. Being thus recovered, and M. M. removed into another Room, the Girl was examined whom she had seen in her last Fit; to which she replied, She had seen the Gentlewoman, tho' in the mean time, she was altogether ignorant of her having been present with her in Person.

That same Day the Commissioners of Justiciary being come to Bargarran, M. M. and the Girl were again brought together; upon which the Girl being in her Light-fit, upon the first Look of M. M. was suddenly seized with severe Fits, and when recovered, accused her as being one of her most violent Tormenters, particularly mentioning such and such Times in which she had afflicted her, after an extraordinary manner; as also what Words she spoke in her hearing whilst in the Fit, and which is yet more remarkable, questioned the Gentlewoman, if she did not some time in December last, when she was tormenting her, remember how she went away from her in great Haste, saying, she could stay no longer, being obliged to attend a Child's Funeral at home. In Confirmation of which, it is very credibly informed, that W.R. a near Neighbour of hers had a Child buried that same Day, and that the Gentlewoman came not in due time to attend the Corps to the burial Place, but the Corps being near the Church-Yard, before she got to the House from whence they came, she returned again to her own Lodging, and so did not accompany the Burial at all.

The Lord's Day, being March 21st, She fell into swooning Fits, complained of a Pain near her Heart, and fell down as dead, not only when the Fits seized her, but also during the Intervals; sometimes singing after an unusual Manner, and informing the Spectators that J. G. constrained her to that Kind of Musick, her own Lips not at all moving in the time, which the Beholders saw to be true; but her Tongue moved, to prevent which, she often put her Hand in her Mouth. At this time when either she her self, or those about her, offered to read any Part of the Scripture, she was violently tormented, declaring, That if she did but so much as hear the Word of God read that Day, she should certainly be extreamly tortured; in Confirmation of which, when some tried to read, Heb. 11. 2. 4. 6. Isa. 40. Psal. 3. She shrieked and cried out horridly, complaining that she was pinched, in Evidence of which, the Prints of the Nails of Fingers were distinctly seen on her Arms; and being thus pinched or bitten, four several times with great Violence and Pain, the Skin it self was torn off those Parts of her Arms and Fingers, where the Marks of the Teeth and Nails were observed; so that the Parts affected fell a Bleeding; and her Blood was both seen and felt by the Spectators.

Whist she was in this sad and lamentable Condition, she seemed to be extreamly affected and oppressed with sore Sickness as one in a Fever; crying sometimes, to remove those dead Children out of her sight, which she frequently repeated from Six to Nine in the Morning. She continued thus the rest of the Day, and it was observed, that some Charms or Enchantments were put in her Mouth as formerly; of which being very sensible, she fell suddainly down on the Ground, putting her Hand to some Spittle which came out of her Mouth, lifting up some Trash which she again cast down to the Ground, so that it made a Noise; yet nothing could be seen in her Spittle, nor elsewhere by Spectators, tho' in her Mouth they could distinctly observe something like Orange-Pills, Whites of Eggs, and Pieces of Chesnuts.

Monday, being March the 22d. The fore-mentioned J. M. or J. G. came to Bargarran's House, and appearing Face to Face with the Girl, asked her if ever she had seen her in any of her Fits, alledging withal that she could be none of her Tormenters, because she was not seized with a Fit; tho' looking upon her, as she used to be, when she looked upon any of her other Tormenters; upon which the Girl being for some time silent, J. M. or J. G. again proposed the same Question; to which the Girl distinctly replied, Yes; upon which J. M. answered, Perhaps you have seen the Devil in my Shape.

In this Conference there are several Things very remarkable; as First, That the Girl upon her answering, Yes, was immediately seized with a Fit. Secondly, That though after Catherine Campbel had touched the Girl, in the Presence of the Commissioners, upon the 5th of February last, she had ever since that time Freedom to touch any of her Tormenters, without being seized with her Fits, as hath been hinted; yet it is true, that in the Room of that Charm a new one took place, viz. when at any time she looked her Tormenters in the Face, at the first Look she was seized with her Fits; which Charm she declared was laid on her by the said J. M. or J. G. and taken off again by her that very Morning before she came to visit the Damsel; and this she said was suggested to her by some invisible Being, speaking distinctly over her Head; and that therefore now the Girl had Freedom to look J. M. in the Face without being seized with Fits, which for a considerable Time before she could not do, when before any of her Tormenters. Thirdly, It is yet more observable, That the same Morning before every J. M. came to visit her, it was told by the Girl to several Persons in the Family, that J. M. had taken off that

Charm, of being seized with Fits when looking any of her Tormenters in the Face; but that she had laid on another in it's Room, viz. That as soon as the Girl should by Words confer with any of her Tormenters, she should be seized with a Fit, which accordingly was verified when she spoke to J. M. or J. G.

On Tuesday, March the 23d, The Girl, being alleep in her Mother's Bed, about Three a Clock in the Morning, was suddainly awakened (having for some time struggled in her Sleep) in great Fear and Consternation, and being seized with her blind and deaf Fits, took fast Hold of her Mother, declaring to her Father and her, that the Devil was standing near the Bed assaulting her, upon which she cried out suddenly, God Almighty keep me from thy Meetings; I will die rather than go to them; I will never through the Grace of God renounce my Baptism; for I shall certainly go to Hell if I do it. Thou sayst I shall go to Hell however, because I am a great Sinner; but I believe what the Word of God says, though I have many Sins, yet the Blood of Christ cleanses from all Sin; and I will not add that great Wickedness to my other Sins which thou art tempting me to. It is no Wonder thou liest to me, when thou liedst to God's Face. I know thou art a Lyar from the Beginning, and the red Coat thou promisedst me, I know thou canst not perform it: And though I should never recover, I am resolved, never to renounce my Baptism. It is God that hath kept me all the time from being a Witch, and I trust he will yet by his Grace keep me, not because of any Thing in me, but of his own great Mercy; and that he who hath kept me hitherto from being devoured by thee, I hope will yet keep me. This Conference continued near the Space of an Hour, her Father, Mother, and others being Ear-Witnesses to the same. And after Recovery the Girl declared, That it was the Devil, in the Shape of a naked Man in a Shirt, having much Hair upon his Hands and his Face, like Swines Bristles, who appeared to her, tempting her as above-mentioned.

Until the Sabbath following she continued in the light Fit, but every Morning and Evening was seized with her severe Fit, and continued still to name M. M. (who was at this Time set at Liberty) the forementioned J. M. E. T a Highland Woman, and others, as being her Tormenters. It is requisite to observe here, that M. M. being set at Liberty upon Bail, the very Day after she went home, she again appeared to the Girl, tormenting her in her Fits, and continued so to do several Days; particularly on the Saturday, March the 27th, after she was set at Liberty, on which Day the Girl was heard to name her in her Fits, and saying to her, wilt thou say God help me poor and mad, or foolish Child, as thou didst the other Day before the Judges? Art thou wishing the Devil to take me? Where is the Habit thou wast cloathed with the other Day?

On the Sabbath Morning, March the 28th, The Girl through God's great Mercy towards her, was perfectly recovered from all her Fits, and became as well, sensible and composed as ever.

If it be questioned, how the Truth of all these Things is attested, there is none of those Particulars, but what had the Witnesses Names inserted at the End of every Paragraph, and are attested before the Commissioners for Enquiry at Renfrew, by the Subscriptions of the respective Witnesses. But since the Placing of them so now would have occasioned the Repetition of several Person's Names, and made the Narrative swell too much; we thought it fittest to set down the Names of the chief Witnesses together, at the End of the Narrative; and rather because those Things fell not out in a private Corner, but Thousands in this Country have been Ear and Eye Witnesses of them, and have been fully convinced of a diabolical Hand in the Affliction of the Girl.

We shall only here make mention of a few of those that witnessed these Relations, as, the Father, Mother, Grandmother, and nearest Relations of the Girl; as also the Servants of the Family, who were always present with her in her Fits. Such of the Commissioners for Enquiry, as of Justiciary, as had Occasion to be at the Place of the Events were as follows; The Lord Blantyre, Mr. Francis Montgomery of Giffen, Sir John Maxwell of Pollock. Sir John Houston of Houston, Alexander Porterfield of Porterfield, the Laird of Black-Hall rounger, the Laird of

Glanderstone, the Laird of Craigers, Porterfield of Fullwood, John Alexander of Blackhouse, Mr. Semple Sheriff of Renfrew, and several other honourable Persons of good Sense and Quality, as the Earl of Marshal, the Laird of Orbiston, the Laird of Kilmarnock, the Laird of Meldrum, the Lairds of Bishopton, Elder and Younger, Gavin Cockburn of Craigmure, William Denneston of Colgran, Dr. Matthew Brisben, &c. and several Ministers who kept Days of Humiliation and Prayer weekly in the Family, and sometimes in the Parish-Church with the Congregation, viz Mr. James Hutchison, Minister of the Gospel at Killellan, Mr. Patrick Simson of Renfrew, Mr. James Sterling of Kilbarcan, Mr. Thomas Blackwell of Paisty, Mr: James Brisben of Kilmalcolme, Mr. Robert Taylor of Houston; and of neighbouring Presbyters, Mr. Neill Gillies, Mr. James Brown, Mr. John Gray, Ministers of Glasgow, whilst the Girl was there, Mr. John Richie Minister of old Kilpatrick, Mr. Alexander King of Bonnil, Mr. Archibald Wallace of Cardross, Mr. John Anderson of Drimmen, Mr. Andrew Turner Minister of the Place, who was frequently there; besides Mr. Menzies of Cammo, and Mr. Grant of Cullen, Advocates, who were Ear and Eye Witnesses to several important Passages of the Girl's Afflictions, and the convincing Evidences of its flowing from the Operation of the Devil, and his Inftruments. The Truth whereof is further demonstrated by the Progress and Issue of the Tryal, at which were present on several Occasions, not only Sir John Hamilton of Halcraig, one of the Senators of the College of Justice, Sir John Shaw of Greenock, Commissar Smollet of Bonnel, Mr. James Stewart Advocate, who were concerned in the Commission with the others before-mentioned. Besides a great Confluence of several of the Nobility and Gentry out of the Country, such as the Earl of Glencairan, the Lord Kilmares, the Lord Semple, &c.

The Report made by the Commissioners appointed by his Majesty's Privy Council for Enquiry: And the Confession of Elizabeth Anderson, James Lindsay, and Thomas Lindsay; transmitted by those Commissioners to the Council, before the granting of a Commission for a Tryal. To which is subjoined, The Sum of the Confessions of Margaret and Jennet Rogers, who confessed, during the Tryal, concerning the rest beyond Expectation. Together also, with an Account of the Confession and Death of John Reid, who made a Discovery agreeable to that of the former Witnesses after the Tryal was over. Lastly, there are added some Passages which fell out at the Execution of the Seven Witches who were condemned.

THE Commissioners for Enquiry having met at Bargarran, in February 1697, chose the Lord Blantyre for Chair-Man, and took the Confession of Elizabeth Anderson, Aged about Twenty Seven Years, as follows.

That about Seven Years ago, She stayed with Jean Fulton, her Grand-mother, and playing about the Door, she saw a Black grim Man go into her Grand-mother's House; after that her Grand-mother came to the Door, called her in, and desired her to take the Gentleman, as she called him, by the Hand; which she did, but finding it very cold, became afraid, and immediately he vanished. About a Month after, her Grand-mother and she being in the House together, the said Gentleman (whom she then suspected to be the Devil) appeared to them, and fell a talking with her Grand-mother, and whispering to one anothers Ears; upon which the Grand-mother desired her to take him by the Hand, being a Friend of hers; but Elizabeth refusing, her Grand-mother threatned, that she should have none of the Cloaths promised her, unless she would obey: Yet Elizabeth refused, saying, The Lord be between me and him, whereupon he went away in a Flight, but she knew not how.

Elizabeth was not troubled for a long time after, till her Father desiring her to go a Begging with him through the Country, and she saying, That she needed not seek for Meat, since she might have Work, her Father pressed her to go along with him, and took her to a Heath in Kilmacome, where were gathered together at that and other subsequent Meetings, Catherine Campbel, Margaret Fulton, her Grand Aunt, Margaret Laing, John Reid, Smith, Margaret and James Rogers, the Three Lindsays, (besides the Two Confessing ones) &c. and several others whom she did not know, and the aforesaid Gentleman with them; he came to her the said Elizabeth, bidding her renounce her Baptism, promising if she would consent to do so, she should have better Meat and Cloaths, and not need to beg; but, as she declared, she would not consent. Then he asked, what brought her thither, she answered, That she came with her Father, whereupon the Devil and her Father went and talked together by themselves, but she knew not what. She declares, in that Meeting was concerted the Tormenting of Mr. William Flemming, Minister of Innerkipp's Child.

The said Elizabeth Confesses, She was at another Meeting with that Crew, above the Town of Kilpatrick, with the aforesaid Gentleman, whom they called their Lord; and that she went with her Father to the Ferry-Boat of Erskin, where the Devil with the rest of the Band, overturned the Boat, and drowned the Laird of Bridghouse, and the Ferry-Man of Erskin, with several particular Circumstances concerning that Affair; as that some of the Crew would have saved the Ferry-Man, but one of them, viz. his Mother-in-Law was against it, because he had expelled her out of his House, a little before the Meeting. She acknowledges she was present with them at the destroying of William Montgomery's Child, by strangling it with a Sea Handkerchief; that having entered the House, they lighted a Candle, which was somewhat blewish; and Agnes Naismith saying, What if the People awake? Margaret Fulton replied, Ye need not fear. She also declares, That five Weeks before, her Father brought her on Foot to Bargarran's Orchard, into which they entered through a Breach of the Wall, and the Persons before named were present, &c. the Devil telling them that no Body would see them, at which they laughed. At this Meeting they with their Lord, contrived the

Destruction of Christian Shaw; some being for stabbing her with a Rapier, others for Hanging her with a Cord, a Third for Choaking her, and some intended to have her out of the House to destroy her; but fearing they might be taken before the next Meeting, their Lord, as they called him, gave them a Piece of an unchristened Childs Liver to Eat; but the Deponent and the other two Confessors avoided the Eating of it, telling them, that though they were apprehended, they would never confess, which would prevent an effectual discovery. And further, several of them being afraid, that the Deponent would confess, and Discover them, as she had formerly served her Grand-mother, they threatned to tear her in Pieces if she did so, and particularly Margaret Laing threatened her most.

After two Hours, they flew away and disappeared, except the Deponent, who went home upon her Feet; she confesses likewise that one Night her Father raised her out of her Bed, and going to the River-side, took her on his Back, and flew with her over, from whence they went on Foot to Dunbritton, and in Mr. John Hardy, the Minister's Yard, the Crew and their Lord being met, they formed the Picture of Mr. Hardy, and dabbed it full of Pins, and having put it amongst Water and Ale mixed together, rosted it on a Spit at a Fire, &c. after which her Father and she returned as they went.

James Lindsay, Aged Fourteen Years, declares, That one Day he met with the deceased Jean Fulton his Grand-mother, at her own House, where she took from him a little round Cap, and a Plack, or 1/3 of a Penny; at which being vexed, he required them from her again, and she refusing to restore them, he called her an Old Witch and ran away; upon which she followed him and cried, That she would meet him with a Vengeance. About Three Days after, being a Begging in the Country, he met his Grand-mother with a Black grim Man, whom she desired him to take by the Hand, which he did, but found it exceeding cold, and his own Hand mightily squeezed; upon which the said Gentleman (as she called him) asked the Deponent if he would serve him, and he should have a Coat, Hat, and several other Things; to which James answered, Yes, I'll do it; after this the foresaid Gentleman (whom the Deponent knew afterwards to be the Devil) and his Grand-mother went away, but he knows not how. He acknowledges he was frequently afterwards at Meetings with the Devil and Witches, particularly those mentioned in Elizabeth Anderson's Confessions; that their Lord came to James at their first publick Meeting; took him by the Hand and forbad him to discover; that they contrived beforehand at the said Meeting the drowning of Bridghouse, and concurs with Elizabeth Anderson as to the Design of saving the Ferry-man, which his Mother-in-Law did divert. He being examined, declared he did not see, J. K. and J. W. at the committing of the foresaid Fact; (and indeed they were then in Prison) That they with a Cord strangled Matihew Park's Child, and that the Person who waited on the Child finding it stifled, cried out, Matthew, Matthew, the Child is Dead. Elizabeth Anderson concurs in this Particular, and tells, that when they had done they took the Cord with them.

This Deponent further declares, That he was present at strangling William Montgomery's Child, with a Sea Handkerchief, and heard Agnes Naismith say, Draw the Knot. That about five Weeks ago, he was carried to them in Bargarran's Orchard, and concurs with Elizabeth Anderson in what was treated of there, as to the Destroying of Christian Shaw, and the Charm against confessing. He likewise acknowledges the Meeting at Dunbritton about Mr. Hardy; and that he hath several times appeared to Christian Shaw both in Glasgow and Bargarran, with the rest that tormented her, and put into her Mouth, Coal-Cinders, Bones, Hay, Hair, Sticks, &c. intending thereby to choak her. That he and they did often prick and stab her in the following Manner, viz. He had a Needle, which if he put in his Cloaths, her Body would be pricked and stabbed in that Place where he fixed the Needle, and if he put in his Hair, that Part of her Head would be tormented; That he saw her void the Pins they had put in, on which time he cried out in these Words, help J. D. who was also then present; That when the Ministers began to pray in Bargarran's House at several Occasions, the Devil and they immediately went away, &c.

Thomas Lindsay being under Age declares, That the same Jean Fulton his Grand-mother, awaked him one Night out of his Bed, and caused him to take a black grim Gentleman (as she called him) by the Hand, which he felt to be cold. And that he having enquired if Thomas would serve him and be his Man, he would give him a red Coat, he consented. And the Gentleman (whom he know afterwards to be the Devil) pinched him in the Neck, which continued sore for Ten Days. That one Day after his Grand-mother's Decease, coming by her House, he thought she appeared to him stroaking his Head, and desiring him to be a good Servant to the Gentleman to whom she had given him; and forbid him to reveal it. He declares, That one Night in Bed in the House of one Robert Shaw, he was a waked out of his Sleep, and carried as if he had flew to Martha Park's House, where were present the particular Persons, named by him, and concurs as to the Manner of strangling of the Child, with James Lindsay his Brother; and that another Night being in the House of Walter Alexander, he was brought to the Strangling of William Montgomery's Child, and agrees likewise in the Manner of it with his Brother, only he says, the Sea Handkerchief with which they committed the Fact was speckled; he likewise concurs as to the Meeting in Bargarran's Orchard about five Weeks ago, and in what was acted there; as also about Mr. Hardy, with this Addition, that he himself turned the Spit, on which the Picture was roasted.

It is to be observed, That as the Three Confessors were apprehended separately upon several Occasions, so after their Obstinacy to discover was abated, they made these Confessions in several distinct Places without Communication, without Knowledge of one another's Confessions. The Commissioners examined them by other trying Questions that were new, on purpose to make Experiment of their Agreement or Disagreement; but still found them to agree in the Matters of Fact (declared by them) particularly in Strangling the Children, the Death of the Minister, the Drowning of those in the Boat, and the Tormenting of Bargarran's Daughter. The Commissioners did also confront them both with Christian Shaw, the afflicted Girl, and the other Persons accused (whom they had caused to be apprehended) and both the Girl and the Confessors did accuse them to their Faces, and convince them by Circumstances, with great Steadiness and Agreement, though frequently brought in. The Commissioners did also try some Experiments, about the Girl's falling in Fits at the Approach of the Accused, as is expressed in the Narrative; and examined her with those who were commonly about her, as to the Particulars of her Sufferings; they tried to cause her to write, since she could not speak the Name of a Person, whom she first called Margaret, or Pinch'd Moggi, and asserted to be one of her chief Tormenters; but upon writing Margaret, and the Letter Z. of her Sirname, the Girl was presently taken with a fearful Convulsion; the Pen was struck out of her Hand, and she fell dead, with heavier Groans than ordinary; after her Recovery, some Ministers shewed her a Passage of the Bible, but as soon as she attempted to cast her Eyes on it, she fell into vehement Pangs; but one of the Commissioners ordering the Book to be closed, she immediately came to her self, In the last Place, the Commissioners called before them, those Persons who had signed the Passages of the several Days in the written Journal of the Girl's Sufferings; and having examined them upon it, transmitted the same with the Declarations of the Three Confessors, and several of the Passages that occurred in the Precognition, to his Majesties Privy-Council, by whom they were appointed to enquire into the Matter.

Besides all this, The signed Attestations of Dr. Matthew Brisben, Physician, and Mr. Henry Marshall, Apothecary in Glasgow; did very much influence them to the Belief of an extraordinary Cause of those Things that befel Christian Shaw.

The Doctor's Attestation.

ABOUT the Twenty Fourth, or Twenty Fifth of October last, The Lady Bargarran brought a Daughter of hers, a Child of Eleven Years Old, or thereabouts, to Glasgow to take Advice of Physicians concerning her. When I was first brought to her, I could hardly be perswaded, there was any Need of me or any Man else of my Profession, the Child appeared so brisk and vigorous in Motions, so chearful, and of so florid, and of so good a Colour, and in a Word, to outward Appearance every way healthful; but it was not long till I found my self obliged to alter my Thoughts of her; for I had not been above Eight or Ten Minutes in the Room, till she arose from her Seat, and acquainted the Company that she was instantly to be seized with a Fit; and so being strait way carried to Bed, I observed a considerable Stiffness and Distention in her left Hypochondre, which falling in a trice, she was taken with horrid convulsive Motions in most Parts of her Body, but her Back and Neck especially. This was accompanied with heavy Groans at the first, which as soon as she was able to frame. Words were converted into a Kind of expostulatory Murmuring against some Women, two whereof she always named; one of them she called Naismith, as I remember, and the other Campbel. All these Symptoms I thought were very reducible to the Effect of hypochondriack Melancholy; and therefore putting her in such a Course as I thought proper against that Kind of Malady, I was in absolute Security as to her Case; the Child having continued free from all the above-mentioned Symptoms, I think, for the Space of a Week, in this Town, and some Eight or Ten Days more in the Country. And I was perfectly surprized, when a Friend of the Lady Bargarran told me, that the Child was returned to Town again, and worse than ever; for now she was in great Hazard of being choaked with Mouthfulls of Hair, which she apprehended the Women above-mentioned to be pressing down her Throat, had not she her self pulled it out.

Having read many such Stories in Authors, and heard the like from other Hands too, but never seen any such Things, I was the more earnest to see the Child again. For some Weeks whilst she staid in this Place, I was frequently with her; observed her narrowly, and was confident she had no human Correspondent to subminister the Straw, Wool, Cinders, Hay, Feathers, and such like Trash to her; all which upon several Occasions, I have seen her pull out of her Mouth in considerable Quantities; sometimes after several Fits, and sometimes without any Fit at all, whilst she was discoursing with us; and for the most part she pulled out all these Things without being wet in the least; nay rather as if they had been dried with Care and Art; for one Time, as I remember, when I was discoursing with her, and she with me, she gave me a Cinder out of her Mouth, not only dry, but hot, much above the Degree of the natural Warmth of a Human body. During the Time she was thus exercised, tho' she had daily not only light convulsive Motions, but two strange Convulsions, such as we call [Greek omitted] to a high Degree, and Rigidity of the whole Body; yet she fancied as at other times, she saw many such People, as have been already named, about her; but the Voiding, or rather Pulling out of the Things above-named, did no sooner cease, but as in all her Fits, when she was able to speak, she constantly cried out, that they were pinching or pricking her. Those Fits were both more severe, and more frequent than before, and followed with an Alienation of Mind for some time. I have seen her too, when free of all other Fits, suddainly seized with Dumbness, her Tongue being strangely contracted, so that it appeared to her self, as she expressed it, as if the People were drawing it down her Throat. This I declare on Conscience, and in most solemn Manner is what I have seen and handled; and were it not for the Hairs, Hay, Straw, and other Things, wholly contrary to human Nature, I should not despair to reduce all the other Symptoms to their proper Classes in the Catalogue of Human Diseases: Written and Signed at Glasgow, the Thirty first Day of December 1696, By me, Sic subscribitur, M. Brisben, M. D.

The Declaration of Mr. Henry Marshall Apothecary. Being desired by John Shaw, of Bargarran, to declare what I know of his Daughter Christian's Condition, I do it as follows.

ABOUT the latter End of October last, She was brought hither, to have Dr. Brisben's Advice about her Health, and I was employed as Apothecary. The Child was about Eleven Years of Age, of a good Habit of Body as far as I could judge; but now and then fell into Convulsions, Swoons, and a little Lightness of Head; and when recovered out of these Fits, she would be perfectly well again, and by the Use of the Means the Dr. prescribed, she seemed to be free of her Distemper; whereupon she was taken back to the Country: but had not been long there till she became worse than before, and was sent hither again, to be under the Doctor's Care; and after her Fits she took out of her Mouth, without any Pressure or Vomiting Tufts of Hair, Straw, long and folded together, burnt Coals, Peices of Bones, Leather, Chips of Timber, and several other Things, several of which she hath taken out of her Mouth and given to me, whilst we were conversing together. And upon the 20th of November last, when I went to see her, I found her in a Swoon, whereinto she had fallen, just as I came to the House. When she had lain so for some Time, she arose in a great Rage, beat all about her, frowning with her Countenance, and expressing a great deal of unknown Language, in an angry Manner. Then she put the Tuft of a Highland Belt, which was girt about her, into her Mouth, and pulled with her Hand so hard, that if we had not cut the Belt with a Knife, she had in all Probability drawn out her Teeth; upon which she tore the Tuft all to Pieces with her Teeth, and afterwards fell a tearing her Cloaths, and her Shoes, which she pulled off, and every Thing she could get into her Hands. Then she fell into a dumb Fit, as she called it, in which all her Body was so convulsed and distorted, that I endeavoured to put her Arms into a better Posture, but found them so stiff, that I could not bring them to their natural Posture without breaking them. Then she arose out of that Fit, and went up and down the Room, and would have gone through the Wall, muttering the former unknown Language. After this she fell head-long on the Ground, as if she had been thrown down with Violence, where she lay for sometime as Dead, but afterwards arose, as if she had been something recovered, and fell a reasoning very distinctly, thus; Ketie, what ails thee at me? I am sure I never did thee wrong. Why should thou trouble me? Come let us agree, let there be no more Difference betwixt us. And putting out her Hands as if she would have taken her by the Hands, she said, Let us shake Hands together; then pulling in her Hand again, she said, well Ketie, I cannot help it, you will not agree with me; and having pronounced those Words she immediately fell into another Fit, and swooned; and out of that into another Rage, in which she bit her own Fingers, and tore her Hands upon Pins that were in her own Cloaths; after which she appeared angry; pulled out all the Pins and threw them away. And after she had been tormented thus for more than half an Hour, without any Intermission, she recovered and became perfectly well. Upon that, I asked her how she was? To which she answered, she had just now a very bad Fit, for during the Fit, she knew no Body, neither took any Notice of me, though I moved her Body, and spoke often to her. I asked her again, what she saw in her Fits? she answered, I saw Catherine Campbel, Agnes Naismith, Alexander Anderson, and others that she did not know. I enquired again, What Catharine Campbel was doing? she told me, she was going to thrust a Sword into her Side, which made her so desirous to be agreed with her. And when she had told me this, instantly she fell into another Swoon, and repeated all that was said before, and much more, which I have partly forgot, and in each of those two Fits she continued Half an Hour. All this I declare upon Conscience, and in most solemn Manner, to be Truth, in Testimony where-of I have Writ and Subscribed this at Glasgow, the First Day of January 1697. Sic Scribitur,

HENRY MARSHALL

Whilst the Tryal was depending, James and Margaret Rogers confessed after this Manner; the Commissioners had adjourned two several Times, and though they were to meet on the Third, yet it was not expected, that they would proceed, till Providence should make the Guilt of the Prisoners appear, by the further Testimonies of those that should confess; but the very Morning they were to meet the Third time, those two Women above-mentioned, confess'd, which was a Surprize to every one that came to attend the Court; since these were not formerly taken notice of as others were; but freely confessed without any Body desiring them, nor had they such Means of Instruction as others had. Their Confessions agreed as to the Meetings and the Things acted in them with those of the three former, and the other Evidences of visible Matters of Fact; only they were so punctual as to name some of the indicted Persons, whom they did not see at those Rendevouzes; and great Care was taken to compare their Testimonies with what had been already discovered, and to try their certain Knowledge by new Questions when they were separated from one another, &c. Thus the whole Matter was so evident, that the Commissioners with the general Approbation of the most intelligent Men in the Country, who came to attend the Court, approved the Proceedings of the Process, and bringing seven of the best known Criminals (for whom an Advocate appeared) to Tryal. Accordingly there were some Days allowed for the Persons indicted, to give in their Informations upon the finding the Bill; and at the Term their was much Time spent in producing Witnesses, an Account of which is referred to another Place.

Upon the 21st of May, 1697, after Tryal of the Seven Witches, there is an Attestation subscribed by Mr. Patrick Simson, Minister of Renfrew; Walter Scot Baily there, &c. of this Import; John Reid, Smith at Inchannan Prisoner, did in Presence of the said Persons and some others, declare, that about a Year ago, the Devil (whom afterwards he knew to be such) appeared to him when he was travelling in the Night-time, but spoke none to him at the first Encounter. At the second Appearance he gave him a Bite or Nip in the Loyn, which he found painful for a Fortnight; that the third Time he appeared as a black Man, and c desired him to engage in his Service, upon Assurance of getting Riches and Comfort in the World; and that he should not want any Thing that he would ask in the Devil's Name; and then he renounced his Baptism, putting one hand to the Crown of his Head, and the other to the Sole of his Foot; thereby giving himself up to Satan's Service; after which the Pain of the Bite or Nip ceased. He said, that hitherto there was none others present with them; but after wards he was at several Meetings, particularly at that in Bargarran Yard, about the Time when there was a Fast for Christian Shaw, where the Devil appeared in the same Kind of Garb as he first appeared to him, and they consulted Christian's Death, either by Worrying or Drowning her in the Well; and the Devil said he would warrant them, that they should neither be heard, seen, nor confess; to which End he gave every one of them a Bit of Flesh; that the Deponent got one of them, but let it fall and did not eat it. He afterwards owned his Confession, in the Presence of the Laird of Jordan-Hill the Minister, Mr. Andrew Cochran Town Clark, and Baily Paterson; and being asked by Jordan-Hill, how they were advertised of their Meetings; he said, that commonly at their Meetings, the Time of the next was appointed; but for particular Warning there appeared a black Dog with a Chain about his Neck, who tinkling it, they were to follow, &c. And being asked by the Minister, if he did now wholly renounce the Devil (for he had formerly told how Satan did not perform his Promise) and give himself to Jesus Christ, and desire to find Mercy in God through him; he consented to the same. It is to be observed, that John Reid after his Confession, had called out of the Prison Window, desiring Baily Scot to keep that old Body Angus Forrester, who had been his Fellow Prisoner, close and secure; whereupon the Company asked John, when they were leaving him on Friday Night the 21 of May, whether he desired Company or would be afraid alone, he said he had no Fear of any thing: So being left till Saturday in the Afternoon he was found in this Posture; Viz sitting upon the

Stool which was on the Hearth of the Chimney, with his Feet on the Floor and his Body straight upwards, his Shoulders touching the Lintel of the Chimney, but his Neck tyed with his own Neckcloth (the Knot of which was behind) to a small Stick thrust into a Hole above the Lintel of the Chimney; upon which the Company and especially John Campbel a Surgeon who was called, thought at First, as he was in an ordinary Posture of sitting, and the Neckcloth not having any drawn Knot, but an ordinary one which was not very strait, and the Stick not having the Strength to bear the Weight of his Body, or the Struggle, that he had not been quite dead; but finding it otherwise, and that he was in such a Scituation, that he could not have been the Actor thereof himself, concluded that some extraordinary Agent had done it; especially considering that the Door of the Room was secured, and that there was a Board set over the Window, which was not there the Night before when they left him.

We shall add but little as to what passed at the Execution of the Seven Witches, because there is no subscribed Attestation of it; and our Design is to advance nothing, but what stands warranted by Testimonies of known Credit beyond Contradiction; yet it is well known when they were going to the Stake, one of the Lindsays was overheard saying to the other, now Brother it is high time that we should confess, since our keeping it up will serve us to no purpose, or the like Expression; to which the other answered, that he should never do that, &c., And Margaret Laing before Execution confessed, that when the Devil first appeared, she knew him not to be such, till afterwards he gave her the sensible Marks found upon her Body, she and laid them in the Corner of the Cellar; and accordingly being searched for, they were found in the particular Place she mentioned. Another such Passage happened to a Friend of Bargarran's, who went with him to sollicit a Commission from the Council: for he having brought along with him these Pieces of Cloth, buttoned up in his Pocket, and secured them, as he thought, they were missing in the Morning; but after Search, found at a good distance from his Pocket, though no visible Thing had been in the Room to open it, or carry them off.

Lastly, it is to be observed, that the Young Girl Christian Shaw, discovers a great Sagacity in her Discourse and Observations, but attended with extraordinary Modesty. She observed amongst other Things, that the Doors and Windows did open and shut, upon the Entry of the Witches, and that there was at no time such a Number of them about her, as the Room might not very well contain, with the visible Persons therein contained; And she likewise observed them to change their Places with a great deal of Agility, when any other came into it, or offered to attack them, upon her pointing where they were. And she often averred, from the Instance of the Spirit that spoke to her above her Head, told their Names, and gave her other Means of discovering of them, &c. that Satan does often contrive their Ruin, by the most indiscernable Methods he can; because if he did it openly, it would scare others from engaging with so faithless a Master.

Two Letters, giving an Account of what appeared most material or curious in the Tryal of the seven Witches.

THE Truth of the strange Things contained in the preceeding Narrative, was at the First only carefully search'd into by private Persons; but at last became so notorious, that upon Application, founded on a Journal of those extraordinary Events, and attested by many of the Gentry in the Country the Privy Council gave a Commission for enquiring into it.

The Honourable Persons to whom this was recommended, did with great Impartiality and Exactness make a Report, which influenced the Government to order the Execution of Justice upon some of those Witches, who other wise might have lurked without being discovered.

Upon this the Council directed a second Commission, for the Tryal of those that appeared to them to be most charged by the Evidence of the Witnesses, produced on the first Commission. Several of the Judges were not only Persons of Honour, but also of singular Knowledge and Experience, and accordingly proceeded with extraordinary Caution; and were so far from Precipitancy in the Affair, that after several Diets of Court they adjourned to a long Term, that in the mean time the Prisoners might be provided with Advocates.

Accordingly an Advocate appeared for them, and managed their Defence with all the Accuracy that could be expected. There were above twenty Hours employed at one Diet, in Examination of Witnesses; and the Jury being shut up, spent above Six Hours in comparing the Evidence; whereupon seven of the most notorious Criminals were convicted and condemned.

The Crimes charged and proved against them, were not meer spectral Imaginations, but obvious and plain Matter of Fact. Viz. The Murders of some Children, and Persons of Age; and Tormenting of several Persons, particularly Bargarran's Daughter; and both these not at a Distance, but contiguously by natural Means of Cords, Pins and the like. Besides the other ordinary Means of Witchcraft, such as renouncing Baptism, entering in

Contract with, and adoring the Devil in a corporal Shape, &c. which could not but be sustained as a sufficient Ground for a Tryal in Scotland, since there is an express Statute, Parliament 9. Act. 73. Queen Mary, ordering such Persons to be put to Death.

To make the Probation the more convincing, it was adduced orderly in three Periods. The First consisted of unsuspected Witnesses, who proved Fact; from whence it was necessarily inferred, that there was Witchcraft in the Cafe. The Second did include unexceptionable Witnesses, who deponed upon Facts, which made it probable, if not necessary, that the Persons indicted were the Witches. The Third comprehended six positive Testimonies, of those who saw and heard the Witches committing the Crimes charged in the Indictment.

The only valuable Subject of Debate, was as to the Import of these last Testimonies; five whereof were by Confessants, who had been at the Meetings wherein the Crimes were committed; and the sixth of Bargarran's Daughter, who was one of the Persons afflicted. The antecedent Part of the Probation was by Witnesses beyond Exception. And the Judges upon Debate sustained four of these Six, cumnota, and Two of them to be examined without Oath. So nice were they in favour of the Criminals Lives, since some of these Witnesses might have been admitted in such a Crime without any Quality, by the most scrupulous Judicatory in Europe. But all Things were carried on in this Proceeding with Tenderness and Moderation. For even the Advocates, who were sent to prosecute the Indictment by his Majesties Council and Advocate, did not act with the Byass of Parties, but on the contrary, shewed an equal Concern to have the accused Persons absolved, if it could be found competible with Justice.

For which Reason it is not doubted, but the two following Letters (one of which contains an Abridgment of the Advocates Speech to the Jury, and the other of their Answers to the Objections of the Confeffants Witnesses) will afford a satisfactory View of the chiefest Part of the Tryal, since the Objections which were or might have been made are therein stated and answered, or anticipated and prevented; and the intended Brevity would not permit at this time to print the whole Process, which being extant upon Record, any who are curious may have easily Access thereunto.

The First Letter.

SIR,

YOU having told me that the odd Passages which occur in the West, have put many of your Neighbours and your self upon reading all the Books you can get that treat of Witchcraft; and therefore desired to transmit to you my Observations at the Tryal; I shall not prepossess your Opinion, by giving them in my own Form, but herein I send to you the exactest Copy of the Advocate's Speech to the Jury that I could obtain, and by the next Post you shall have something more curious, viz. a Collection of their Answers to the Objections against the Six last Witnesses, that were brought for concluding the Proof; having these you will want little that could be agreeable to such an accurate Palate as yours is.'

The Speeches to the Jury were to this Effect.

Goodmen of the Jury,

YOU having sitten above Twenty Hours in hearing the Evidence, and being now to be enclosed, where it is like you will take no small Time to reconsider and compare it; we shall not detain you with summing up the same in particular; but shall only suggest some Things whereof it is fit you take special Notice in your Perusal of it, viz. First the Nature of your own Power, and the Management of it. Secondly, The Object of this Power which lies before you; wherein you are to consider in the first place, whether or not there hath been Witchcraft in the Crimes libelled; and in the next place, whether or not, these Prisoners are the Witches.

    As to your Power it is certain, that you are both Judges and Witnesses, by the Opinion of our Lawyers and Custom; Therefore you are called out of the Neighbourhood, as presumed best to know the Quality of the Prisoners, and the Notoriousness of their Guilt or Innocence. Your Oath is, That you shall all Truth tell, and no Truth conceal; which plainly implies, that you are to Condemn or Absolve, according to your own Conscience. Such is the excellent Constitution of Juries in England, and ought more especially to hold in this circumstantial Case, where there is such a Chain of different Kinds of Probation concurring against the same Prisoners, as will appear by the Review thereof in its proper Place.

    We are not to press you with the ordinary Severity of threatning an Assize of Error, in case you should absolve; but wholly leave you to the Conduct of God and your own Consciences, and desire you may proceed with all the Care of the Prisoners Lives that is possible for you, as the Honourable Judges have set you a Pattern, by their great Caution in this Matter.

    As to the Probation it self, you see that it is divided into Three Parts, viz. the Extraordinariness of the Crimes; the Probability of the concurring Evidences; and the Clearness of the Positive Probation.

As to the first Part, The Crimes, or Corpora Delicti, are proved by unexceptionable Witnesses, to have fallen out in such an odd and extraordinary Manner, that it points out some other Cause than the ordinary Course of Nature, to have produced those Effects.

For clearing of this, particularly in Relation to Bargarran's Daughter, you may consider, not only the extraordinary Things that could not proceed from a Natural Cause, which is proved before you; but also several other Matters of Fact, which is notorious, have been seen by some of your selves, and lie here in a Journal of her Sufferings; every Article whereof is attested by the Subscription of Persons of entire Credit, before the Honourable Commissioners appointed by his Majesty's Privy Council, for making Enquiry into the Matter.

This Girl's throwing out of Hair, Pins and Coals of greater Heat than that of her Body or Blood; as also so dry that they appeared not to have come out of her Stomach; nor had she any Motions to Vomit at the same time, and she declared the same to have been put into her Mouth at the same time by her Tormenters, is Deponed by Dr. Brisban, in his Opinion not to appear from a natural Cause.

She was not tormented by any of the Criminals after their Imprisonment, except two Nights by Catharine Campbel, which being a Surprize, it was afterwards discovered, that these two Nights, the Jaylor's Wife had let out Catherine Campbel to Spin in the House.

She having been speaking with one of her Tormenters as present, (though invisible to the Standers by) and asking how her Tormenter had got those clouted Red-Sleeves, she suddainly gets up, takes hold of them, and the Company heard the Noise of the Cloaths tearing, and she pulls away two Pieces of the Red-Cloath, which all the By-standers beheld with Amazement in her Hands; nor was there any other Piece of this Red-Cloth to be found in the Room at that time.

She told, that her Tormenters were giving her a Glass of Sack, and Orange-Pill, &c. (thereby ensnaring her to accept of a

Favour from them) and accordingly she was seen to move her Lips, and to have the Orange-Pill betwixt her Teeth, though there was no visible Hand that could have done it.

She advertised before-hand, that one of her Tormenters was to be at the Door at a particular Hour, and that another of them was in the Kitchen, before any Body told her of it, which accordingly fell out; and these being brought to her Presence, became obnoxious to the ordinary Ways and Means of Discovery.

When her Glove fell down from her, at a time that several Persons were about her, it was lifted up again by a Hand invisible to them.

She was not only transported through the Hall and down Stairs, without perceiving her Feet to touch the Ground; but also was hurried in a Flight up Stairs, and when a Minister endeavoured to retain her, he found a sensible Weight, besides her own Strength drawing her from him.

When she complained that her Tormenters had Bitten and Scratched her, the Marks of the Nails and Teeth were seen upon the Skin, with Blood and Spittle, about the Wounds, which were above Twenty Four; which neither her own nor any other Teeth that were visible, could have done.

She was most vehemently distorted upon attempting to tell, or even to write the Names of her Tormenters; yet that ceased as to any of them, as soon as that Person was accused by any other; and particularly she had Liberty after many painful Attempts to accuse Margaret Laing, as soon as the Charm of Hair to restrain her (which Margaret had left behind the Door) was found and burnt, the Girl having told it to have been lost, as mentioned in the Depositions.

She threw out no more Hair, after the finding and burning of a Ball of Hair, of the same Colour and Kind with that thrown out by the Girl, in Catherine Campbel's Pocket with Pins in it.

After Agnes Naismith had prayed for her, she appeared to her, but did not torment her.

She foretold that her Tormenters had concerted to throw her, at a certain Hour, in a Fit, (which they forewarned her of, with a Design to frighten her, to renounce her Baptism by the Terror) and had left one of their Number to execute it; and accordingly there was a Woman with a Red-Coat, seen under the Tree in the Orchard; and the Torment was brought on at the time appointed.

When she told that there was something tormenting her under the Cloaths, the Spectators saw the Bed-Cloaths move in an extraordinary Manner, after the Girl had been raised out of them. When she complained that she was beaten, the Standers by heard the Noise of the Stripes.

She cried out at a Time, that her Thigh was hurt, and one of the Company having searched her Pocket, found a clasped Knife, but unfolded; however having folded up the same, and put it up, a second Time she cried out of the same again; and upon the second Search (though secured by the Spring) it was found open, to the great Wonder of the Beholders; since they watched that no visible Thing could have possibly opened it.

She told of a Charm under the Bed, and accordingly it was found in the Shape of an Egg, which melted away it being put into the Fire. She told also, that her Sister that was boarded abroad, had Charms put about her in the House, and would not recover of the decaying Sickness till she was brought out of it, and accordingly the Child being brought home, straight way recovered. She told of their meeting in Bargarran's Yard, to consult about the destroying of her; and accordingly the Confessants have deposed, that they did meet and consult her Ruin in that Place.

The Story about her telling, that the Commissioners, though at Three Miles distance, had granted a Warrant to the Sheriff to apprehend One of her Tormenters; her giving so perfect an Account of the Sheriff, and of Mr. Guithrie who was with him, whilst her Eyes were sealed and fast; her being in Excessive Torments (as she foretold) till that Person was apprehended, and immediately thereupon, though at many Miles distance, her telling that her Tormenters were now taken, betwixt Twelve and One a Clock in the Morning; and the Sheriff when he returned, declared the Seisure to have been about that Time, is so notorious and so well attested, that we need only to be put in mind of it.

Her falling in Fits upon the Sight or Touch of her Tormenters, was no Effect of Imagination; for she was fully hood winked with a Cloak, so that she could see no Body whatever; yet upon the Approach of her Tormenter, she immediately fell down dead; whereas she did not so much as startle upon the Touch of another. Which Experiment was tried for ascertaining this Method of Discovery.

In the last place, she is naturally sagacious and discovering, and shewed her Integrity in the Face of the Court. For when the President asked, whether or not she knew one of the Prisoner's Names that was to be pricked, she answered, that though she knew her well enough of her self, yet one had told her the Name of this Prisoner when she was sent for to appear with her Face to Face; so far did the Girl discover her Aversion from any Thing that might seem intended to aid the Natural Evidence of Truth unfairly; and her Firmness to the utmost against Temptations of becoming a Witch; particularly against the last Assault of Satan, wherein he at least perswaded her to go to their Meetings; and she answered, That she would not follow such a base fallen Creature; and he rejoining, that she would go to Hell however for her other Sins; and she answering, That he was a Liar from the Beginning, and the Blood of Jesus would cleanse her from all Iniquity; upon which he disappeared, and she recovered the Sabbath Day following, when a happy End was put to this fearful Tragedy of Witchcraft, and convincingly confirmed the Reality of it.

As to the Murthering of the Children and Minister, charged in the Indictment, you may observe several extraordinary Things appearing in them; particularly the Witnesses depone, the Minister to have been in excessive Torments, and of an unusual Colour; to have been of sound Judgment, and yet he told of several Women about him, and that he heard the Noise of the Door opening, when none else heard it. The Children were well at Night, and found dead in the Morning, with a little Blood on their Noses, and Blewness at the Root of their Ears, which were obvious Symptoms of Strangling; besides the Mother of one of them cried out Matthew, Matthew, the Child is Dead. And the House of the other was whitened with Sifting of Meal the Night before; both which Particulars were told and discovered by the Confessants, before the Witnesses, which now concur with them in it, were examined.

Secondly, The second Part of the Probation consists of several admirable Things, and corroborating Evidence proved by unsuspected Witnesses, which lead us to suspect those Prisoners to be Witches, as so many Lines drawn from a Circumference to a Centre, and positively confirming the positive Probation after added to them. In general we need not mention all these accessory Circumstances, but refer you to the Probation which is so full concerning it; only you will be pleased to take notice, that it is clearly proved, that all the Accused have insensible Marks, and some of them in an extraordinary Manner: That most of them have been long reputed Witches, and some of them in 1687, by a Confessing Witch, which Subscribed Confession hath been produced. You see that none of them shed Tears, nor were they ever discovered to do it since their Imprisonment, notwithstanding their frequent Howlings; so that it is not a suddain Grief or Surprize. And finally that the Girl fell in Fits of Torment upon the Prisoners Approach to her, and that she named them all frequently either in or out of her Fits.

In particular, you see how Catherine Campbel was provoked, by this Girl's discovering her Theft; whereupon she hath brought in the rest of her Confederates to act the following Mischief; How upon this Campbel did Curse and Imprecate in a terrible manner; how she stayed out of her Bed at Night, and was frequently drowsie in the Morning; how she was named by the Girl, particularly the two Nights she was out of Prison; The Ball of Hair was taken out of her Pocket and burnt, upon which the

Girl ceased to void Hair at her Mouth; she could not express one Word, even when she was on her Knees, of Prayer for the Girl's Recovery; and the insensible Marks on her were very remarkable.

Agnes Naismith did not torment the Girl after she had prayed for her; she was reputed a Witch and hath the Marks. She came early in the Morning to Bargarran's Yard, when by her refusing to go in, it appeared she had no Business; Yea it is plain, that she had a Resentment because she had not a greater Alms the last time she was there. The Girl declared, that Naismith asked about her Health and Age which in these Circumstances, was a shrewd Presumption of her ill Design; and she acknowledged her self to have done this, when she asked the Age of another Child, where in by Providence she was fooled; since that which she thought would have been an Excuse, tended to discover her Guilt. And lastly, after this Appearance of Agnes Naismith, the Girl took her first Fit, and nominated her amongst the first Tormenters.

Margaret Laing, that great Impostor, had been a Masterpiece of the Devil; she hath Confessed unnatural Lust', which is known to some of your Number. She sat near the Door where the Charm of Hair was found. which the Girl declared kept up her Tongue; and upon burning the same, it was loosed. The Girl fell in Fits upon her Approach, she hath notable Marks; particularly one which the Confessants declare she lately received, and by Inspection it appears to be new. When she came from her private Conversation (no doubt with the Devil) she raged as if she had been possessed, and could not but declare, that she expected a violent Death. She looked in the Face of James Miller's Child, and asked her Age, whereupon that Child sickened the same Night, and named Margaret Laing on her Death-Bed. It appears she was ready to show to James Laird a Sight of her Mother, who had been dead Three Years. And finally, she hath been taken in several Lies and gross Prevarications; particularly you may remember, how Six Hours ago, when the Witnesses were Examined on the Ball of Hair found on Catherine Campbel, a Gentleman, Mr. Stewart of------, heard her whisper Catherine in the Ear, this is well bestowed on you, you would not put it away when I desired you, &c. which the said Mr. Stewart did openly Confess in court upon Oath. Notwithstanding which this impudent Wretch had the Confidence to deny it, though

Catherine Campbel also confessed, that she had pulled her, and had spoke somewhat to her, which she did not give Ear to, which was no wonder, the Witnesses deponing at the Time, being close upon Catherine.

Margaret Fulton was reputed a Witch, and hath the Mark of it; and acknowledged in presence of her Husband, that she made use of a Charm, which appeared full of small Stones and Blood. That her Husband had brought her back from the Fairies, and her Repute of being a Witch is of old Date; besides her being named often by the bewitched Girl.

As to the Lindsay's they all have the Mark; and were all of a long time reputed to be Witches. John Lindsay of Barlock, was accidentally discovered by the Girl's falling into a Fit, upon his coming into the House. John and James Lindsay's were accused by a confessing Witch Anno 1687. which Confession is publickly read before you, and there was Money given to the Sheriff deputed, for the delaying of the Pursuit. James Lindsay appeared to William Simpson suddenly, and flew about like a Fowl, for an Opportunity to strike him, in revenge of the Quarrel mentioned in the Deposition, and at last prevailed to strike him dead over a Wall. And finally, which is a Remarkable Indication both of Truth and Providence, the very Witnesses brought in the Defence of the Lindsays, deposed so clearly against them, even beyond the Prosecutors Witnesses, that their Advocate was surprized at it, and thereupon desisted from calling any more Witnesses to be examined in their Defence.

It is true some of these Indications may be in one and others of them in another, either from Nature or Accident, and yet that Person not be a Witch: But it was never heard nor read, that all these Indications, which are so many Discoveries by Providence, of a Crime that might other wise have remained in the Dark, did ever concur in one and the same individual Person that was innocent: Yea, on the Contrary, they by the Wisdom and Experience of all Nations, do as convincingly discover a Witch, as the Symptoms of a Leprosy concerted by all Physitians, argue the Person affected with the same to be leprous; yet granting they are not sufficient of themselves, yet their Tendency and Meaning being clearly applyed to their proper Cause, by a plain and positive Probation, there wants no more to determine you as to the Prisoners Guilt. And therefore,

Thirdly, As to the Third Part of the Probation, we remit the positive Depositions of the Confessants, and against whom they do concur, wholly to your own Perusal, and Examination. Only be pleased to take Notice, First, Some things which very much add to the Credibility of their Testimonies, arise from their Examination in Court: Secondly we shall explain to you the Import of the Word Nota, which is added to the Decree of the Judges, admitting these last Witnesses.

As to the First.

Elizabeth Anderson is of sufficient Age being Seventeen, yet so young and punctual, that her Deposition appears to be no Effect of Melancholy; she accused her Father to his Face when he was a dying in the Prison; as now there are two of her Aunts in the Indictment, which certainly must proceed from the Strength of Truth, since even Dives retained a natural Affection to his Relations. She went on Foot to the Meetings with her Father, except only that the Devil transported them over the River of Clyde, which was easy to the Prince of the Air, who does far greater Things by his Hurricanes. She tells that Montgomery's House was Mealy when his Child was strangled; and she declares that she never renounced her Baptism, but was carried along by the Compulsion of a Parent, so that nothing can be objected against her Testimony, in any Judgment, much less in an accepted Crime.

James Lindsay, it is true is of less Import, yet by his weeping, when he came in and was admonished of the Greatness of his Guilt, it appears he had a Sense of it; He hath a natural

Precipitancy in what he speaks, yet that is commonly the Concomitant of Ingenuity, as importing his Expressions not to be fore-thought. He concurs in most Things with the Others, and yet he declares he saw not Margaret Fulton at Dunbarton, &c. which implyes that he does not foil the Prisoners at Random, but tells what occurred to his Senses, &c.

Jennet and Margaret Rogers, are Instances of a Singular Providence; for they did confess the same Morning that the Court did last fit, of their own proper Motion, there being neither Ministers nor Judges at that time by them. Agnes Naismith is Jennet's Relation, and she tells that she never saw Catharine Campbel, as Margaret declares she did not see John Lindsay of Barlock; which plainly demonstrates, that they tell only the Dictates of their natural Conscience arising from Discretion and Knowledge of the True Matters of Fact, they both professed their Repentance last Sabbath in the Church, and do persist with a great Firmness, and you see their Deportment in their Depositions to be agreeable and exact.

Thomas Lindsay and Christian Shaw being under Age, we did not press their being put to an Oath, yet you saw that they did declare in Court against these Criminals, in such an Harmony with the rest of the Deponents, and gave such a Cause of their Knowledge, that it is certain, that their Youngness of Years adds a great Deal of Credit to their Testimony, because thereby it is incredible they could have contrived or executed the acting so by Concert.

As to the Second,

Since these Witnesses are admitted by the Judges, it necessarily implies, that they meant them to be Probative; only they added the Words cum Nota, that is, you must take notice, or Notandum est, that there must something else concur to prove the Guilt of the Prisoners, besides the Depositions of any two Witnesses such as these; but so it is that all the circumstantial Evidence on which you have seen Probation led, for more than Sixteen Hours of your Time, are strengthning Evidences of those Witnesses Credibility, and cannot but have been taken Notice of by you, as inferring the same Things which they Deposed, whereby the Nota is fully taken off by the Concurrence of Four other positive Testimonies, agreeing with that of Two of these Witnesses, by the Extraordinariness of the Deceased Persons; by the Probability of Circumstances, and finally by the whole Chain of this Affair, and the Sparkles of an infernal Fire, which in every Place hath broke out.

It is true, there are some few of the Circumstances, that are proved only by one Witness; but as to this you may consider, First, That a Witness Deponing concerning Matter of Fact, is in Law credited more than any other single Witness; and this is the present Case as to some of the Circumstances. Secondly the Antecedent, Concomitant and Subsequent Circumstances of Fact do sustain the Testimony, and make the single Evidence more full. But thirdly, The other Circumstances, undoubtedly proved by concurring Witnesses, are of themselves sufficient; and therefore you saw us at the Desire of the Judges, forbear to call the far greatest Part of our Witnesses; because the Time had already run to so great a Length, and it was thought that Presumptions enough were already proved; for it may as reasonably be imagined, that the most reasonable and curious Scheme had emerged from the fortuitous Concourse of Atoms, roving without Rule, as that so many Indications should concentre against each of these Prisoners, and yet they remain Innocent of Witchcraft.

Now upon the whole you will take Notice, that Presumptions being vehement, make a more certain Probation than Witnesses; because Presumptions are Natural Emanations of the Thing it self, which cannot be bribed; whereas Witnesses are obnoxious. So in our Law there was One condemned for Theft, another for Falshood, and a Third for Murthering of a Child, merely upon Presumptions, as Mr. Mackenzie relates in his Criminal Treatise; much more may Presumptions add to the Credit of, and take off the Nota, from, positive Witnesses; for it is a gross Mistake, that several Proofs, which have each of them some Import, may not be joined to make a full Evidence, the same way as two small Candles in a dark Room will not suffice; yet several others being added to them, will make a sufficient Light to discover the Murtherer; Two Boys will be able to carry a Weight which one of them would not be able to sustain, as two Units make a full Number. One Witness of whatsoever Dignity proves nothing; yet out of the Mouth of Two or Three Witnesses, every Truth shall be established; and finally though one Coal make not a Fire able to do the Work, yet several Coals added to it encrease the Flame, which is hoped will be sufficient for the Operation.

We shall therefore leave you with this Conclusion, that as you ought to be cautious in Condemning the Innocent, and ought to incline to the safest Side; so if these Prisoners be proved legally Guilty, then as to what is past, your Eye ought not to spare them, nor ought you to suffer a Witch to live; and as to the future, in doing otherwise you would be accessory to all the Blasphemies, Apostacies, Murthers, Tortures and Seductions, &c. whereof these Enemies of Heaven and Earth shall hereafter be Guilty, when they are set at Liberty. So that the Question seems simply to come to this, whether upon your Oath you can Swear, That the Prisoners, notwithstanding all that is proved against them, are not Guilty of Witchcraft? In the Determination whereof we pray, God may direct you to the right Course.

The Jury being enclosed near Six Hours, brought in their Verdict to Court, that they found the Indictment.

I am, &c.

The Second LETTER.

SIR,

I Have collected according to my Promise, what appeared to me most Specious in the Reasonings, either in Court or private Conversation, about receiving the Confessants as Witnesses. You are not to imagin that the Prisoners were condemned on the Credit of these; for I do believe the Probation by unexceptionable Witnesses, led antecedent to this last, was so pregnant, that the Prisoners might have been condemned on it; though these last had not been adduced.

 I may have missed the Energy of the Argument sometimes, in a Case which in it self is so abstruse; however you have it in such a manner as I was able to comprehend it, as follows.'

 In order to the more satisfactory answering of the Objections made against the last Witnesses, we shall first lay before you the State of the Case; and then clear up the Determination of it.

 As to the First, The Question is not whether Partners in the Crime, or others mentioned in the Objections can be a concluding Proof in themselves, though two of them should concur as to the same Act of Witchcraft: But whether the Bodies of the Persons Deceased appearing already to imply Witchcraft, and the extrinsick Presumptions being so Strong and Pregnant, to infer that these Prisoners are the Witches? There concurring such Characters, as by the Observation of all Ages and Nations are the Symptoms of a Witch, particularly the Marks, Fame, not Shedding of Tears, &c. which are Providential Discoveries of so dark a Crime, that like Avenues lead us to the Secret of it. And finally, when Six Persons of different Ages and Stations, Five Confessants, and the Girl, do, when separately examined, agree in their Answers to every Material Question that is put to them though it be even new; so that it could not be concerted; we say, in such a Case whether or not Witnesses may be received to compleat the Evidence by a Positive Probation, of a Matter of Fact which is the Object of Sense, though otherwise they be liable to Exception; if such Extraordinariness of the Persons who suffered, Clearness of the Circumstances, and of the Diagnosticks of the Witches did not precede them, as you have seen it proved that they do.

The Case is not, whether these Witnesses would be good in an ordinary Crime, which commonly happens to be exposed to other Witnesses, than those concerned in it; but whether they can be received in this Extraordinary occult Case, and excepted Crime of Witchcraft; in which there are two special Cases to be considered, Viz. sometimes the Acts thereof are open, and admit the Choice of Witnesses, such as Charms used in the Day time, when the Actor is visible. But that Part of Witches whereby Witches meet in the Night time, adore their Lord, contrive their Mischievous Designs, and accordingly afterwards put them in Execution, when other Witnesses are a-sleep, or the Witches themselves are covered from Sight, we say, this can be no otherwise proved than by these that are privy to it, joined to the positive Proofs and Presumptions before mentioned.

We do not alledge that Persons altogether destitute of Knowledge, and Natural Conscience are to be admitted in any Case; such as Infants, Mad, Foolish Persons, &c. neither do we contend that Thomas Lindsay, Christian Shaw, who are under Age should be put to their Oath; but they are only to be examined separately before the Court, upon Queries, by which it may appear, whether or not they agree with the Four other Confessants that are to Depone before them; and this is the Prisoner's Advantage in Case of Disagreement: But we insist that any Person above Nonage, giving Evidence of considerable Knowledge and Natural Conscience (which is a sufficient Fund for all the Credit we want in this Case, which is already almost fully proved) is to be received as a Witness.

As to the Second, we shall make this as clear as Noon-Day; First from Reason and the Nature of the Thing: Secondly, the unanimous Judgment of Lawyers in all Nations and Ages:

Thirdly, our own Customs and Decisions: And Fourthly the Singularity of this Circumstantial Case.

As to the First, The Going to and Coming from Meetings, especially on foot; the falling down and Worshiping the Devil there, under a Corporal Shape (which he had when he tempted our Saviour to do it;) The usual Murthering of Children, by a Cord and Napkin, and the Tormenting of others by Pins, &c. are plain Objects of Sense; and therefore the Senses are to be believed concerning them; for as Reason hath Things Intelligible, and Faith Things Supernatural; so the Senses have Things Corporeal to their Object, in respect of which they are to be trusted, until it be proved, that the Appearance is impossible, or that the Witness of it is an Impostor. It is Part of the Witches Purchase from the Devil, that they cannot be seen on some Occasions; so that the Abominations committed then would remain unpunished, if such Witnesses were not admitted. It cannot be thought that Witches (who of all Criminals are most backwards to Confess) would venture the Loss of their own Lives, by deponing against others, against whom they have no special Pique, yea for whom they have particular Affection, as several of the Prisoners are some of the Witnesses Relations. Nor hath the Devil any peculiar Interest to instigate them thereunto; for several of the Prisoners have confessed other execrable Crimes, whereby it cannot be supposed, that Satan would be divided against himself. God in his ordinary Providence hath taken such Care of publick Judgments, that the Enemy of Justice's special Power ceases as to that; as appears by the Witches either being not able either to do more Harm, or to escape, after God's Ministers begin to act contrary to Satan's Instruments by Imprisonment: And finally the Oddness of the Crimes, the Concurrence of the Presumptions, and the Existence of Matters of Fact, wherein these Confessants (though not knowing the same otherwise) do agree with other unexceptionable Evidences, &c. which sufficiently add to their Credibility: But as Falshood being a Crime is never presumed; so a Person found true in many

Things, is still presumed to continue such, till the contrary be evinced.

As to the Second, Socius Criminis, &c. admittitur si delictum sit nefandum, Men. A. J. Q. l. 2d. l. C. cas. 474. N. 27. Seq. aut occultum and veritas aliunde haberi non possit. Mas. Vol. I. Con. 466. N. 6. aut difficilis Probationis, Farin. lib. 2. Op. Criminalium, Tit. 6. Q. 63. N. 28. Mas. Vol. 3. Con. 1360. N. 4. Menoch. lib. 2. Cas. 116.1. I. Q. 58. nocturno tempore commissa quæ difficilis dicuntur Probationis. Boer. decis. 68. N. 6. Menoch. D. Cas. 116. N. 14 Ideoq; non solum præsumptio and conjecturata probatio sufficit, verum inhabiles admittuntur, Farin I. 2. Tit. 6. Q. 55. N. 40. Mas. I. 2. Con. 1124. N. 13. Idem in delictis commissis in Eremo, Nemore, Monte aliove loco secreto. Gomez. Var. res Tom 3. I. 12. N. 21. Far. D. Tit. 6. Q. 62. N. 55. Sed occultum non dicitur, quod actu non Intervenerint, at quod de Natura delicti vel Ratione loci and temporis alii testes habiles intervenire non poterint: ut est Maleficium in quo socius Criminis admittitur. Men. I. 2. Cap. 5. Cas. 474. N. 33. Campeg. te teste Reg. 86. Fallew. 6. Crotus de Test. Part. 4. N. 97. Oldindorp. de Test. tit. de Personis test. N. 21. In a word, all Lawyers who have writ particular Treatises on Witchcraft, in Germany, Italy, Levain, France and Spain, &c. do conclude, that inhabil Witnesses, and particularly Companions are to be admitted in Witchcraft, only the strictest of them do think, that this Admission is to be cum Nota, or as Delrio, in the Place cited for the Prisoners expresses it; ex his solis, upon this Evidence alone, the Judge is not to Condemn, nor do we require it.

As to the Third, We have the Testimony of our Famous K. James the VIth, Demon. lib. 3. C. ult. telling us, That it is our Law, that Boys, Girls, Infamous Persons, &c. are not to be rejected any more in Witchcraft, than in human lese Majesty, though they assert others to have been present at Imaginary Meetings; because this supposes their having entered into a Precontract. He says, that Satan's Mark, and the Want of Tears are Pregnant aids to the Discovery. He gives an Instance of a Girl, who having named several Witches in her Fits, they were all Condemned upon other concurring Presumptions.

This is not a common Author, but a Man, who, as curious, was exact; and as Prudent did not publish such Things, without the Approbation of the best Divines and Lawyers; and as a Prince is to be credited about the Law of his own Country, and as a King hath determined any Doubt that might have remained in this Point, as far as the Law of our Government will permit.

But further, our Lawyers and Judges have followed his Majesty; for in all the Processes in the Journals, Fame, and Accusation, and the Mark, are still sustained as most Pregnant Presumptions; upon which, and a very small Foundation besides, Witches have been frequently condemned. So in the Processes against the Bewitchers of Sir George Maxwell of Pollock, and Hamilton of Barns, Anno. 1677. One that was a Companion in the Crime, though under Age, is sustained to be a Witness. And Witnesses are adduced before the Jury for proving, that the Mark was found upon some of the Witches. Women and Minors have been received by Multitudes of Decisions cited by Mc. Kenzie, Tit. Prob. By Witnesses and Tit. Witchcraft. And he also cites Decisions, where, in parallel Cases, Companions in Crimes, and others inhabile were admitted, particularly in Treason and in Falshood; and all Lawyers conclude, that Witchcraft is as much an excepted Crime as these.

As to the Fourth. Whatever Inhability these Witnesses might be under, it is fully made up, and they rendered unexceptionably habile, by the Train of this whole Business. It is true one Man, through the Concurrence of Corrosive Humours, may have an insensible Mark; another be enviously defamed; a Third may through suddain Grief or Melancholy, not be able to Weep, &c. A foruth may be loaded with Suspitious Circumstances, when extraordinary Things fell out in the Country; and a Fifth may be Deponed against by two False Witnesses; tho' none of these separately may be truly Witches. But by the known Observation and Experience of Mankind, none except Witches have had the unhappy Medley and Concourse of all or most of these, and commonly and for the most part Witches have them: So that since the Rules of Justice are established upon that, which for the most part happens, that prevails till an Exception be apparent in a special Case; the Conjunction of these, does as plainly give his Character, as the most certain Symptoms of the plainest Disease, being universally Concerted in all Parts of the World, point out to us that the Person Affected is truly afflicted with that Disease, whereof he hath the Diagnostick Symptoms concurring. In a word, one or other of these may occur in the Innocent; but no Writers do attest, that all of them have concentered in any other Person but a Witch. And on the other hand, their taking Place in a Witch, through all Parts of the World must proceed from a Common, and not from a peculiar Humour or Cause.

The Specifick Aptitude of some of the Nicest-Indications, which appeared from the Probation already led, to discover a Witch, do serve to clear the Ground of the World's Observation concerning them. Particularly the Devil, as aping God, imprints a Sacrament of his Covenant. Besides that, commonly this Mark being given at the first. Meeting, does by its intolerable Pain, force the Witch to a Second Meeting or Rendezvous for curing it, at which the poor Wretch being under this furious Necessity, sixes the Bargain by renewing it with Deliberation, having been diverted in the mean time from considering the Horridness of the first Engagement by the Pain. The Inability to shed Tears, may be a Characteristick of hardening, though not always in the Case of Christians, yet in these that have ceased to be such, lest the Devil giving them such Words of Scripture and Prayer as many have, it should be impossible to discover their Hypocrisie; and that is not Satan's own Interest, since by this Discovery Occasion is given to buffoon the Profession of Holiness. A Report often arises without Ground, but a constant Report that keeps footing, implies for the most part a surer Cause; especially when it is of Persons below Envy, and by Persons above Calumny. The Girl's falling in Fits at the Appearance of the Prisoners might appear from Antipathy, arising from the Poisonous Steams of the Witch accustomed to produce that Effect, through a vertue affixed thereunto by the Devil, by Conjunction of Natural Causes, (the same way as the invisible Pestilence operates) or his Promise of casting the Girl in Fits at the Witches Presence, might have been general; whereby the Witch was in Event buffooned and discovered, as it often falls out; but Satan envies even their Temporal Felicity, and fears lest by continuing here, they should be plucked out of his Hands by Conversion; when they come to perceive the Delusion of his Promises to make them Rich, &c.

There was one Thing further which was tried before their Lordship's, viz. none of the Prisoners who were tried (though most Sagacious and Knowing, and perfect in Memory, so that it could not proceed from Ignorance or Forgetfulness) could make out the Attempt of saying the Lord's Prayer, which may either be a Secret Judgment for renouncing their Lord, from whom it is peculiarly denominated, or by Restraint of their new Lord, who may think that too special Homage to his Adversary.

But we have been too tedious in that which may seem not so necessary; for this being an incontrovertible Law and Custom, there is no need of Philosophy to support it; since Legislators reason, but Subjects must obey; and both the Fool and the Lazy (who have neither Read nor Thought enough to understand this Subject) are to be left to their own Chimera; yet lest they should insult, we shall Answer briefly such Objections as the Prisoner's Advocate thought any ways worthy to be repeated in this Place.

Whereas it is Objected, that Delrio Sect. 5. Less. 4. says, That Companions are not to be admitted Witnesses in respect of Condemnation, especially considering that the Probation ought to be, clearer than the Meridian Sun. It is answered, That the Place it self confutes this Inference in the present Case; for it says, That this Evidence is not sufficient to warrant Condemnation; I know the contrary is commonly maintained and practised, &c. So that it is evident, First, That the common Opinion and Custom is contrary; even when there is no other Proof, but by the Partners of the Crime. Yet, Secondly, We are not so straitned, but presume in his very Words, that by this Evidence alone, we desire not that the Prisoners should be condemned. But your Lordships see, that the Witnesses we bring are not only such as were Concomitants of the Fact; for the Proofs brought these last Sixteen Hours are so many Concomitants and Discoveries of Providence, which make up any Defect in their Credit that can be desired. Hence, Thirdly, The Meaning of that Axiom, (which is Metaphorical, as appears by the Words, clearer than the Meridian Light) is fully answered, and takes Place in the present Case. Form the Extraordinariness of the Persons Afflicted, the Pregnancy of the Presumption, and the Punctualness of the positive Proof being joined together, there is not a Clearer Proof upon Record in any Nation, than that to which, it is hoped, these will amount.

Whereas this Allegation is enforced, by pretending it were of dangerous Consequence to allow such Witnesses to prove Meeting with the Devil, since Satan might have represented others by their false Shapes.

It is Answered,

First, That we are not straitened in this, because there are many Articles proved, which could not have been falsified. But if we give some scope to Reasoning, even in this Point it is to be considered, that the Rules of Judgment are established upon that, which for the most part still prevails; and Rules are to be followed, till an Exception be proved in a particular circumstantiate Case. But so it is by the Experience and Observation of the Wisest Divines, Lawyers, Philosophers, Physicians, States-Men, Judges and Historians, at Home and Abroad (that are too Wise to be imposed upon, and too Ingenuous to deceive us, when they all concur in the same Matter of Fact) besides the Testimony of Witches themselves every where, makes the Apparitions of Witches to be commonly and most real. So Delrio tells us, Lib. 5. Sect. 16. It seldom happens that they are deceived: And therefore the Testimony of the Senses is always to be credited concerning them, till it be disproved. For single or few Instances of false Representations to the Senses esteeming them to be true, or a Possibility of Appearance being false, can no ways invalidate the Rule established upon Experience, which is common, and for the most part, whereby no Exception is to be proved in a special Case; since a Wonder does not subvert the Proof drawn from the common Course of Nature.

Logick admits not to argue a particulari, or from Possibility to Existence. Law puts the Burthen of proving Simulation on the Affirmer, and that which seldom occurs is not considered by Legislators.

For illustrating of which it is further to be considered, that for the most part and commonly, Witches are personally existent in the Places where they appear, because it is more easie for the Prince of the Air, to transport them in his Hurricanes, which he can raise, as is plain in the Instance of Job (who was put in his Power) forming a Fence upon their Face, by which the Violence of the Air may be diverted from choaking them, than to form the Curious Miniature of various Transactions on their Brain: The Difficulty whereof is the greater, that all their Extasies are not disposed at all times the same way; and they have not the Seeds of this Work, unless they had once acted it in Reality. It is both the greater Crime and Pleasure to act in Reality, which therefore the Devil and Witches do rather chuse (unless the Place be far distant, or the Person indisposed) and this in Fact is attested to be so, by the Writers and Witches in all Nations and Ages.

Secondly, Notwithstanding the Rule must hold, till an Exception to make it void be evinced, as to a particular Person, by making it evident, that the real Appearance was in that special Case, a true Mistake; yet this Exception is for the Safety of the misrepresented; since the same Providence which hath permitted the Affliction, will order the Out-gate and Way to make it void; either by the Aerial Bodies not abiding the Touch, or some other Distinction; as Providence commonly allows the Devil to personate only with Cloven-Feet; or that the Apparition was only to one single Person, who cannot be a Proof, or that the Innocent can prove this otherwise; or finally the known Character of a

Samuel will purge and dispel the Aspersions of Satan, contrived on purpose to discredit the Evidence of Sense, by which alone his Instruments can be discovered. Especially this Character being joined to the other Circumstances of the Providence; such as when Men are disguised, they are most passive in the Scene and Presumptions. Whereas Witches are personally active in their common Life by such Words and Deeds, as (in Conjunction with these Appearances) conspire to make us know and distinguish them from the truly Good; since these Witches ape Prophaneness, Naughtiness, and undiscerned Hypocrisy, being made evident by Fame, sealed and confirmed by the Mark, and the other Discoveries of the Presumptions, which lye proved before you, still make a Land-Mark betwixt the Children of Darkness and Light. So Delrio Lib. 5. Sect. 16. N. 5. tells us of St. Athanasius and St. Germanus against whom Proof was brought of Sorcery; but Providence disproved it. It is a famous Instance of Susanna represented by the Elders, which though not in the Case of Spectre, yet agrees in point of Reason. The Representation by Pharoah Magicians had Concomitants by which they were discovered and confounded. But lastly, Suppose that God in the Depth of his Wisdom (to convince the Error of too much self Confidence) should permit all necessary Probation to concur against an Innocent Person; yet the Judge following the Faith of Proofs, established by Divine and humane Laws, is altogether Innocent. And since this Case is very rare, the Evil is less than the establishing of a Principle, by which most of all these Monsters could not be cut off.

Upon the whole 'tis certain, that though often times false Witnesses set on by the Devil, have taken away a harmless Life, by accusing it of Crimes; yet the Testimony of Witnesses must still be credited, till they be made evident; so these Apparitions of Witches, with the other Specialities before mentioned, being proved, ought to be esteemed real, till the Fallacy be made evident, especially since there are Examples in Antient and Modern Histories of Satan's representing the best of Men, as commiting Murther, &c. in their proper Shape. So Delrio Lib. 5.

Sect. 16. N. 5. relates, That St. Sylvanus was represented by the Devil, committing Common Capital Crimes, and the like of a Monk Whereof there are several Modern parallel Instances, yet this cannot weaken the Rule and Faith of publick Judicatures, founded on no more than the like Appearances; and any Argument against the Proof in Witchcraft, will equally hold against the Proof of any other Crime whatever. Wherefore the Rules of them both must be common, as to believing the Senses fortified as above, till their Error be individually discovered.

Finally, the Certainty is no ways diminished by the Extraordinariness of the Appearance to the Senses; for in Law and Nature, Reality and not Simulation is presumed, till the contrary be made appear, by proving the Thing not possible in Nature, or though it be possible that it is actually false. This is Answer enough to those who place a great deal of their small Wit in a Nonsensical arguing against all Divine Authority. But Writers further illustrate, that the Extraordinariness of a Matter of Fact, does not exclude its Reality from being the Subject of the Testimony of Witnesses, in our Saviour's Transfigurations, Miracles, walking on the Waters, standing in the Midst of the Disciples whilst the Doors were shut, and arguing Assurance by their Senses, that a Spirit had not Flesh and Bones, though indeed, the surer Word of Prophecy put these beyond Doubt.

Nor could it be alledged for the Prisoners (though they had the last Word, as perhaps they have not, in Objection against Witnesses, since therein they were Actors, by attacking the presumed Hability, of the Legality of the Witnesses) that it is not conceivable how the Girl or Witnesses could see what the Standers by could not behold. Besides the Impossibility of the Real Bodies entring at close Doors and Windows, or not intercepting the Sight of what is at its back.

For to this it would be answered,

First, Proved Facts must not be denied, though Philosophers are not yet certainly acquainted with the Invisible Manner of their Exiftence. So in Nature, the Load-stone draws the Iron, the Compass turns always to the North-Pole, &c. in

Scripture the Angels (and the Devil was once such, retaining as yet his Natural Powers) smote the Sodomites, that they could not see the Door, though they saw the House. Balaam's Ass perceived the Angel that stood undiscovered to himself; and the Rod thrown down by the Magicians of Ægypt was no doubt seen by themselves, though invisible to the Standers by; which obscuring of their Eyes, Interpreters explain to have been done by Natural Means; and yet the manner thereof is certainly difficult. However it is also certain, that if a possible way can be proposed, the Reality of a proved Fact is not to be contradicted; and this can be done in the present Case.

For Secondly, Satan's Natural Knowledge and acquired Experience makes him perfect in Opticks and Limning; besides that, as a Spirit he excels in Strength and Agility, whereby he may easily Bewitch the Eyes of others, to whom he intends that his Instruments should not be seen in this manner as was formerly hinted, viz he constricts the Pores of the Witche's Vehicle, which intercepts a Part of the Rays reflecting from her Body; he condenses the inter-jacent Air with grosser Meteors blown into it, or otherwise violently moves it, which drowns another part of the Rays. And lastly, He obstructs the Optick Nerves, with Humours stirred towards them. All which joined together may easily intercept the whole Rays reflecting from these Bodies, so as to make no Impression upon the Common Sense. And yet at the same time by a Refraction of the Rays, gliding along the fitted sides of the Volatile Couch, in which Satan transports them, and thereby meeting and coming to the Eye, as if there were nothing interjacent, the Wall or Chair behind the same Bodies, may be seen; as a piece of Money lying out of Sight in a Cup, becomes visible as soon as the Medium is altered by pouring some Water on it. Several of the Persons present knew, that the Girl declared, that she saw and heard the Doors and Windows open when the Witches entered, when no Doubt Satan had precondensed a soft Stoppage on the Eyes and Ears of others, to whom that was unperceived.

So Apolinus escaped Domitian's Sight, and Giges became invisible by his Magical Ring. John of Salisbury tells us of a Witch, that could make any Thing Invisible, and Mejerus tells us of another that had the like Power. Some Italian Witches of greater than ordinary Wit confessed to Grillandus, the Devil's opening Doors and Windows for them, though the more Ignorant by a Fascination, think themselves Actors of it. Whence it ought not to be doubted, by any Reasonable Man, what in all Times and Places is such undeniable Fact.

Finally, The Prisoners could not insist, that those Confessants are to Depone only on their Imaginations, which can prove no more against themselves or others than a Dream.

For still it is to be minded, that there are other Proofs, to which this is only accessary, as a Consonant Circumstance. But further, for Argument sake it is answered; That all the Allegation is a Mistake, seeing they declare plain Matters of Fact, obvious not only to one, but several of their Senses. Some of them went the greatest Part of the way to these Meetings on Foot; they there saw and touched their Confederates; they heard their Combinations to destroy the Infants, the Girl, and the Ministers. They returned on Foot again, and even when they were carried there, or back again, they knew on the next Day, that it was no Dream, by the same way that all other Mortals discover the Difference; but moreover this was confirmed by some reall Effects of a Personal Presence, as you have seen in the Probation; and it is yet further cleared by the Journal of Bargarran's Daughter's Suffering's, which was attested before the former Commissioners; and is known in the Country; particularly the Glass of Sack and Orange-Pill; the Pieces of the clouted Sleeves; the Words expressed suddenly; the Murther of the Child by the Woman that looked after it; which are constantly told by some of the Confessants, as also the Houses being strew'd with Meal that Night. The Girl's falling in Fits, though hood winked, at their Approach, &c. And others which shall be pointed at to the Jury, conjoined together, can be ascribed to no other Cause but the real Existence of the Witches Persons in the Place; unless it be said, that Satan might possibly have foisted and suborned all those, and thence it be concluded that the Devil did actually so; in case the Objectors are the Persons that found their Opinion on Imagination, without any positive Ground of the Reality of what they fancy, yea against positive Grounds of Belief in the contrary; which arguing from Possibility to Existence, is already sufficiently exploded.

Whereas for strengthning the Objection it is alledged, That the Confessants having been in the Devil's Service, and renounced Christ, they are not capable of making a Religious Oath;

It is Answered,

First, In the Rules of Charity, &c. the Confessants, tho' once Witches, have now, at least the Majority of them ceased to be such, having had the Use of Means, by the Ministers and Word, and effectually declared, their Repentance and the Devil's ceasing to molest them; particularly Elizabeth Anderson was only carried along violently by her Father, and stood out, to the last, the renouncing her Baptism, or consenting to those Crimes, which were contrived in their Meetings. Jennet and Margaret Rogers do testify a great Remorse, and avowed the same, last Sabbath, in the Face of the Congregation. So those Three are sufficient, whatever might be said against the other Two; especially if we join the Improbability, either of hazarding their own Lives, or the Devil's sending them out against these Prisoners, or their destroying their own Relations, as was remarked before.

But, Secondly, Whether they remain Witches or not, it is certainly Reason and Experience, that the Devil's peculiar Influence ceases, when they are brought to Judgment by the common Course of Providence; and therefore the Authors before cited, admit Witches whether Penitent or not.

Thirdly, All the supposed Defects of their Evidence is supplied, and the Entireness there of compleated by their Testimonies, being so wonderfully confirmed; particularly the Confessants are constant from the first Discovery; uniform in such various Circumstances, not only with themselves, but with the Girl. They declare nothing but what is probable, most of the Prisoners having been reputed Witches; all of them having the Mark; and one or other of them (to whom their Associates who delighted in Mischief, never failed to join) having had particular Provocations to take Revenge by the Torture and Deaths mentioned; besides the other Presumptions of Guilt, already proved before you. The Confessants were threatned to retract by the Prisoners themselves and their Friends, besides the bad usage from others in the Country.

They concur with the bewitched Girl's Testimony, and amongst themselves, even when examined singly, and upon new Things, as several have tried the Experiment. On this Head Delrio Lib. 5. Sect. 16. N. 5. wisely observes, Though it would be easy for a Dæmon to deceive more than one, yet it is not to be thought that God will equally permit it, lest Judges should be wholly at a loss in using their Reason in the Tryal of others, which would be contrary to the Methods of Divine Providence. The Reiteration of the Acts which they declare, as to some Persons that they never saw, except in these Congresses, and yet whom they knew now on the first Sight, is unaccountable, if they were Cheats. And that they are not such is further confirmed, by some of the Prisoners being accused by a confessing Witch in the Year 1687. And you know, that others accused by these Confessants, were lately brought in Guilty by the Verdict of a former Inquest, &c. which are so many joint Proofs of the Witnesses Integrity, and make a Chain of Evidence and moral Demonstration, both against Error in themselves, and Delusion in Relation to others, &c.

There are some Things also objected from the Law of Scotland, which we shall give some brief Hints of.

Whereas it was alledged, That those that were indicted for capital Crimes, and so under the Prosecutor's Power, cannot be admitted to be Witnesses; conformable to a Statute in Regiam Majestatem;

To this it was answered, That we need not say, that these Statutes have the Force of Law, except so far as they are received by Custom, and are conformable to Law. A Lay-Man cannot witness against a Clerk, and on the contrary, &c. nor need we make use of that which is obvious, viz. That these Statutes are only common Rules in ordinary Crimes; which have their Exception in Occult and excepted Crimes, such as Witchcraft, &c. Not every Rule is to be overthrown, and particularly this Rule is so restrained in the Case of Witchcraft, by the Opinions of Lawyers and the Customs afore-mentioned, which are the best Interpreters of Laws; for if this Application should hold, a Companion in a Crime could never be admitted: But we positively deny that those Confessants are under our Power or Influence; seeing Elizabeth Anderson is not Guilty of Witchcraft, for any Thing that does appear; The Lindseys were never Indicted for it, and the Indictment against Jennet and Margaret Rogers was dropped; as the whole Commission is to expire against the first of June, betwixt and which Time, they are to proceed no farther than this particular Tryal; so that this Objection vanishes.

Whereas it is pretended that the Rogers's cannot be received, because not given out in the List of Witnesses, conformable to the Regulation, whereby the Prisoners might have proved their Objection by their Exculpation:

It was answered,

First, This Objection ought to be rejected; because, besides that the Act speaks only of criminal Libels and not Indictments; which with the List of the Witnesses may be given in far shorter Time, than the additional List hath been given to the Prisoners indicted, being Prisoners: This Act as interpreted by the common Custom of the Justice-Court, of giving additional Lists after the first, upon shorter Time than this hath been given; as is particularly attested by James Guthry Macer, who gave them; and being a Person in Office, his Testimony is to be credited in what relates to his Office; so that the Old Custom confirmed by a Decision, August the Third, 1661, where Alexander Forrester was cited, apud Acta, against a Witch, continues as to this Point, as is related by Mr. Kemple, Pag. 529.

Secondly, Any Objection that the Prisoners pretend against these Witnesses, is in jure, or may instantly appear.

Thirdly, The Case is altogether Extraordinary, and Circumstantiate; for these Witnesses had not confessed; and so were not Existent under that Reduplication, when the Principal List was given out; whereby the Act of Parliament can only be understood of Witnesses that were then Existent.

And finally, The Prisoners got a general Warrant of Exculpation for citing of any Witnesses they pleased, and they have had several Days since they got this general List, so that they might have cited Witnesses to prove their Objections, were it not true, that they have none besides these that are common and before answered.

Thus we have given some Hints, which your own Reason may improve and apply, so as to dissolve the Quibbles which Petty Wits, who have not Soul enough of themselves to penetrate into the Depth of that which is abstruse, may raise against it: Their common Talent being either to pass over Things supeficially, or else to attack some of the slightest Outworks, and then to triumph as if they had obtained the Victory.

I confess none could be more Sceptical as to the Truth of some odd Things I had heard, and more inquisitive into the Reality, than I was before my Attendance at Bargarran's House, and the several Dyets at Court; and my Conversation with some of those-concerned in the Matter. But now, after all that I have seen, reasoned and heard, I acknowledge my self intirely captivated by the Dictates of Natural Understanding and Common Sense, into a firm Belief and Perswasion, that as there is such a Thing as Witchcraft, so it was evident in it's forementioned Effects, and that the Seven Prisoners were some of the Witches.

I have troubled you little with my own Observations, yet lest you should think me too Lazy, I shall make one; and that is, that I do not think the greater Part of the condemned Prisoners will ever fully Confess; for which Conjecture I have two Grounds, viz. that they are neither Ignorant nor Melancholy, but on the contrary, some of them would seem to have been once enlightned, before they fell away, so that if this be a Sin unto Death, there is no Appearance that they will glorifie God by a Confession.

Several of them are Persons of singular Knowledge and Acuteness, beyond the common Level of their Station; particularly Margaret Laing made Harangues in her Defence, which neither Divine or Lawyer could well outdo. Yet I thought, that when they spoke in a Matter of any Concern, their Eyes stood asquint and fixed, as if they had been turning their Ears and attending to some invisible Dictates. Their Answers to the Trying Questions put to them, were surprizingly subtle and Cautious, though indeed by the Industry of some of the Judges and Lawyers, they were sometimes catched in Lyes, Prevarications and Contradictions, which might have proceeded from either Natural or Preternatural Causes. Some of them were esteemed in the Country, to be very sagacious and exact in their Business; Margaret Laing having been a Noted Midwife; and one of the Lindseys having acquired a considerable Fortune by his Tillage and Trade. Yet it was observed, that there did commonly break out in their Hypocritical way of Living, something odd, either of Iniquity or Affectation; and Lindsey did cunningly enough get off from the Sheriff, when he was formerly accused in the Year 1687.

Melancholy Persons are lovers of Solitude, Witches of Society and Feasts. Those are commonly Pale and Heavy; many of these Corpulent and Voluptuous. Witches, are hard to Confess, as knowing their Guilt: The Melancholy delight to discover their horridest Damps, because they think them no Crime. The Confessions of the one are every where Uniform; The others Phantasms are as various as their Humours. Finally, Witches teach their Trade, whereas Conceits would Dye with the Melancholy, and can no more be conveyed by them to others, than the Humour which is the chief Cause thereof. As these distinguishing Characters do hold in General, so in this particular Case there are several others; so as most of the Prisoners were of a middle Age. One not much above Twenty, and the first Confessants are known to be Young; so that Dotage or

Melancholy are the less to be suspected; yea, was morally impossible in many of their Cases. For the Facts which the Confessants had formerly declared before the Commissioners for Enquiry, were sworn to by other unquestionable Witnesses before the Commissioners for the Tryal; and their Circumstances were such, that one of them could not know, what the other had Deponed. As it is already manifest, that the real Effects in several Passages of Bargarran's Daughter were not possibly producible by any Imagination of Humour, and it is special in this Case, that neither the Prisoners nor Confessants, were distempered by being kept from Sleep, tortured or the like, which were too usual in former times; but all the Measures were strictly observed, that are requisite to a truly Impartial Judgment.

There is no Need to insert the Copies of the Depositions themselves, because it is not denied that they are such as represented in the Pleadings, the chief Question being about the Legality of the last Deponents. Nor is there any Need to insert the Defendants Part of the Debate separately by it self, in respect that it is faithfully repeated or implied in what is here contained.

Upon the whole I do believe, that there is scarce a more remarkable Providence of this Nature to be found in any true History; nor was there ever a more exact Caution in any Enquiry or Tryal of this Kind: A clearer Probation, without Confession of the Prisoners themselves, or a juster Sentence, puting together all Circumstances upon Record.

I am, what you have made me,

Yours, &c.

CHAP. V.

Containing a brief Narrative of the Surrey Dæmoniack. The Testimony and Information upon Oath of several Persons who voluntarily offered themselves concerning Richard Dugdale of Whalley, in the County of Lancaster, Gardner; taken before Hugh Lord Willoughby, and Ralph Egerton Esq; Two of his Majesties Justices of the Peace for the County of Lancaster, at Holcomb in the said County, the Nine and Twentieth Day of July, 1695.

THomas Dugdale, Father of the said Richard Dugdale, maketh Oath, that he consulted one Crabtree in Behalf of his said Son, then under a strange Distemper, and had his Answer; that if there was Money enough he could effect the Cure; whereupon this Deponent seeing his Son's Body much weakened with the said Crabtree's Physick, and his Fits more violent, applied himself to Mr. Jolly a Neigbouring Minister, and others of his Brethren in the Ministry. And this Deponent says, he hath seen his Son Vomit up Stones, several times and other Things. Once he declared, he must either Vomit up Gold, Silver or Brass Rings, and Hair-Buttons, and accordingly did so. At other Times he vomited great Stones, also blue Stones like Flints.

One time he vomited a Stone an Inch and a half long, and an Inch and a half broad, having Blood upon the Edges, which this Deponent and others standing by him, apprehended to be painful to him.

And further this Deponent maketh Oath, that one Day a little before Night, walking by his said Son then in a Fit, it growing dark, a Candle being brought in, the Deponent looking upon him, there was a great Stone laid upon his Belly, weighing about Twelve or Thirteen Pounds, this Deponent, not knowing how it came there, nor were there any such like Stones about the House. Besides Stones have been thrown at the Barn-side, falling very thick upon the Door, yet this Deponent could, never discover the Hand that threw them, nor any Person employed therein, although this Deponent's Wife was hit with one of them, but without any Hurt. At other times the said Richard Dugdale would cast Goose-dung at this Deponent, and others standing by, which he seemed to fetch out of the Barn-side; altho' neither this Deponent, nor those that were with him could find any there, nor discover any one that brought it, nor were there any Geese kept at the House, nor other Geese came near it. And lastly, this Deponent saith, that his said Son would run upon his Hands and his Feet together, as fast as most Men could run upon their Hands alone, and his Body would sometimes be so heavy, that Two or Three strong Men could hardly lift him up; and at other Times as light as a Bag of Feathers.

John Walmsly of Harwood, in the said County of Lancaster, Saddler, Deposes, That he hath seen the said Richard Dugdale in a Fit, held in a Chair by Six Men. And whilst his Feet were off the Ground, he hath leaped up in the Chair for Two or Three Hours together, as fast as a Man can ordinarily count any Thing, and hath so sweated through his Cloaths, that it hath stood like a Dew upon them. Moreover this Deponent hath taken the said Richard Dugdale by the Shoe, betwixt this Deponents foremost Finger and his Thumb, another taking him at his Head, and so lifting him up, this Deponent could not think he weighed Six Pounds.

And further this Deponent says, that Mr. Jolly the Minister, sending Word by him to the said Richard's Father, that the Ministers would be at his House called Surrey on such a Day; this Deponent going the same Day he was spoken to with his Errand, the said Richard declared it before this Deponent mentioned it; as likewise what Ministers would be there.

And further, this Deponent upon his Oath says, That the said Richard Dugdale in some of his Fits, opening his Hand hath received written Papers into it, none of the By-standers knowing how they came thither; which the said Richard Dugdale hath given People that were about him; also the said Deponent hath seen him shuffle Rushes like Cards, and play Games on them, as though he had been playing with some other Person, with whom he had Child about the Casts, Cursing and Swearing about his Play, and then said, Do not Gamesters thus? He likewise played with Rushes as if they had been Dice, using exactly several Expressions belonging to that Play, saying, People think this is laid upon me for my Sins, but I never was a Gamester in my Life, neither know I how to Play at such Games, when out of my Fits. And the said Richard Dugdale did likewise play at Bowls, making Bowls of Rushes; and when he had thrown the Jack, he said, I must now throw my Gill; then running a good way, as if he had been running after a Bowl, Swearing, Run, Run, Flee, Flee, Hold a Biass; and sometimes he catched up Rushes as if they had been Bowls, Swearing, Sirrah, stand out of the Way, or I'll knock out your Brains; adding, I never was a Bowler, But don't Gentlemen do thus.

And this Deponent says, That the said Richard Dugdale had several Fits, after his being threatned with his being brought before a Justice of Peace. And once being in his last Fit, when this Deponent was present, he declared his Fit was thro' Obsession, and in a Combination which should never be discovered whilst the World endured. And this Deponent hath seen him in a great Fit, as in a great Agony, with something he could not see, and then hath been taken up and thrown backwards, set upon his Head, and so stood till he was pulled down by one Jahn Fletcher. As also this Deponent hath heard him Curse and Swear, his Gesture being so terrible, it would have frighted a Man to come near him, and yet in a Moment's time after, in such a Fear that he sought to creep into any Hole, or behind any Rody to have hid himself, and so lamented himself, as moved the Standers-by with great Compassion. He would at other Time; have told when his Fits would begin, when he had Two or Three in one Day, or Three or Four Days asunder, wherein he was never disproved, that he knew of, which Fits commonly began with the Calf of his Leg, and wrought upwards into the Chest of his Body, and then he was thrown down, where he would lye for a good while as Dead, or Breathless; and then would have a strange Noise in his Mouth and Nose, and there would to his Apprehension be something like Whelps in his Bosom before he rose, after which sometime he would be very furious, sometime more quiet.

William Loond of Harwood, Carrier, in the County of Lancaster maketh Oath, that he hath heard the said Richard Dugdale Curse and Swear, his Gesture being so terrible, it would have frighted a Man to come near him, and yet in a Moment of time after, in such a Fear, that he hath sought to creep into any Hole, or behind any Body to have hid himself, and so lamented himself, as moved the Standers by with great Compassion. He would at other Times have told when his Fits would begin, when they were Two or Three in one Day, or Three or Four Days asunder, wherein he was never disappointed that he knew of, which Fits commonly began in the Calf of his Leg, and wrought upwards into the Chest of his Body; and then he was thrown down, where he would lye for a good While as Dead, or Breathless, and then would have a strange Noise in his Mouth and Nose, and there would be in his Breast like Whelps before he rose; after which sometimes he would be very furious, sometimes more quiet.

Wiltoughby.
Ralph Egerton.

John Livesy of Clayton, in the County of Lancaster, Skinner, maketh Oath, That he the Deponent being at home with him, the said Richard Dugdale, he Cursed and Swore, making Answer to something at the Window that he could not see, whom he called Nicholas, saying he would go with him. And this Deponent being with him at the Chappel Door, he then being in a Trance, this Deponent observed there would be such a Noise in his Breast, as went in Course with the Peoples Voices Singing Psalms within, Singing, or turning as they did, and ceasing when they ceased; and whilst his Eyes were close shut, he told a Woman she had a Pipe in her Pocket, which proved very true. Also this Deponent hath seen him run over Three or Four Stiles with his Eyes closed, and hath heard his Voice as in his Ordinary

Discourse, when the Deponent hath been above a Mile distant from him.

Nathaniel Waddington, of Altham, in the County of Lancaster, Husbandman, upon his Oath saith, That he hath carried the said Richard Dugdale in one of his Fits, for the Space of Eight Roods; that in the Beginning of some of his Fits, he would be as light as a Feather-Boulster, but before he came out heavier than a Load of Corn. That sometimes this Deponent hath taken him off the Ground by his Buttons with one Hand, and to this Deponent's Thinking, he hath weighed but twenty Pound. And further this Deponent saith, That in some of his Fits, a Swelling as big as a Man's Hand in one of his Legs, moved towards his Knee. That in some of his Fits he had more Strength than six Strong-Mer.

John Dorrel, of Wismall, in the County of Lancaster, Husbandman, maketh Oath, That he hath seen the said Richard Dugdale Dance upon his Knees, without touching the Ground with his Toes, with his Body bowed forward, and that for the Space of a Quarter of an Hour, with as much Activity, as though he had been upon his Feet. And hath also seen him Dance upon his Toes, quickly changing to Dance upon his Knees, and so hath leaped up again upon his Feet, and hath seen him in his Fits, have Motions of Dancing Antickly, being kept down in a Chair.

William Seller, of pendleton, in the County of Lancaster, Husbandman, maketh Oath, That he heard the said Richard Dugdale in his Fits, utter Words which this Deponent understood not; in one of which Fits, Twelve Men could not hold him, but with ease he could throw them a good Distance from him. And another time the Deponent being told by Mr. Jolly, he expected the said Richard Dugdale would have a Fit about Seven a Clock next Morning, wished this Deponent to see the said Richard Dugdale, giving this Deponent Five Shillings for him; but before this Deponent could come up to the said Richard Dugdale, he cried, here is a Man will bring Money to Day, and fell a leaping and dancing in the Barn, as a Token of Joy, but after a while seeming to be displeased at something, he said, Dick,

Dick, Thou shalt have Meat enough, and not long after fell down Dead, and then in a little time turned on his Back, and seemed to fall a Eating; at which time this Deponent, with Richard Dugdale his Unckle, lifted him up twice, and found him to be as Light as a Hat or a Walking-Cane. And when he was sensible, this Deponent demanded of him the Occasion of his Distemper, and whether he had not made some Contract with the Devil; who answered, saying, would you have me to lye. This Deponent also maketh Oath, that at a Meeting in one William Waddington's House in Altham, the said Richard Dugdale made such a Noise, as terrified several People, in so much that they left the House; and at the same time this Deponent heard two distinct Voices at once come from him the said Richard Dugdale, the one being a very hideous Noise, which running through the Crowd, put some People into horrible trembling, so that some of them said, They thought the Devil went out of him.

Willoughby.
Ralph Egerton

Lawrence Roberthshaw, of Harwood, in the County of Lancaster, Woollen-Weaver, Deposeth, and saith, upon Oath, That he heard one of the Ministers then present, and the Devil as he supposeth, in the said Richard Dugdale, talk one to another. One Passage this Deponent well remembers, viz. The Minister said, Satan thou hast made a Tryal both of Heaven and Hell, which of them likest thou best? To which an Answer was given by Satan (as this Deponent supposes) saying, Hell is my Palace and Paradice, where I'll have thee shortly. Upon which the said Richard Dugdale shivered as if one Joint would have fallen from another, and many other Sayings could this Deponent Report, if he was required.

Willoughby.
Ralph Egerton.

Thomas Booth, of Hay-House, in the County of Lancaster, Carpenter, maketh Oath, That he heard several Voices come from the said Richard Dugdale his Lips not moving, and his Tongue appearing to be strangely rowled on a Lump, and his Eye-Balls turned inwards, at the Time when the several Voices came from him. And further this Deponent saith, That in the Time of his Fits, the said Richard Dugdale was of an exceeding Lightness, and again of an extraordinary Heaviness; sometimes as light as a Chip, and again as heavy as a Horse, and all in one and the same Fit. In the light Part of his Fit, this Deponent hath taken him up about his Hips, betwixt this Deponent's Hands, and he was so light, this Deponent thought he could lift Twenty fuch.

Willoughby.
Ralph Egerton.

These Depositions were taken at the Time and Place aforementioned, upon the Holy Evangelists.

Willoughby.
Ralph Egerton.

The Informations of divers Persons taken before the said Justices of Peace, at the Time and Place aforesaid, declaring themselves ready to do it upon Oath, when required.

JAmes Abbot, of Whitberk, in the County of Lancaster, Dyer, declares, That he went, on purpose, to see the said Richard Dugdale at Surrey, the Place of his Abode, having no Acquaintance with him, nor had he any Knowledge of this Informant, as this Informant verily believeth. When this Informant came, the said Richard Dugdale being in one of his said Fits, said, Abbot, Thou thinkst no Body knows thee, but I know thee well enough; thou must go into Cheshire and Staffordshire; when as this Informant says, He had not so much as a Design of such a Journey to his Remembrance; but accordingly it happened, that this Informant went that Journey soon afterwards.

John Fielding, of Harwood, in the County of Lancaster, Joyner, declares, That being with the said Richard Dugdale in one of his Fits, this Informant to his Thinking heard something within him like Piggs Sucking of a Sow; and also like the Barking of a Dog.

John Whally, of Harwood, in the County of Lancaster, Hair-Cloth-Weaver, informs the same which John Fielding does; and further, informs the same with John Walmsly, as to the said Richard Dugdale's Carding, Diceing and Bowling. And moreover informs, That he this said Informant, being with Richard Dugdale in one of his Fits, he said, There were Lapideers a coming; and presently after came a Stone, which this Informant took up, and felt it to be very warm. And he further Informs, that the said Richard Dugdale in his Fits commonly told when the next Fit would come.

William Livasay, of Whalley, in the County of Lancaster, Shoemaker, informs, That he being in Whalley, desired several Young Men to go along with him to Surrey (above half a Mile distant) but they refused; when the Informant came to the Barn, where the said Richard Dugdale was, the said Richard Dugdale told this Informant, that he had desired several Persons to come along with him, but they had denied him, naming Ned Dean in particular. And he further Informs that the said Richard Dugdale, on his Feet, Three Yards from the Wall of the Barn, was as soon as he could turn himself, set straight upon his Head, and was as stiff as a Tree.

    John Grimshaw, of Clayton, in the County of Lancaster, Woollen-Weaver, informs, That the said Richard Dugdale being in a Fit, he said, Nicholas, Art thou there? What seest thou for? Come up. Then said, Seest thou where my Mother sits? Then something came to his Shoulder, and several Parts of his Body; and the said Richard Dugdale seemed to be much afrighted with it. And he further informs, That he coming to the Surrey one Night, he the said Richard Dugdale told Mr. John Grimshaw, that he the said Informant Grimshaw, was coming before he came. And this Informant leaving his Horse at a considerable Distance from the Place, where the said Richard Dugdale was, and going into the Place, the said Richard Dugdale meets him with a great Noise, and faith, How now? calling him Grimshaw; adding, art thou there with all thy Knives, (this Informant having Three or Four Knives about him) telling this Informant likewise that he could not go on Foot. And this Informant further says, That when the said Richard Dugdale was in his Trances (as they called them) and lying upon the Ground, he was sometimes as light, to this Informant's thinking, as his Shoes and Stockings, and sometimes as heavy as a Man could lift.

    The Informations aforesaid were
taken at the Time and Place
above mentioned before Us,

Willoughby.
Ralph Egerton.

And, Lastly, We the said Justices of the Peace, do Certify, that the said Thomas Dagdale, Father of the said Richard Dugdale, did make Oath before us, That he knew not of any Design or Combination betwixt his said Son, and any other Person, which might occasion the aforesaid strange Fits and Disturbances. Nor that he the Deponent was any way privy to it; nor knoweth he of any Cheating or Deceiving Practices for Gain, or any such End, Purpose or Design whatsoever.

Willoughby.
Ralph Egerton.

The Information of several Persons, who voluntarily offered themselves, concerning Richard Dugdale, of Whally, in the County of Lancaster, Gardener, before Thomas Braddil Esq; and Ralph Egerton Esq; Two of his Majesties Justices of the Peace for the said County, at Derwin, in the said County, on the Twentieth Day of July, 1695.

John Fletcher, of Harwood, in the County of Lancaster, Husbandman, declares, That he hath seen the said Richard Dugdale in many of his Fits, wherein he hath barked like a Mastiff Dog, being then as strong, as Ten Men: For this Informant hath been of the Ten, that have undertaken to hold him. Also that this Informant one Time found him in the River of Calder up to the Neck in Water, crying out, and saying, Wilt thou Drownd me? striking at the same time upon the Water with Two Sticks. Whereupon this Informant, with the Help of others, by a Rope, drew him out of the Water. The said Dugdale being then in a Dumb Fit; which began in the Water, and continued near Four Hours after. And further this Informant saith, he found in the Barn where the said Dugdale lay, a round Hole in the Hay like a Hen's Nest, wherein were Seven Stones laid together. And this Informant hath taken up several Stones cast by the said Dugdale, running upon his Hands and Feet, Barking and Howling. And the said Dugdale being fat down, he hath seen him, several times, thrown Five or Six Yards from the Place.

John Whitehead, of Bankbey, in the County of Lancaster, Labourer, declareth, That being at Surrey with the said Dugdale in one of his Fits, he found him lying upon the Barn-floor like a Dead Man; at which time, Mr. Ainsworth the Apothecary, and another Apothecary from Manchester coming in, both of them felt the said Dugdale's Pulses, which did not beat, and then they laid their Faces to his Mouth, to try if he breathed, but could not perceive it. And further this Informant says, that at Mr. Jolly's House, the Informant endeavouring to hold the said Dugdale, in his Fit, by the Wrist of his Arm, could by no means do it, for this Informant's Fingers were no sooner closed but they opened again.

John Smallwood, of Harwood, in the County of Lancaster, Cooper, declareth, That he hath seen the said Richard Dugdale in Twenty or Thirty of his Fits; sometimes lying on the Floor, for the Space of Four Hours very stiff and heavy, in so much that this Informant with Three more have carried him out of the Barn, but on his coming out of his Fit, his Head and Part of his Body hath been lifted up by this Informant's Daughter, a Child of Seven Years Old.

The Informations aforesaid were taken,
at the Time and Place afore-mentioned,
before the said Mr. Braddil, and me the said

Ralph Egerton.

The Informations of divers Creditable Persons which were, and are ready to give in upon Oath, before the said Justices of the Peace, or others at the Places aforesaid, or elsewhere if desired to do it, as they voluntarily offered, and declared unto Mr. Jolly, and others of sufficient Credit and Cautiousness.

John Fletcher, further says, I was one Night in Bed with Richard Dugdale, and I felt something come up towards my Knees; then I felt it creep up till it came towards my Heart, than I got hold of it, and it was about the Bigness of a little Dog or Cat, and it slipped through my Hands as if it had been a Snig; and when we were in Bed, very often there hath been something in Bed knattering, as though there had been Mice or Rats, and we searched the Bed, but it was not harmed; and Things have seemed to our thinking to have fallen in the House, as if all had been broken, yet in the Morning nothing stirred; and one Sabbath Day there was a Knife length-ways in his Mouth, none knowing how it came there, where it was held so very fast, that I with much ado pulled it out, and asked the Company, whether any of them wanted a Knife. They all said no, till one Jeremy Webster, that was newly come in said, I had one when I came in, and I think he cannot have got it out of my Pocket; but he finding nothing but a Sheath in his Pocket, claimed the Knife, and it was certainly his. John Fletcher further says, That when the said Richard Dugdale was in a Fit, about Five a Clock in the Night, John Hindle pricked a large Pin in his Feet, and he neither stirred nor complained at all. Besides in one of his Fits, I heard him tell, that he must vomit a Hair-Button, and a Curtain-Ring, which I saw him do within an Hour. I have seen, as John Darwin before testified, Richard Dugdale for a Quarter of an Hour together Dance upon his Knees, with as much Activity as any one on their Feet.

John Fletcher.

John Hindle says; These strange Things I have heard Richard Dugdale do and say; I was by when he told, that he should vomit a Hair-Button and Curtain-Ring, which I saw him do within an Hour. Likewise I have lifted at him, when I could not lift as much as his Head for my Life; and at other times I have lifted at him, and could lift him with as much ease as if it had been a Child. I was present when Richard Dugdale was in a Fit, about Eight a Clock in the Night, and I pricked a Pin into his Foot, and he neither stirred nor complained at all. I was present at all which William Loond Swears to, in the first Part of his Oath.

John Hindle.

Thomas Core, saith, I have seen several times the Lump on his Breast or Belly, as big as a Man's Fist, and heard strange Voices coming out of it.

Thomas Core.

John Fielding, saith, That the said Swelling of the said Richard Dugdale, when it rose from the Thick of his Leg, was about the bigness of a Mole (or a Molewarp, as they call it) and worked up and down like such a Creature, towards the Chest of his Body; that it got up into his Shoulder, and then he was in the worst of his Fit. He also says, that the said Richard Dugdale did, in several of his Fits, take several Things out of the Hands of several Persons, and would by no means part with the said Things, but to the Person to whom they belonged, having his Eyes close shut all the while; also he says, That they which attempted to force the Things out of his Hands, could not force them out, how strong soever the Persons were, so that they might sooner pull the Things in Pieces, than get them from him. The said Fielding also saith, That the said Creature, rose under the said Richard Dugdale's Skin, as he does verily think. Also, he says, That the said Richard Dugdale did in his Fit lift up several lusty Men, and the Chair wherein they held him, though the said Richard Dugdale is but of ordinary Strength of Body when out of his Fit.

James Fielding, Jun.

John Smalley further says, (and John Fletcher witnesses the same, in which he agrees with several other Witnesses, as well as in other Things) that he saw Richard Dugdale ly Four Hours in one Fit, as if he was stark Dead, and as stiff as a Board; also when his Shoes were fast buckled to his Feet, they flew six Yards, and hit the Skel-boos in the Barn with great Force: also he said that Richard Dugdale was in the same Fit, as light as his Cloaths, and as heavy as a Sack of Corn.

John Smalley also further says, That upon Occasion he went to the Abby in Whalley, and whilst he was there, the said Richard Dugdale said, that Smalley was taking Liquor at the Abby, and he takes it freely, it costs him nothing. This he said to Thomas Dugdale as he also testifies.

John Smalley.

Edmund Haworth of Rhushton, Carrier, testifies, to the Passage about Jeremy Webster's Knife, as aforesaid; also to these Passages about Richard Dugdale's Vomiting several Stones, Hair Buttons, Curtain-Rings, &c. He moreover testifies, that the said Richard Dugdale, in one of his Fits, told him, with his Company that came along, what they had been Eating at home, what they discoursed of by the Way, what Stiles they went over, how they stumbled; and that the said Richard Dugdale threatened Robert Turner, to send his Sister (as he called his Spirit) to give him a Fall at such a Fields End; which fell out accordingly, so that it set all the Company a trembling; and that he and Three or Four more were coming towards Surey, and that Richard Dugdale in a Fit said that such were a coming, but he would send them back again, which fell out accordingly; for they turned back, near Harwood Church. He also testifies, That a Voice spoke in Richard Dugdale, besides his own Voice, without his Lips moving; and that another Voice, as they apprehended, spoke out of the Earth in Answer to him, and that he hath been one of the Seven or Nine to carry him, and yet so many have been hard fet to do it, and that he, and some others were coming, and such a Fear came on him, that he durst only go betwixt his Company, and that when he came to Surrey, he found Richard Dugdale in a Fit, who asked him Questions concerning his Fear in such a Place, and told him, that his Sister, as he called the Spirit, crossed him in the Way, but had no further Power than to put him into that Fright.

Edward Haworth.

Henry Page, of Harwood Magna, Felt-Maker, certifies, That he saw Richard Dugdale Dance on his Knees a good while together, not touching the Earth with any thing but his Knees. Further, that he saw the same Person Bowl with a Bowl he had made with Rushes; and that he heard him Bark like a Mastiff-Dog.

Henry Page.

Grace Whalley, of the same Place testifies, that she heard Richard Dugdale Snarl and Bark like a Dog; that she also heard (as she and others thought) a Noise out of his Belly, as if a Litter of Young Dogs had been Sucking there. And she further testifies, that she helped to hold his Head, the time he vomitted a Stone, weighing Three Ounces as she thinks. Further that she hath seen Richard Dugdale Gallop round the Barn on his Hands and Feet, for half an Hour together, as cleverly as any Horse; she hath heard him Whinying like a Horse, and as eating Provender. She further Declares, That she hath seen the said Richard Dugdale Dance on his Knees, not touching the Earth with his Toes; and that she heard Richard Dugdale tell, in one of his Fits, that there would come Three Lapiders at a certain Time; accordingly at the Time he foretold, there were thrown Three Stones, some distance of time from each other, which were as warm as New-Milk. These foresaid Passages she saw, heard and observed, when Richard Dugdale was in his Fits. Also she asked Richard Dugdale, when out of his Fits, whether he knew of any Thing spoken or done by him, whilst in the Fit, which he utterly denied. Also she testifies, that coming with her Brother and others to the Surey, to see Richard Dugdale, she being behind the rest, and coming over the Hippens, she unaccountably slipped off one of the Stones into the Water, and could not get out till her Brother came to help her; at the same time several Persons came out of the Barn, upon some Words spoke by Richard Dagdale at the same time, being in a Fit, viz. Sister Ekel, Put the hindermost into the Water.

Grace Whalley.

Surrey, July the Thirty First, 1695.

THomas and Anne Dugdale, Parents to Richard Dugdale, with Mary and Alice, Sisters to Richard Dugdale, testifie, That Richard Dugdale's Fits began soon after St. James's Day, when they went first to a neighbouring Doctor for Help, who prescribed several Things, which were observed without Effect; whereupon the Doctor was desired to take Richard Dugdale to his own House, but refused, acknowledging that he had done what he could, yet promised to Ride his Horse a Hundred Miles if that could help him. After this Richard Dugdale's Fits were more violent; soon after we consulted Dr. Crabtree, who undertook to Cure him. Upon which Thomas Dugdale went along with his Son Richard to Dr. Crabtree, where they stayed a Fortnight, and upon Richard Dugdale's Fits abating they came home; but within a few Days after his Return, his Fits were more violent than ever. A Fortnight after Thomas Dugdale and his Son Richard went to Dr. Crabtree the Second Time, where they stayed not so long as before; the Reasons were two; First, Richard Dugdale was tired with the Methods prescribed by Dr. Crabtree. The Doctor confessed that he gave the Patient Physick enough at once for Six Men, which weakened Richard Dugdale so much, that he had Strength little enough left to carry him cross the House; yet in his Fits Seven strong Men could not hold him. The Second Reason was the great Charges we were at, for it cost us more than Three Pounds Ten Shillings in a little time more than Three Weeks, which was insupportable, considering our Indigency, and no encouraging Signs of Help: But the Doctor's Words to his Neighbours were at first, that if the Father would bring Money enough, he would cure Richard Dugdale; yet said at another time, that if the Spirit in Richard Dugdale was a Water Spirit, there was no Cure for it. Some time after we consulted Mr. Jolly, who, with others in the Ministry, upon our Request, were much concerned for Richard Dugdale, Praying for him near Twelve Months, in which time he had many strange Fits; sometimes vomited Stones, a Curtain-Ring, a large Hair-Button;

in Fits would be lighter than so many Feathers. In the Beginning of several Fits would gape and catch with his Mouth (as a Dog at Flies) Ten or Eleven times together, and at the last would open his Mouth as often; when we thought Spirits might come into him or leave him. In many of his last Fits he told the People, that he might be killed or cured before the 25th of March, which proved true; for on the 24th coming from his Work on Hindfield-side, his last Fit seized him, and when he came Home he was in the Fit, his Face as black as a Coal; upon which he fell down, and lay a While, and then recovered out of his last Fit. After this Richard Dugdale had no Fit; though once when he had got too much Drink, he was after another manner than drunken Persons usually are.

Thomas Dugdale.
Anne Dugdale.
Mary Dugdale.
Alice Dugdale.

Altham, August the 4th. 1695.

NAthaniel Waddington, further testified, First, That he had seen Richard Dugdale gallop round the Barn several times together; and heard him Whinying much like a Horse, and making a Noise as if a Horse had been Eating Provender. Secondly, That he told Things in his Fit, which neither he nor any could by Lawful Art. As one time the said Nathaniel Waddington, and his Neighbour Joseph Hargreaves, going to Surrey, to see Richard Dugdale, they called at a House of a Neighbour of theirs, to desire the Master to go with them; but a Relation's Averseness prevented him. Richard Dugdale was in a Fit at the same Time and spoke it, before a great Number of People, that Nathaniel Waddington, and Joseph Hargreaves were coming; that they called on such a One whom he named, and told further how that Good Man's Wife hindered him. The latter Part, viz. The Discovery they met with from several which were with Richard Dugdale in the Barn, being sure that the Circumstances of Things were such, that Richard Dugdale could have no Intelligence. And further, Richard Dugdale's Relation was so particular, that it could not be an uncertain Guess. Further, That a certain Person going to see Richard Dugdale, took some Bisket, and a Piece or some Pieces of Gold, on purpose as the Person said to try whether Richard Dugdale could discover it. Soon after the Party came to Surrey, the Relator saw the Person standing upon a Seat to take a fuller View of Richard Dugdale in his Fit. Richard Dugdale immediately treated her so very rudely, discovered the Bisket, and said, I'll play at Cards with thee for those Guineas in thy Pocket, &c. These Words the Relator heard Richard Dugdale speak in his Fit. And further, John Feilding, Joyner, related in the hearing of the said Nathaniel Waddington and others, that he the said John Feilding was working at his Calling, above Thirty Miles distant from the Surrey; and that Richard Dugdale in one of his Fits said, John Feilding is this Day at such a Place Working, and further named the Piece of Work he had in Hand at that time. The said John Feilding coming over to see his Relations, several Persons who had heard. Richard Dugdale speak these Words, and relate such strange Circumstances, came to the said John Feilding to know whether it was true; this he acknowledged, being much surprized at their Relation. Thirdly, That he asked this Richard Dugdale, when he came out of his Fits, whether he could give an Account of any of those Things which passed in the Fit; this Richard Dugdale denied: yet once related a strange Passage; That in his Fit he thought he had distinct Sight of a Person, and told the Posture he thought he saw him in, and the Place where, many Miles from the Place where Richard had his Fit. Which Things concerning that Person were found true upon Enquiry.

Nathaniel Waddington, further testifies, That Richard Dugdale in his Fits, would sometimes pretend that a good Spirit was in him, and that Richard Dugdale then would in a long Discourse speak against several Sins, viz. Drinking, Gaming, &c. bringing several similar Texts of Scripture; naming Book, Chapter, Verse, either whole or Part, as much as was pertinent Mr. John Grimshaw examined the Places, and found them true, and that Richard Dugdale in his Discourse would use many pretty Similitudes.

Joseph Hargreaves, Neighbour to Nathaniel Waddington, testifies, that coming to the Surrey, and finding the Boy laid on the Barn-Floor, he the said Joseph Hargreaves lifted Richard Dugdale from the Ground more than once, and thinks at the most, that Richard Dugdale did not weigh above a Stone and a half; and further that Six strong Men could not hold him in a Fit, but that he hath drawn them all a great Way, and been forced from amongst them, hanging upon him at a Table a Yard high; and that he saw the Lump upon his Leg, about the Bigness of a Turkey-Egg, rise towards his Body, and that he and others have endeavoured to stop it, by tying a Boot-Garter above it, and beneath the Knee, and by grasping the Part with their Hands, yet could not prevent its rising into the Chest of his Body; but this to his thinking crept up his Leg like a Bat; sometimes being in Motion, and sometimes at a Stand; Joseph Hargreaves testifies, the first and second of Nathaniel Waddington's Depositions.

Richard Chrichly, under his Hand testifies, concerning Richard Dugdale's Strength.

Several other Testimonies as to Richard Dugdale's Case, are as followeth.

WE whose Names are Subscribed, being Ministers of the Gospel, having read or heard the Affidavits and Depositions taken before the Right Honourable Hugh Lord Willoughby, and Ralph Egerton Esq; Two of his Majesties Justices of the Peace, for the County Palatine of Lancaster, concerning one Richard Dugdale of Surey, in the Parish of Whalley, do verily believe the Truth of the same, and that the strange Fits of the said Dugdale were by a Diabolical Power.

Given when we met at Blackburn,
in Lancashire, on August the 6th. 1695.

> Thomas Crompton.
> Peter Aspinwall.
> John Crompton.
> John Parr.
> Samuel Angier.
> Nathaniel Haywood.
> Samuel Eaton.
> Nathaniel Scholes.

I do hereby testifie (as many more will if there be Occasion) from my own Observation as an Eye and Ear Witness, at the Meetings concerning Richard Dugdale, that I verily believe, he was then under a Diabolical Possession or Obsession. I do also testifie, That he is now delivered from that Super-natural Malady; and that no other probable Means of his Deliverance may be assigned, but the Word of God, and Prayer with Fasting; which Spiritual Means was made use of by several Ministers with great Faithfulness and Diligence, for a considerable time together.
Witness my Hand the
Tenth Day of June 1695.

> Robert Whiteaker Physician.

Concerning Richard Dugdale's Certificate, which is voluntarily Subscribed before James Gregson and my self, with others, which is elsewhere mentioned, the Words in the Original are as follows.

July the 10th 1695.

I Richard Dugdale, Son of Thomas Dugdale, of Surrey, near Whalley, in Lancashire Gardiner; do Certifie all to whom this may come, That my former strange Fits, were not any of them by any Cheat, or Art of Man, that I know of, but, as I do verily believe, were caused by the Devil; from whom and from my terrible Fits, I do verily believe my Body was cleared, through the Ministers Prayers, at or about Lady Day, 1690. After which I never had any more such Fits, whereupon I went and took some Physick, for the clearing of my Body from any ill Humours, it might have gotten by my said Fits. Signed in the Presence of,

Witness my Hand,

James Gregson.
Thomas Jolly.
Richard Dugdale.

We whose Names are subscribed, were present at many of the within mentioned Meetings, concerning Richard Dugdale, and so were Eye and Ear Witnesses to many of the Things within mentioned, and do verily believe the rest, not doubting but that the said Dugdale's Affliction was through Possession or Obsession, by Combination, or some secret Judgment of God; from which he was delivered, as we are fully perswaded by the Gospel Means within mentioned.

William Cross.
John Durden.
Laurence Walmsly.
John Baxon.
John Bayly.

Christopher Duckworth.
Leonard Bayley.
John Marsh.
James Whiteaker.
William Waddington.

George Cockshut.
Samuel Hey.
Charles Rily.
James Hindle.
Nathaniel Hindle.

Richard Jackson.
William Barton.
Christopher Tatterfeill.
Richard Sudal.
Nicholas Grimshaw.

On the Occasion of some Reflections Alexander Haworth gave the following Certificate.

I Alexander Hayworth, of Top-Royal, in Bury Parish in Lancashire, Yeoman, going with the Reverend Mr. Pendlebury, to see Richard Dugdale in his strange Fits, at the first time, upon my asking him his Opinion of the said Dugdale's Fits, he answered, That he questioned whether the said D. might not be acted, by some Bodily Distemper in the said Fits. But when the said Pendlebury had been with the said D. a second time, I asked him his Opinion again in the Case, and then he had altered his Perswasion concerning D. having such Things in him, as he judged more than natural, and he gave such Reasons for it as altered my Judgment as well as his.

Decemb. 25. 1697.
Alexander Haworth.

To these we shall add further Informations, as to the Case of the said Richard Dugdale, taken before the Right Honourable Hugh Lord Willoughby and William Hulme, Esq; Two of his Majesties Justices of the Peace, and Quorum, for the County Palatine of Lancaster, taken at the House of Richard Sharples of Blackburn, in the County aforesaid, the 15th, 16th and 17th of September 1697; where the Informants were examined by the said Justices, upon the Account of several Passages, in a Book called the Surrey Impostor.

The Confession of Richard Dugdale, of Whalley, in the County of Lancashire, Gardiner; taken before the Right Honourable Hugh Lord Willoughby, and William Hulme, Esq; two of his Majesties Justices of the Peace and Quorum, for the said County, taken at the House of Richard Sharples, of Blackburn, in the County aforesaid, the 15th Day of September, Anno Dom. 1697.

Impr.

THE said Richard Dugdale, answers and says, That he was in Health of Body and Mind, at the Age of Eighteen Years or thereabouts. About the Nineteenth Year be says, he was a hired Servant with Thomas Lister of Arnald's-bigging, in the County of York, Esq; and begging Leave of his said Master, to go to a Rushbearing at Whalley, and being in Drink, fell out at Whalley with a Man, and fought abundantly that Night about Dancing. He says afterwards he went to his Father's House. The Day after he went from his Father's House. The Day after he went from his Father's House to Arnold's-bigging, and on the Road being troubled in Mind, he thought that he saw several Apparitions, but could not tell the Resemblance thereof. The Day afterwards, he says, he went to make Hay, and he found himself clogged with some Heaviness, that he could not Work or Stoop; from thence he went to a Well, about a Field's Breadth from the Hall aforesaid, and saw a Gallon or Pail standing at the Well, and that he laid himself down to drink at the Well, and as he was Drinking, there came up to him a Neighbouring Woman of good Repute, and advised him not to drink so much Water, but rather to go up to the Hall, and get Drink; and told him that so much Water was enough to ruin him; and he says he took her Advice, and went up to the said Hall, and getting some Drink from the Cook-Maid, he went up into his Chamber, and being after some time laid down upon the Bed, the Chamber-Door opened of it self, as he thought, and there appeared something to him like a Smoak or Mist, which presently vanished, and afterwards there came partly a Fear upon him. Immediately after, he thought there came unto him, the Likeriess of a hard favoured Man, which at that time he thought had been one Hindle, a fellow Servant, whose Hair seemed to be clipped close to his Ears, and lay very heavy upon his Breast, so that he asked him what he would do with him, which suddenly after speaking, he thought the Vision turned into the Likeness of a Naked Child; he says he thought, he got hold of the Naked Child by the Knee, and that the Child turned into the Likeness of a Filmet, and went away with a Shrill Schreak. All this was done when he was awake as he is now, to his thinking. Immediately after this, he says, that he was very rude and troublesome, so that two Women could scarce hold him, and that he raved of one Dr. Chew, and desired the Woman to send for his Unkle, to go with him to the said Doctor, who was the first and last Physician he had Physick from. He says, to the best of his Knowledge, he thought he had little Advantage by the first Physick, but whether he took all or no he cannot tell, After the first Time of taking Physick from Dr. Chew, he went to Dr. Crabtree, and says the Doctor Blooded him several times, the first of which was as black as Ink, and that Blood, was got with very great Difficulty. Afterwards he went to Dr. Crabtree a second time, and was blooded, and took Physick as before; and whilst he was with Dr. Crabtree, he says he was for some Two or Three Days, and sometimes a Fort-night without any Fit, and had sometimes Two or Three Fits in a Day. He says, his Senses were sometimes taken away from him in his Fits. He says, sometimes he could remember some Passages. After this he believes one Robert Martin advised his, the said Dugdale's Father, to advise his Son to apply himself to one Mr. Jolly, to desire his Prayers, where he fell into a Fit, but remembers no Discourse he had with Mr. Jolly. He the said Richard Dugdale says, he believes he was not possessed with an Evil Spirit. And he says likewise, that he had a Fit on the 24th of March last at Evening; and on the 25th of March in the Morning he took Physick from Dr. Chew, and says that the Physick worked well with him, and since that time, he says, he never had any Fit, but says, that the strange Things that befell him, occasions him to believe that the Disease was not.

Ordinary. And he likewise says, that he was not in any Combination with any Person, or Persons whatsoever, and that there was no Cheat in any Thing, to his Knowledge. He cannot remember that he could play any more Tricks than the rest of the School-Boys; and he denies that he ever spoke any such Things as are laid to his Charge, to the School-Master about the Money, and says, that he is no Latin Schollar, nor knows any of those Sentences charged upon him, neither by Heart or otherwise. He says, he wrote a Letter to Sir Edmund Asbton, but remembers no Latin Sentence therein. He says likewise, that he never wrapped himself in a Blanket, in order to fright any Person. He says likewise, that after the Ministers left Surrey, he had not Fits so often as before, but they were more violent than ever before.

Taken before Us
Willoughby.
Will. Hulme.
Richard Dugdale.

Some Remarks concerning Richard Dugdale's Testimony.

IT does not seem strange, that he does not mention several Particulars, mentioned in the Narrative; particularly about the Beginning of his Fits, and when we began with him, and when we left off Meeting at Surrey; and when his Fits left him, &c. for he might easily forget the said Passages in Seven or Eight Years time, or be straitned by the Presence and Influence of some there present; but some of us noted down the said omitted Passages all along, and can satisfie any Sober Person, that all was true that is expressed in the said Narrative. He declared such Things to us, and desired such Things of us from first to last.

Neither should it seem strange that he does not expresly own the true Cause of his strange Fits, nor the only proper Means of his Deliverance (though he hath freely owned both, more privately, and under his own Hand;) for he is apparently over-awed by those, on whom he hath his Dependance, as to his Livelihood, and by his Neighbours; alledging in his Excuse, that he is a poor Man; hath a Wife and some small Children; a Temptation that might put a strong Christian to it to conquer it.

Yet does he by the foresaid Information fairly overturn the Objector's Foundations, for he owns himself sound in Body and Mind, when these Fits first seized him, and disowns them as any Ordinary Disease; and though in his Information, he says, he believes he was not Possessed with an Evil Spirit; he is partly to be excused, because he himself little knew how he was in those Fits; but when he heard how it was with him from others, and considered of it, he acknowledged that his strange Fits were caused by the Devil. And so must any one who exercises his Reason, and is not blinded with Passion. He solemnly disowns any Thing of a Cheat, or Combination, that he knows of, in the Case, as his Father also doth; so that if it be not any ordinary Disease, nor Cheat, nor Combination, What must it then be? And what must there follow? Especially when all the Informations are well weighed; so that any sober Person may easily judge of the Malady, as well as the Remedy.

For as much as the Informations both Private and Publick are called over again before Authority, it is to take away all Suspicion of Private or Unfair dealing; and what he now acknowledges, confirms and adds to what was said before.

John Walmsly confirms what he formerly testified, and adds, I have heard Richard Dugdale in his Fit say, That he had a Familiar, Or how should I tell such Things as I do? I have seen Richard Dugdale stand upon his Feet with his Arms open, and I have swayed at his Arm and Hand, till I have been afraid of breaking it, and could not stir either his Body, or a Joint of his Arm or Fingers. And when it was reported, that Mr. Bradil would send him to the House of Correction, I have seen Richard Dugdale use scornful Expressions towards him, calling, John, John, Come you must make a Mittimus! I will send him away, (or Words to this purpose;) then he would cast up his Shoulder like Mr. Edleston, and appear as if he would have Written with his Finger in the Ball of his Hand, with scornful Language and Laughter. I have seen him in his Fits at Mr. Walmsly's, Mr. Cronbook's and Mr. Braddil's, so that any of them might have seen him coming forth of them. They at Surrey have come for us, at our House, to assist them; and we have gone, and Robert Turner along with us, and taken Ropes and tied them about Richard Dugdale's Middle. Robert Turner hath gone to the Hedge to get a Stake to beat him with; but Richard Dugdale hath managed the Matter so, that he hath broke or slipped the Rope, so that we have been forced to lay hold of him. And Robert Turner hath been satisfied, that contending with him would do no Good. Besides, I have seen Dugdale make towards Robert Turner, when in a Fit, and offer to pull the Skale-boos down to come to him; and that Robert Turner hath gone back, lest he should have gotten hold of him; and I never perceived, that Richard Dugdale ever valued I'ersons or Place wherever he was. I have seen him likewise have his Arms about his Neck; and they have been so fast that no one could pull them asunder, till opened of themselves. I likewise once came behind him when he was Dancing, and pushed him off the Place where he was, and he turned at me again, and his Father offered to help me, but they all could not so much as open a Finger of Dugdale's Hand, but he held me there, till his Fingers opened of themselves. I likewise put up my Hand to open his Fingers, but found that I could do no good; to my thinking, I might as well have offered to have broken a Bar of Iron. I verily think it was no Cheat of Dugdale. As to hearing his Voice, I told Mr. Braddil it was betwixt the Surrey and Mill-Lane-Head, which he and Mr. Barlow took to be a Mile and a Half; but I have enquired of Neighbours since, and we conclude it to be two Miles. Besides Surrey stands in a Bottom, and I believe any unbiassed Man, cannot but think, that one might have heard him Four Miles another Way, as well as that Two; for Surrey stands close to a rough River which makes a great Noise; besides Woods and all against the Hand. As to Dugdale's School-tricks, I learned when he did, I believe Three or Four Years; and I never saw or heard such Things as Edward Slayter relates.

John Walmsly.

This is further added to the former Confession, taken before Us, the 16th Day of September, 1697, at the House of Richard Sharples in Blackburn.

Memorandum. Some Passages in Walmsly's Information are thought fit to be waved, having Reflections on some, and not to be made use of, unless there be special Occasion for them.

Willoughby.
Will. Hulme.

John Livesay, of Clayton, confirms what he had before testified, and further testifies, That Richard Dugdale was seemingly Dead, or in a Trance, when he heard singing of Psalms, as if from the said Dugdale's Breast, exactly tuneable, and in Consort to the singing of psalms in the Meeting-House, before the Door of which, he lay as Dead. He also says, he heard the

Voice of Richard Dugdale a Mile and a Half distance from the Surey, exactly such as it used to be, when he was with him. He says also, That at Wiswel Eues, near Mr. Walmsly's, he saw him in an outragious Fit, before several Gentlefolks, not leaving his Fit for fear of them, and saying to their Maid, Nasom, Give me the Pipe out of thy Pocket; and she chanced to have one.

John Livesay.

Dr. Whiteaker, testifies, That it was proposed to him, to undertake the Cure of Richard Dugdale by Physical Means, which he declined, he concluding it to be more than a Natural Distemper.

Robert Whiteaker.

John Fletcher, of Harwood, testifies, That he knows nothing of any Papers, that were laid in any Place for Richard Dugdale to take, when he was Frisking about, as Mr. T. suggests. Nor did he know that Richard ever took any Stones from any Place in his said Friskings. And he says, He believes that there was no trick of Legerdemain about Webster's Knife, as appeared from his and John Mercer's best Observations. And he says, that he saw a large Pin pricked, not into the Lump on his Body, but directly into his Heel, not aslope, but directly downwards into the Flesh towards his Toes. And he says he knows nothing of any Bodies teaching him to call Richard's Fit, a Dumb Fit. And he confirms the Information which he formerly gave to be true.

John Fletcher.

Edward Haworth, of Rushers, confirms the Information he formerly gave, concerning Richard Dugdale to be true; and particularly that about Robert Turner. Edward Haworth. The *Confession of John Fielding, of Harwood, a Conformist; taken before the Right Honourable Hugh Lord Willoughby, and*

William Hulme Esq; Two of his Majesties Justices of the Peace, and Quorum; taken at the House of Richard Sharples, in Blackburn, the 16th Day of September, 1697.

Impr. John Fielding confesses, and says, That being impowered by his Lease to cut down Wood, for House-boot, Plough-boot and Cart-boot, and Hedge-boot, he did however ask Leave of his Land-Lord to cut down Five Trees, for repairing his House, which were by his Land-Lord's Orders marked out by one Edward Ryley, all growing on his own Tenement; one of which being a Handful too short, he cut it not down, but one taller though worse in its stead, which Wood not sufficing for the said House Repair, he bought more to make it out; not withstanding which the Land-Lord sued him about the said Trees. Whereupon he, by the Advice of his Neighbours and Friends, tendered his Land-Lord Five Pounds, in hopes of having it all returned back again, but his Land-Lord kept it all, and afterwards struck him. He likewise says, That having lived for many Years in Lincolnshire, where he was Nicknamed Lancashire Fielding, which is Threescore Miles distant from this Surrey; yet coming to Surrey, to see the Dæmoniack, he in a Fit cried, There comes Lancashire Fielding. He also says, That the Certificate shewed before us, about his being no reputed Thief, was verily Subscribed by his Neighbours, many more of whose Hands he might have got, had he desired them.

John Fielding.

THomas Booth, of Hay-Houses, Confesses at the same Time, and declares, That his former Examination was true, and further adds, that he and another striving to lift him up, could not stir him off the Spot, and yet within a Quarter of an Hour after, he alone laid hold upon him about the Hips, and lifted him up about Three quarters of a Yard high, and held him for a considerable Time, and felt him to be no heavier than his Stick, and his whole Body was straight and stiff; after which he having laid him down, saw him in his Dead Fit half an Hour longer, without any Motion from Richard, either as he lay or as he was lifted up.

Thomas Booth.

These Informations were taken before Us, the 26th Day of September, 1697. Willoughby. Will. Hulme. John Smalley, of Harwood, testifies, That his Information formerly given about Richard Dugdale was true, and he is sure that Richard's Shoes mentioned therein were buckled just before they flew off, nor had he any Hand himself in loosening them or helping them off, nor knew of any other Person, or outward means confederate, or assisting in their flying off. John Smalley. Lawrence Robertshaw, of Harwood, testifies, That the Information he formerly gave in the Surrey Dæmoniack was true. Lawrence Robertshaw. William Livesay, testifies, That the Information he formerly gave in the Surrey Dæmoniack is true; and says, He saw two Stones thrown into the Barn End, which Richard foretold were a coming, which he took up, and felt them more than ordinary warm. Nor did he go up and down to pick up company to go to the Surrey, nor knows he of any Spy that went over the Fields, or any other-ways to give Intelligence.

William Livesay.

These Informations were given before Us, the 16th Day of September, at the House of Richard Sharples of Blackburn, 1697.

Willoughby.
William Hulme.

John Jolly, testifies, That the private Information of Thomas and Anne Dugdale, Parents to Richard Dugdale, with Mary and Alice Dugdale, Sisters to the said Richard Dugdale, which is mentioned and Printed in the Surrey Dæmoniack, was freely declared to him by the Parties aforesaid, at Surrey, July 31, 1695. And that the Information aforesaid was by him put down in Writing in their own Words and Meanings. And that all the said Informations were distinctly read over to the Parties aforesaid, to which they voluntarily put their Marks.

John Jolly.

This was affirmed before Us, the 16th Day of September, 1697.

Willoughby.
William Hulme.

James Abbot does under his Hand testifie, That when Dugdale had told me of my Cheshire and Staffordshire Journey. I came home and told our Folks, that I wondered what I might go into Cheshire for, we none of us having any Occasion thither; we had afterwards a Letter which came to inform us from Beverly, that one Elizabeth Gundy would come over to see her Grandfather, and from thence into Cheshire to Knulsford; but in all this I never thought of Staffordshire, nor had I never been there, nor ever thought that I should have gone there; yet when it fell so out, I called to Remembrance, that Dugdale told me of it.

James. Abbot.

This is further added to the former Confession taken before Us, the 16th Day of September, 1697, at the House of Richard Sharples of Blackburn.

Willoughby.
William Hulme.

Joseph Hargreaves, testifies, That his former Confession in the Surrey Dæmoniack is true.

Joseph Hargreaves.

Nathaniel Waddington Confesses and Testifies, That the Information he formerly gave, concerning Richard Dugdale is true, except what is mentioned about Fielding, and likewise what was mentioned about the Gold and Bisket, which he only heard by Report. he further says, He was present when Dugdale accused the Gentlewoman of having Bisket in her Pocket, and challenged her to Play at Cards, for the Gold she had in her Pocket; but says, he cannot tell whether she had any or no; but it was generally reported that she had both in her Pocket.

Nathaniel Waddington.

William Fort, of Altham, confesses and testifies, That he saw Richard Dugdale in one of his Fits at his Father's House in Altham, and that for half a Quarter of an Hour together he stood straight up, and was as one Dead, and breathless. He says, That he himself and others, all the While held a Candle to his Mouth and Nostrils, and could not in the least perceive, that he had any Breath in his Body. Before this, whilst he was in his Fit, he says, he saw his Body rise up from the Ground Five or Six times, being stiff and straight, Three quarters of a Yard above Ground, and that he did not bend in any Joint whatever; but with sudden Motions was thrown from his Back to his Belly; and so likewise from his Belly to his Back, rising Three quarters of a Yard from the Ground as he turned himself. He likewise says, that he heard him sing some Verses of a Psalm in Latin; and some Scholars that were present said it was true Latin.

William Fort.

These Informations were taken before Us, the 17th Day of September, 1697.

Willoughby.

William Hulme.

The further Information of William Sellers, of Pendleton, Husbandman, concerning Richard Dugdale, which he is ready to take his Oath upon, when he is called to it, and it be within compass, considering his great Age and Bodily weakness. Whereas I did heretofore make Oath, as to several Particulars of Richard Dugdale's Case, before the Right Honourable the Lord Willoughby, and Ralph Egerton Esq; two of his Majesties Justices of the Peace for the County of Lancaster; I do now upon Occasion more particularly express and explain my said Testimony as follows.

I did lift up the said Richard Dugdale several times; and because I thought it very strange, that he should be so light, I do well remember, that I did once my self, without any help, lift him up by his Legs all at once, about a Yard from the Barn-floor, and held him up so long as I could well judge of his weight, Richard Dugdale's Unkle being present, when he was as light as a Hat or a walking Cane, and as straight as a Cane. He was then in a dead Fit, and continued therein some considerable time, after I had laid him down again; all this I do faithfully testifie.

Witness my Hand,
William Sellers.
John Birch.

This Paper being read before the Right Honourable the Lord Willoughby, and Will Hulme Esq; was approved by them, as delivered by John Brich to them, but could not be subscribed in William Seller's Absence.

John Hindle testifies further, That he and John Walmsly were present when Richard Dugdale had his last Fit in Surrey-Barn; where in his Fit Richard Dugdale said it was Obsession, and in a Combination, and that he might never have more Fits, and it should never be discovered whilst the World endured.

John Hindle

As to the following Informations, they were brought to me, after the Meeting at Blackburn; and much more might be given in to the same purpose, if there were need for it; and that we made it our business to seek further Testimony, though the Thing happened so many Years ago; and that the Informant's testifying thereunto, be so much against their Worldly Interest.

ANNE Whiteaker, who at that Time, when Richard Dugdale had those strange Fits, was Servant to Major Rowel of Morton, next House to Surrey. She Testifies that Richard Dugdale told her, that his said Fits began at Westly-Hall, as it is commonly called, as he was making Hay; upon which he came into the said Hall, and laid himself down upon a Bed, according to the Advice of a Servant there. Then he said, That Five or Six Evil Spirits appeared to him; and then the Appearance of a Black Man did grin at him, and pressed very hard upon him. Then both the Spirits and the Man danced upon the Floor, and then vanished in a Flame of Fire.

She also testifies, That at a certain Time, when a Fit was coming on him at Morton, he fell a Dancing and Roaring hideously; then he fell to the Ground, and had something rising under his Cloaths as if it were quick; and that it begun in the very Part of his Body, where he said that Grim Man pressed him so hard at the first. Also, that whilst he lay in the said Fit, he sweat so much, that one might wipe it off his Cloaths; and all the Flaggs under him were wet with it. She also testifies, That she often saw Richard Dugdale in his Fits at Surrey, and that he was much after the same manner.

The said Anne does also testifie, That Mr. Batton Shuttleworth, being at the said Morton, upon Occasion, he followed her to Surrey, she her self then not knowing of his following her; yet Richard Dugdale told of Mr. Batton's coming, tho' Richard Dugdale could not see him, nor did any one tell him of his Coming. He did also in a Fit tell several Young Persons of their Resolution to go to an Ale-House, and what they Spent (viz. Two-pence a-piece). This one of the Parties did Confess to the said Anne, and that it was indeed so as Richard Dugdale had told.

The said Anne does also testifie, That her said Master had oft Occasion to make use of all the Surery Family, about his Worldly Affairs; and that she never perceived any Thing about any of them, that might give the least Occasion of Suspicion, as to their being Guilty of Witchcraft, or of any cheating Practices.

Anne Whiteaker.

Nicholas Haworth, of Altham, Miller testifies, as followeth. I have seen Richard Dugdale in his Fits, run about the Surrey-Barn on all Four, as fast as any Man that I ever saw, could run upon his two Feet I have seen the Lump in Richard Dugdale's Leg rise upwards, and although I have endeavoured to keep it down, by girding it with a Belt or Boot-Garter, a little above it, yet never could; for it still would shoot under. I have heard Richard Dugdale harr and bark like any Mastiff; so that I have been very much afraid of him. I have heard Richard Dugdale whisper at the Wall of the Surrey-Barn, and to my thinking refuse to do something. He hath fallen flat upon his Back as if something had tripped up his Heels. After he had lain a while he would have risen as soon as a Man can turn his Hand; and his Rising was so sudden that one could scarce perceive it.

Nicholas Haworth.

John Hindle, of Altham, testifies as followeth; I have seen Richard Dugdale ly on the Surrey Barn-floor in some of his Fits, and very suddainly he was set on his Feet, without the Bending of any Part of his Body, that I could perceive; I could liken it to nothing but one's Raising a Stick on an End. I have also seen a Lump on Richard Dugdale's Shoulder, about the Bigness of an Hen's-Egg, and have offered to hold it down, but could not. One time standing behind Richard Dugdale, he being then in a Fit, I heard him say to Mr. Carington, Thou shalt be Porter of Hell-Gates, Thou'st have Brewis and Toad-Broth.

John Hindle.

Joshua Thomason, of Entwisle, in the Parish of Bolton, in the County of Lancaster, Yeoman, witnesses as followeth.

It was publickly reported about us, That a certain Young Man called Richard Dugdale, living at Surrey, was possessed with the Devil; upon which several of my Neighbours concluding to go and see the said Dugdale, I went with them; and coming to Surrey it happened to be a Day appointed by the Ministers to be spent in Prayer, and other Religious Exercises for the said Dugdale, Mr. Jolly, one of the Ministers present, being earnest in Prayer for the Party Afflicted, That the Lord would free him from so sad an Affliction. Dugdale being then in one of his Fits in the Surrey-Barn, with a loud Voice, said many times over, O thou crying Jolly, thou shalt never cast me out. In the same Fit, the said Dugdale cried out, O Carlile, Carlile, Carlile, (so he called Mr. Carrington.) After this as Mr. Jolly was ending his Prayer, and was ready to dismiss the Assembly, Mr. Carrington came to the Barn Door, where kneeling down he pulled out a little Bible, and looking in the same, Dugdale cried out several times, Carlile read upon the Wall; Mr. Jolly and the other Ministers feeing Mr. Carrington, desired him to go to Prayer Whilst Mr Carrington was at Prayer, Dugdale still cried out in a Language unknown to me, when Mr. Carrington had done Prayer, he applied his Discourse to Dugdale, and said, Thou declarest thy self to be an Unclean Spirit, thou art such a Reviler. Dugdale and Mr. Carrington continued their Discourse together a long time; one while Mr. Carrington spoke, then Dugdale, then Mr. Carrington. I could understand Mr. Carrington very well; for he, as I suppose answered Dugdale very soberly, and with some Texts of Scripture: But I could not understand one Word of Dugdale's Discourse to Mr. Carrington, and I find several Sentences that Mr. Carrington spoke, are Printed in a Book called the Surrey Dæmoniack.

At Night Mr. Jolly, Mr. Waddington and Mr. Carrington examined Dugdale whether he had made any Contract with the Devil or not, either by Writing, Word or any other way? To which Dugdale answered, That there was no such Contract as he knew of. Whereupon the Ministers told him, that if he had any Contract or Bargain with the Devil, they could not help him, except he would first make an Ingenuous Confession. Dugdale's Mother upon this with seeming Earnestness said, I pray thee Richard if thou hast made any Bargain or Contract Confess it. Thou had'st better Confess it now: To which Richard answered somewhat faintly, I know of none. Mr. Jolly then asked Dugdale how then can thou answer several Questions, and tell many Things which cannot be done by lawful Art, thou having seemingly whispered with something at a Hole or Corner of the Barn? Mr. Jolly said further, how couldst thou Name those Persons that came from Haslingden, and tell them at what Ale-House they called, and how much they drank; out of what Vessels, Cans or Cups; what every one Paid, whether Silver, Half-pennies or Farthings, and how many of each, and so particularly what Change was returned to any of the Company? To these Dugdale answered that he could not tell any of these out of his Fit: But in his Fit it seems, he going to the aforesaid Hole or place in the Barn, a Voice declared to him all the Answers proper to the several Questions that had been asked him, and further told him what Things had been done by the Persons aforesaid at a considerable Distance from Surrey.

Likewise the Ministers examined Dugdale about an Elephant-Hafted-Knife, which was found in his Mouth in a Fit, how he came by it? Dugdale said he could not tell.

Another Time when I came to see Dugdale, I found him out of his Fit, and entring into Discourse with him, he told me how his Fits began with him at the first. Several then present also told me, that still in his foregoing Fit, his Spirit foretold when his next Fit should come, and how long it should continue. I asked how he knew when his Fit began. Dugdale said, always when my Fit began. I lose my Sight, yet to my thinking an Old Man, in a

Black-Mantle appears in the Beginning of my Fit, and goes before me over the Green, and leads straight way into the Barn, and if I be not there, I cannot but follow him. At the End of this Discourse, Dugdale suddainly rose up from his Seat in the House, and went into the Barn, where he fell flat upon his Back. When he had lain a While, he was turned on his Belly; as he lay, something in the Calf of his Leg leaped up very often. Upon this I took his Leg betwixt my Hands, yet still it leaped and sprinted, as if I had a small Chicken in my Hand, especially when I strove to hold it down. After this he was turned on his Back again, and still I perceived that leaping in the Calf of his Leg, and it jutted out as far as his Stocking could stretch. This after some time rose up, and went up his Thigh to his Breast, and as it went a long, it thrust up his Cloaths the Height of one's Fist. This Lump rose as high as the Collar of his Doublet; and then (though at other times his Face and Neck were of a White or Pale Colour) his Neck and Face were as red as Blood. I could not see any Eyes that he had, but the Holes were the same Colour with his Face, upon this he was set on his Feet in a trice, without the Natural use of Arms and Legs, and without Bending any Part of his Body, as one raises a Stick or Board to an end very nimbly; and then he went to the aforesaid Hole, at the End of the Barn, and laid his Mouth a While to the Hole.

  Soon after he turned him about to the Company, and reeling down the Barn came to the Ring where he used to Dance, and said I have a Message to deliver to you all. In the First Epistle to the Thessalonians, Chap. 5. Verse 16. Rejoyce evermore. This Verse he Expounded very handsomely and seriously, shewing what it was to rejoyce evermore, and in what way we must do it; He spoke to this Verse a long while in good Order and Words; and from other Scriptures proved what he said. Yet when he had done, he fleeringly said, But which of us does so? Then he came to the Seventeenth Verse, and shewed what it was to Pray, and what to Pray without ceasing, and this he did as well as the former, then ended it, saying, Which of us does so? He also Expounded the 18, 19, 20, 21, 22, Verses, and ended the

Exposition of every Verse with, but which of us does so; and besides that, at the End of the last said, Ha! Ha! and then danced very cleverly.

After this Dugdale with his Hands and Arms drummed on his Side, and with that and a Noise that he made in his Throat, any one, who had not seen or known his Fashions, would have taken it to be a Drum: I heard a Man there present, who had been in Ireland say, That Dugdale did then beat a March exactly, which was used by the Irish, which he never heard in England. Then he danced again, after that fell flat on the Floor, and as he lay on the Floor along, a lusty strong Man who had been Fellow Servant with Dugdale, came Hectoring into the Barn, and said, Come Dick, They say thou art Possest, if thou be, I can get thee Help, but I think thou art not, for thou wast always a good Lad. This Fellow would needs shake Hands with Dugdale, and talked over him a long time, till being perswaded, he sate down at the Barn-side. Soon after Dugdale leaped up, and ran to the aforesaid Hole, and as he turned him about, he called the Man by his Name, and said, Art thou come to see me? Thou hast got a Bottle of Ale in Whalley, and hast left thy Horse there. The Man said, If thou can tell that (Dick) thou art Possessed, and I can get thee Help. Dugdale said further to him, Thou thinkst to have another when thou goest back, and a Wheat-Cake, and I'll fill thy Wheat-Cake with Sparables, and in such a Lane I'll break thy Neck. The Man said, I fear thee not, and all the Devils in Hell to help thee. After this Dugdale stooped down and gathered up a deal of Rushes, which he would but could not make a Thumb-Rope of; however he drew them out a pretty Length, and got them about the Man's Neck, with which Dugdale hurled him about, as if he had been a little Dog; and the Man could not with all his Strength get loose, till the Rushes broke. The Man after this was extream tame and quiet.

Dugdale discovered many Things of several Persons, particularly a Woman, who came from towards Burnly. Dugdale came up to her, and smelling at her, called her by her Name, and said, O! Art thou there? thou got some Stone-Fruit at such a Place (which Dugdale named) as thou came, and thou intendest to have more. The Woman Blushed and slipped away.

Then Dugdale fell flat on the Earth again, and as he lay he began to draw himself on a Heap, and then harred and snarled like a Mastiff-Dog. A Mastiff which then lay in the Cow-House, harred and barked fiercely at Dugdale again, and had leaped at him if some had not put him out. Much more I could have told of him; but through Distance of Time, it is now slipped out of my Memory.

November, 12. 1697.
Joshua Thomason.

Some Remarkable Passages which were taken Notice of from the first, as to the Case of Young Dugdale, of Surrey, near Whally, in Lancashire, Aged about Nineteen or Twenty Years.

UPON the Twenty Ninth of April, 1689, in the Morning, Richard Dugdale came to my House, desiring the Liberty, and I having granted it; he had signified his Mind to that Purpose, a quarter of a Year before; but the Messenger failed to give Notice, until a Day or Two before he came.

He and his Relation that came along with him, gave such an Account of his Case, that I saw Cause to suspect he was Possessed by an Evil Spirit; and I was further satisfied concerning it, whilst we were at Family Duty, at which he was present.

The Fit did then seize on him, partly whilst I was reading, and opening the Word, but much worse whilst I was at Prayer. His Motions in his Fit were very strong, particularly turning the Sight of his Eyes inward, and thus making him quite Blind, whilst his Eye-lids were open, with other Motions preternatural. He had also such strong Motions as were above his natural Ability and Agility; but I was more confirmed by that Rage he was in, against the Ordinance of God, especially when Christ was solemnly named, and his Condition was earnestly commended to the Lord. Then he raged as if the Devil had been in his Bodily Shape, though he manifested other Inclinations to the Word and Prayer when he was not in his Fit. And he was in Health of Body to all outward Appearance at the same time.

Other Means he had used, both Lawful and Unlawful, so that Prayer and Fasting seemed to be the only proper Means in his Case. Accordingly he desired that we would keep a Day of Prayer and Fasting on his behalf.

Accordingly we met at the Sparth, upon the Eighth of May. Before we began to Exercise (the Pastor of another Society being present to assist in the Work) we examined the Parents and the Young Man himself: as to the Occasion of the Affliction they at that time confessed, that both Father and Son were in Drink at Whalley Rush-bearing upon the James-Tide before; that they then had a Scuffle with a Young Man, whom they suspected, or his Partakers to be Instrumental in this Mischief.

We also enquired as to the means they had made use of already, and convinced them of the Evil of some unlawful Means they had made use of. One Instrument they made use of was mr. Grabtree. We also the wed them that these Means we were about, were appointed by Christ in this Case, and that they might hope for a Blessing in this Way. Multiplying of Prayers and other Services being in vain, if there be not Repentance and Reformation withal. God regards not to answer in Mercy, where there is a secret Regard to an Iniquity. We see to whom the Promise of Mercy belongs, Prov. 28. 13. Viz. Those who confess their Sins, and forsake them, through Divine Grace.

We then proceeded to the Word and Prayer, the Scripture insisted on being Acts 26 18. To turn them from the Power of Satan to God. The Power which Satan hath in Particular and in General is Matter of Lamentation and Supplication. The Lord rebuke Satan, and rescue Sinners from his Power. He had two dreadful Fits in the Time of the Exercise. He also confessed several Apparitions he had upon the Riot at James-Tide, and Offers of God to him, &c.

One Sabbath he was quiet under the Ordinance all the while; another Sabbath he was extream rude all the while. He commonly attended at our Meeting under his Affliction.

Upon their Desire we kept another Day, the 28th Instant, on his behalf. The Concourse of the People was much greater; and he was extreamly rude in his Fits all the while; yet we continued in the Word and Prayer all the while as before. Thus the Providence of God puts his Servants upon Tryal, and withal put his Spirit into them, that they may be more Instant and Importunate with him in Prayer: He needs not intreating; it is we that need exciting; and we are humbly bold to say, the Lord did graciously help us.

Our Third Meeting on his behalf was at Surrey, and because of its Vicinity to Whally, we acquainted Mr. Jea the Vicar with the Occasion, that he might take no Offence. All the

While the Evil Spirit worked in the Dæmoniack, yet it broke not out into a Fit; but afterwards the Evil Spirit broke out in a most violent Manner, and discovered more than ordinary Rage against Mr. Waddington; and the Subject insisted on was, Ephes. 6. 12. The Rulers of the Darkness of this World, shewing the dark Regions where the Devil rules.

This Surrey, the Place of the Party's Habitation, was recorded and certifyed according to Law. Providence set as upon the publick Stage, that the Thing might not be done in a Corner.

On the following Sabbath there was yet a greater Concourse of People; many came to see him, but heard something that affected them also; the Sermon being to shew, that many are under the Power of Sin and Satan, in a less sensible, and therefore in a more dangerous Manner. We were without Distraction from the Dæmoniack all the While.

Another Subbath he was very ill, through all the Time of the Exercise; and afterwards as I stood by him, he spurned at me with great Violence, grinning, and spitting at me in a strange manner, but he hurt me not. I could little think of any ill Intent therein of his; I only took it for the Devil's Spite at me.

With respect to the Sabbath before; God hath his Ends as well as Men have theirs; we designed it not to draw People to our Meeting, nor indeed perhaps did many design to hear the Word, much less to get Good thereby. It was far from Onesimus's Design in fleeing to Rome, that he should there be converted by Paul's Ministry. Christ's End for the Conversion of the Woman of Samaria, was not her Errand to Jacob's Well.

The next Day upon this Occasion, was at Surrey, upon the Fifth of July; the Lord was gracious to the Assembly and Party also, in freeing us sometimes srom those grievous Distractions, which at other times we had upon this Occasion. the Lord pittied us partioularly with respect to the Lord's Day, that Day of Rest, that we might the better sanctifie it. Yet had we Spiritual Rest, whilst in our Way and at our Work; when he was at the Worst, we were helped to wait on the Lord without Distraction within, however. He was a very present Help.

The next Meeting on this Occasion was on the 16th Instant, though the Youth knew nothing of it upon the Lord's Day before (nor any of the Family) concerning this Meeting; yet in a Fit upon the said Lord's Day, he foretold of this Day, and told of the Number of Ministers, viz. Five, when as none of the Ministers themselves knew it would be so. The Devil raged exceedingly at this Meeting; it may be the great Confluence of People on this Occasion enraged him the more; had not the Lord helped us mightily, we had been outdone by him. He played upon the Younger Ministers very severely, until they got above him.

As the Evil Spirit filled the Jews with Envy, Contradicting and Blaspheming, when they saw the Multitudes flocking to hear the Word of God; so in this Case. Yet were not the People affrighted, but followed on; yea the Concourse was still greater.

On the Sabbath following we were Mercifully freed from Disturbance by the Dæmoniack, until the Close of the Exercise.

We were in our Place at our Work; we should not hinder the People from coming, nor give place to the Devil; but the Lord was pleased as he thought fit, to make him give place to us, being met together in the Name of Christ. It is he that rebuketh Satan; It's through him only that the Weapons of our Warfare are mighty. Alas! we are meaner, weaker than others, than any.

On the 25th Instant we had another Opportunity on this Occasion. The Young Man was detained from us most of the Time, by Reason of several Trances he was in. The Multitude of the People was very great, so that it caused great Distraction and Danger. Also a Hay-Loft in the Barn being broken down by the Weight of the People: Yet through God's special Providence there was no further harm done. This Meeting was in Altham.

We were forced many Times to meet in Out-Houses, the Crouds of the People being so very great, our Chappel also being rather at an Outside from the Ordinary Congregation. We did for their Ease sometimes meet elsewhere, having Christ's Example and Encouragement thereunto; all the Places of Meeting being also Licensed according to Law.

The next Day on this Occasion was at Surrey, the 1st of August, and then the Youth was quiet all the While. Here the Young Man dwelt with his Parents. His Father and he were Gardiners; it being about a Mile from Whalley. Should there not have been some Respite sometimes, it had scarce been possible for the Man or us to have held out. We mention it, that others may see the Lord's Mercy, as well as our Infirmity. We would not so far offend others, as to meet at Surrey upon a Lord's Day, it being so near Whalley, yea all our Meetings were ordered as inoffensively as might be.

Again at the same Place on the 23d Instant, the Devil raged in the Young Man exceedingly, discovering himself more than ever, by the Dæmoniack's Discovery of several Things in his Fit, which could not be discovered but by a Diabolical Means. That Subject, John 16. 8, 9, 10, 11. was several Days insisted on there, and also at our Lord's Day Meetings.

In my Absence Mr. Waddington and the Rest of our Society, had a Day in Read upon this Dugdale's Account, though he was not present. Indeed he was mostly present at the Meetings, whether on his Account or not, though not always. I was absent at this Time only, and so I have no further Advantage of giving an Account of this Affair.

Upon the Third of September, we again met at Surrey on Young Dugdale's Account. As I went to the Place of the Meeting he gave me Notice by a little Paper, which he put into my Hand; that, as his Spirit told him in his Fit, he must be Dumb and Deaf whilst we Prayed; immediately upon his Delivery of the Note to me, he became both Dumb and Deaf all the while that the Exercise continued. Note, That he sometimes out of his Fit discovered what he heard, and saw in his Fit, being done at a great Distance, at the same time: As the Prophet would by Means of a Good Angel tell what was done at a great Distance. But commonly he, out of his Fit did not know what happened in his Fit. We would deal plainly on the one hand as well as the other.

We were but few to carry on the Work, so that we continued not so long as at other times. They shewed us at that time a large Button, and Curtain-Ring; but especially a large cornered Stone; all which the Young Man had vomited to the Astonishment of all. Also we had an Account of several Latin Words and Phrases which he uttered, though he knew nothing of them; his natural and acquired Abilities being but small.

Upon the 5th Instant we met at the same Place, upon the same Occasion. The Lord brought in more Ministers for our Help, and the Meeting was very full. Satan was chained up, and the Dæmoniack gave us not much Disturbance.

We met in the same Place in the same Manner, upon the Tenth Instant; the Concourse of People being as great though the Weather was very bad. Satan was silenced this Day also. It seems the Dæmoniack was told by his Spirit in his Fits, that he must not be delivered as yet, but be as Lot's Wife, a Warning to others.

Mr. Waddington and my self, were on the 19th Instant called to Surrey. The Occasion was; The Devil, in one of the Young Man's Fits, had signified something of a Contract which the Youth had made with him, for a certain Time, by Subscribing to a Parchment. A Jade (as he stiled her) taking one of his Hands out of the Bed, and putting One or Two of his Fingers to the Writing. We were also informed, that the Youth had written to Sir E. A. their Landlord, to signifie to him that he got no Good by our Prayers, and so he seemed to grow weary of our Pains. It concerned us to hear these two Things; but he was then in a Fit, and continued so as long as we staid, so that we could not examin him as to the former. As for the latter, he dealt very unworthily with us, considering the Care and Charge we had been at for his Relief every way. Had he not manifested himself free, and forward for our Proceedings thus far, we had desisted before this. We had upon this desisted, had not the Youth confessed his Fault, and his Father desired us to go on.

On the 26th Instant, we again met at the Surrey, upon the same Account; and the Reverend Mr. O. Harwood came in also on that Day to our Help. The Lord sent us that suitable Word by him, I John 3. 8. I thought it requisite to say something also, as to our Call to the Work, and Conduct therein, as to the

Case and present Circumstances also. The Truth is, we were then in great Doubt and Distress; for as we are Men subject to the like Infirmities with others, so our Temptations were then more than ordinary; in so much that it was very necessary for us to look very narrowly into the Case, our Course, and Carriage also. We had need to be satisfied from our selves, when we had so little Satisfaction from others.

Upon the Desire of Young Dugdale, the Junior Minister of the Company staid with him that Night. The Devil (it seemed) in the Dæmonaick did still further declare, that there was such a Contract; and the first time he got Hold of him, was upon a vain With he had in the Abby-Hall, That he might excel all others in Dancing. That the Contract was for Eighteen Months. Out of his Fits he would Confess what a Fancy he had for Dancing; and that he could not refrain from Dancing, after the said James-Tide was a Twelve Months, when he danced most Artificially in the Fits we saw, though he said, and others testify, he could not Dance at all before, nor then out of his Fits. The Youth out of his Fit would not Confess any Thing of a Contract with the Devil, that he knew of. But it is too probable there was a Confederacy, because the Devil was so ready to gratifie him; not only in such Artificial Dancing, but to tell many Things which could not be known without such hellish Help: yea those Discoveries being frequently upon whispering with something in a certain Corner. That it is the Devil that speaks in him seems very plain, speaking strange Languages which the Youth never learned, and with another Voice than his own; yea with two Voices at once, and sometimes speaking when the Organs of Speech were not made use of. Also his saying that he was God, and requiring to be worshipped; yea using many such Words and Gestures as are most dreadful; though the Youth can tell nothing of them when the Fit is over; yet at some other times in his Fits, he declaimed much against the Sins of the Place and Times.

Upon the 11th of October we again met at Surrey, in the same Manner and upon the same Account, the People still flocking to the Meeting very much, and many were much convinced and wrought all along; the Lord working by Providence and Providence together. Being desired, I staid to see his Fit over, though that was not till about Eight a Clock in the Evening. Some of the Time was spent in Discoursing, Expounding, Singing and Praying. The Youth was very attentive all the while, and at the Close of the Exercises his Fit began and lasted about an Hour; in which Fit the Spirit said, That the Young Man was his own, declining any Discourse with me, and insulting at Mr. Carrington's not appearing that Evening, as he had done the Night before, for then Mr. Carrington had baited the Evil Spirit sufficiently. His Language in his Fit seemed to be but a Sort of Gibberish, at that time; or he spoke his Words so thick that I could make nothing of them; there was a great Number of People even in the Night, and they were very rude; so that some Harm was done to the Place, and likewise to some Persons.

We met again at Surrey, on the 18th Instant, and the Croud of People was very great, tho' the Season was very wet; it was some Distraction amongst our selves, that one of the Ministers, whilst he was Praying, turned his Speech to Satan as we thought, which some took to be an unwarrantable Apostrophe; though the Dissatisfaction was privately managed, yet the Devil took Notice of it, and reflected on some for it.

Upon the 22d Instant we met again at Altham, upon this Occasion; a great Concourse of People being there also, though we divulged not the Opportunity, but changed the Place on purpose to conceal it the more. He had a Fit in the Time of the Exercise, in which Fit two Voices spoke in him at the same time; and in a strange Manner, the Devil threatned what he would do this Day, and said, How narrowly the Youth escaped being hoisted quite away in the Air, as he came to the Meeting. Some would say, that it was a Bodily Distemper or Cheat; also that there was an Agreement of Thomas Dugdale the Father, with a Popish Priest; but Thomas disowned it, and the Event disproved it. Tho' some will not believe, yet it is as evident Testimony against the Prophanity and Vanity of the Times (whereof this

Family had been very Guilty) as also against the Sadducism and Atheism of many. Yea some testifie their Envy against God's Servants, and their Enmity against his Way; as others are much convinced, and their Prejudice quite removed upon this Occasion. We could do no less, than with the Good Samaritan take Compassion when the Priest and Levite passed by.

However upon the 31st Instant we met again at Surrey upon this Occasion; the Evil Spirit had so tormented him the Night before, that his Limbs were taken from him, as to the Use of them, and he continued in great Pain; so that before we began the Exercise, he broke out into a Fit of Impatience, resolving that this should be the last Prayer Day, and that he would take another Course for his Help. Had his Parents been in the same Mind, we had then desisted. But his Parents entreated us to go on. The Youth was somewhat eased, and very quiet all the Time of the Exercise. In the Close he thanked us, and wished us to go on in the same Course.

So that it seems altogether Improbable by this, and several other Passages, that there was any ill Design or Cheat in the Party or in his Parents, though some have been apt to charge them to that purpose. Charity would rather offend on the other hand, especially when the Charge is so Criminal.

On the Seventh of November we met again at Surrey upon the same Account; and found Young Dugdale in a much better Disposition, and carrying it better than formerly. The Young Man seemed all along to us to be naturally of a plain Spirit; neither having the Art, nor being apt to dissemble the worse, nor the better. Here a Christian Candour appeared to us.

Again at Surrey upon the 14th Instant, since our last Meeting, a great Stone about Fourteen Pound Weight, as I suppose, was laid upon him in one of his Fits, yet without Harm to him. Neither the Family nor the Spectators knew whence it came, nor how it came there; no such Stone being there about.

The Day after he was extreamly hurried in his Fits, ridden about and chafed on his Head, as if it were a Horse hard ridden, and of a very rank Smell. Yet the Spirit confessed in his

Fit, there was good News for Dick (as he called the Youth) but ill News for it self, viz. the Spirit; meaning some Respite the Dæmoniack should have from his Fits for some considerable Time. The Youth fasted for Three or Four Days together, being always full, when he should come to his Meals; this seems unaccountable to us in a Natural ordinary Way.

Upon the 21st Instant we met again at Surrey, upon the same Account; our Number of Ministers and others was but slender, the Lord's assisting us (without any other Abatement of our Exercises at home and abroad) appeared both as to our Spirits and Bodies; for some of us found that we could well Fast Twenty four Hours, notwithstanding extraordinary Pains, besides on this Occasion.

The Youth's being lighter by more than the half, and heavier, or as heavy again as at other Times; yea, this in the same Dead Fit; is altogether unaccountable, when the Sadducees of the Times have studied and said their utmost. Upon the 28th Instant we met at my House, this being one main Occasion of the Day; the Youth was quiet and attentive all the While; yea, very devout, both now and at other Times. Indeed sometimes his Carriage under the Ordinances, and at other Times, gave us some Hopes towards a Change, as to his Spiritual State; which would be much better to him, and more desirable to us; yet a partial Change as to that, and a perfect Change as to his Body, are signal desirable Mercies.

As he returned from the Meeting on the Lord's Day following, he had a Fit, in which, as some credible Persons said who were with him, he repeated the Heads of the Sermon, and the Proofs also. The Return of his Fits after many Days Discontinuance, must needs much Exercise us; but Psalm 31. 3. to 8. was of good Use to some of us in that Case. Yea, we were as fresh to Work as at the first, the Lord anointing us with fresh Oyl of his Spirit to enable us.

On the 5th of December we again met at Surrey. We were but two Ministers to carry on the Work. He told me of some private Discourse and Passages betwixt him and Sir E. H.

On the 12th, we met at the Sparth on the same Occasion. We were but few, and the Dæmoniack was detained at home by a Fit. In that Fit the Devil told him he would find him somewhat else to do, than to Eat Bread and Cheese, with Cottom-Cass of Sparth, as he had done Twenty five Weeks before. He also told what Distress Ireland was in, and that England must Pay the Piper, as he termed it, notwithstanding its present Security. We have by sad Experience found the Truth of the Dæmon's Predictions in this, and other Instances. The false Prophet could foretel Evil, Deut. 13. 18. O that any Warnings might awaken us, That though our Iniquities have brought us very low, they may not be our Ruin. In his Fit of the Day following he told us of some Money coming, before the Messenger came, by whom I sent some for their Relief; The Family being taken off their Calling, put to Charges, and very much Impoverished on this Occasion.

Upon the 20th Instant our Meeting was again at Surrey, upon this Account. We had but little Company. His Fits were not so frequent and violent as formerly; several Scriptures besides those before-mentioned had been insisted on in these Meetings, on this Occasion, viz. Ephes. 6. 12. Mat. 17. 21. I Tim. 5. 15. I Tim. 1, 13, 14, 15, 16. Mat. 11. 28, 29, 30. All which were directed for the satisfying of this Occasion to the Family and Country; that all might be Sanctified to us by the Word and Prayer, not only that the Devil might be driven from the Dæmoniack.

January the 1st at Surrey, my Brethren the Ministry being all taken off by other urgent Occasions, I turned this Meeting to an Exercise, there being a Likelyhood of a Temptation. As to the Success of Prayers, in this and other Cases, I took Occasion from Heb. 5. 7. to clear the Providence of God, concerning that Point of the Answer of Prayer.

It was near Twelve Months we were almost Weekly employed upon this Account, in most solemn Prayer with Fasting, some of us coming many Miles. Had not some of us been long enured in hard Service, it could not have been so well endured.

Upon the 9th Instant we again met at Surrey as formerly. Before the Exercise began I dealt particularly and plainly with the Family. We had apparent Cause to judge that the Work did stick on their Part, considering how Popishly they had been brought up, and what Prophane Lives they had led: Yea, how little Sense some of them had of their sad Case, and how slow they were at Confessing what might be the Cause thereof. Some of my Brethren thought it requisite yet to deal more roughly with them, there being some Suspicion of a Contract with the Devil, or of Witchcraft amongst themselves. I confess I was somewhat shy as to further Proceeding, lest we had not ground to go upon; lest we should exceed the Bounds of our Calling; lest we should give the Man Occasion of Offence; yet they offering themselves to Tryal, some Tryal was made, and further was intended, that the Thing and themselves might be cleared. And in Case of grounded Suspicion as to Witchcraft or Imposture, the Matter must be put into the Magistrates Hands, who is the Judge in that Case, and must do as he sees Cause. We in the Use of Spiritual Means are concerned so far as it is a Possession. We would have proper Means used; and we would keep our Place.

Upon the 23d Instant we again met at Surrey, on the same Occasion, and after the same manner. I thought the Work must be wholly devolved upon me, but one of my Brethren came in to my Help about the Middle of the Exercise. I had laboured to work some Sense upon the Youth as to the Nature of his Case; but alas! to little Purpose, so that I much feared the Total and Final giving him up to Satan in the worst Sense. The Devil acted him very strangely in his Fits, so that he did Feats much above his own Skill and Strength; and it is altogether wonderful his Head was not dashed in Pieces, and his Spirits quite spent; yet his Body was then in as good a Case, if not better than ever. The Doubt and Distraction about our Duty in this Case did much exercise me; Law Severities being so Foreign to my Spirit and Calling.

Upon the 6th of February we again met at Surrey upon the same Account. I was then wholly failed by my Brethren, through their other Occasions, as I suppose, but the Lord helped in all the Work. The Youth had been free from any considerable Fit a Fortnight, so that they seemed to be wearing off. In his last Fit he further spoke of Things done at a Distance, and at the same time when they were a doing.

Upon the 20th Instant there was again a more full Meeting of Ministers at Surrey, upon the Occasion aforesaid. Though the Discouragements from many others were very great, I then finished that Discourse upon 2 Cor II. 3. At the Close of the Exercise, we found the Youth something more Ingenuous towards us, though his Father shewed more Disingenuity. The Youth took Occasion to Confess further to me, that after the aforesaid Drunken Fit, upon James-Tide was Twelve-Months, and the dancing Humour he was then in, he had the Apparition of a Man's Head all along in the Way he went to Westly-Hall, and the Week after. When he came thither he wrought hard at the Hay, and was taken with a universal Merriness in the Evening of the same Day. He made himself Drunk again as he confessed, and in his Drink he was transported into such a Height of Prophaneness as astonished the Standers by, so that they concluded the Devil had some extraordinary Power over him. He also, as himself said, had an Apparition of the Devil, pointing at something he had lately done, so that then we concluded, the Devil in his Drink drew him into a blind Consent and Compact to satisfie his Curiosity and Dancing Humour. He also confessed to me since, that when he had thought to Confess something to this Purpose, his Mouth was stopped, so that he could not; and then he had a check for Confessing so much. Sometimes he refused to do what the Devil moved him to, and then it appeared he was tossed strangely.

Providence now seemed to call us off from attending upon this Surrey Case, laying before us Occasions and Opportunities of more publick Concernment. It seemed also to take us off from meeting at that Place, the Land-Lord being stirred up against the Family there, his Hedges being damaged by the Concourse of People; so that had we persisted in meeting there, it might have been prejudicial to them, they having much

Dependance on him, as to their Worldly Affairs. In those Circumstances the Ministers, and others generally, rather halting in their Work also, as Jacob even when he prevailed for the Blessing. The Lord was pleased to give some visible Encouragement, as to the good Issue of this Affair in some sort; for upon the 24th of March he had a most terrible Fit, and in that the Evil Spirit took his Leave of him. As it is said by several Witnesses, it lest him with a strange Kind of Vomiting, yet nothing visible appearing.

After that Time he told me, he did not find that manner of Working in his Body as heretofore, so that he hoped he was delivered. I told him, that at the present we did not meet at his Father's House as formerly, for the Reasons aforementioned; yet we did continually remember his Case both privately and publickly. He owned the Spiritual Means, as the Cause whereby he had this Help, and desired our continuing of the Use thereof. He hath been altogether freed for these many Weeks (now Years) only once he had some Threatnings again as to a Fit, being then in Drink; this he was troubled for. He hath Cause to be troubled, remembring what Advantage Satan got against him by that Sin at first, dreading lest the Unclean Spirit should return, and his last estate be worse than the first, Luke II. and the Lord smote him with his immediate Hand, which I endeavoured to set in with. Thus far Minutes were kept in a Diary, as to this Case.

This short Journal of the said Affair might seem necessary to give the World an Account of this surprizing Case.

FINIS.

www.ingramcontent.com/pod-product-compliance
Lightning Source LLC
Chambersburg PA
CBHW071434300426
44114CB00013B/1431